THE NORMAL CHILD

THE NORMAL CHILD

Some Problems of the First Five Years and their Treatment

by

RONALD S. ILLINGWORTH

M.D. (Leeds), F.R.C.P. (Lond.), D.P.H., D.C.H.

Professor of Child Health, The University of Sheffield.
Pædiatrician to The Children's Hospital Unit
and The Jessop Hospital for Women,
The United Sheffield Hospitals.

SECOND EDITION

With 69 Illustrations

LONDON

J. & A. CHURCHILL LTD.

104 GLOUCESTER PLACE W.1.

Reprinted

1959

First Edition 1953
Reprinted 1954
Second Edition 1957
Reprinted 1959

Printed in Great Britain

PREFACE TO THE SECOND EDITION

When I completed the first edition of this book I felt that from the nature of the subject many years would elapse before sufficient alterations would become necessary to justify a second edition. I soon discovered how wrong I was. There seems to be an increasing interest in the problems of the normal child—certainly an increased recognition of their importance—and a large number of relevant papers have been published in the last three years. These have been studied and digested, more than 200 new references being added, obsolete ones being removed.

The title of the book has been changed to include the first five years, and the contents have been modified accordingly. Many sections have been rewritten, and new ones inserted, so that the whole text has been brought thoroughly up to date. By rigid pruning it was found possible to avoid materially lengthening the book.

The index has been completely rewritten.

R. S. Illingworth.

Sheffield, 1957.

PREFACE TO THE FIRST EDITION

It has long been recognized that a knowledge of anatomy and physiology is a necessary basis for the study of medicine and every medical student accordingly has to learn about the structure of the human body and how it works. It is notable, however, as Ryle pointed out some years ago, [365] that while one would have thought that the study of health would seem to be the proper preliminary to the study of disease, health has no special place in the curriculum. Ryle said "It is surely an omission that so little attention has been paid by the students of disease and their teachers to that state from which deviation or departure must occur before the existence of disease is recognized." In the case of Pædiatrics, it certainly cannot be said that a knowledge of the normal child, of his growth, mind and development, is regarded, in England at least, as an essential basis for the study of the sick and diseased child. Yet it would seem obvious that a knowledge of the normal should precede the knowledge of the abnormal. Individual variations in the anatomical, physical, mental and biochemical make-up of the normal healthy child are so great, that a thorough grounding in the normal and in the normal variations which occur, is an essential preliminary to the fuller study of disease.

In some teaching schools, there is too much emphasis on the rare and the "interesting," and too little emphasis on the common conditions which form the large bulk of family practice. In the case of children, many of these common conditions consist of variations from the normal which hardly amount to disease, but which cause a great deal of anxiety and concern to the parents. The doctor may leave the medical school ill-equipped to deal with them. He learns a great deal from his own children, but lacking that knowledge of the normal and of normal variations which he should have learnt as a student, he is liable to read far too much into his experience with his own family and to make unwarranted generalizations which will prove harmful when applied to his patients.

It is the responsibility of the teacher to interest the student in the common rather than the unusual, the important rather than the rare, in persons and people rather than in cases, in health as well as in disease, in prevention as well as in cure. He must instil in him a thorough knowledge of the normal, as an essential basis for the study of the abnormal.

It is because I felt that this knowledge of the normal is not easy to acquire from the available textbooks that this one was planned.

This book is intended to describe the problems other than disease which arise in the normal child in his first three years. It is not intended to be a handbook of child management, to give a description of the normal child, or to discuss biochemical and other laboratory investigations. The variations in the normal biochemistry of childhood are so great and the interpretation of the findings so difficult that, if properly covered, such a discussion would fill a book in itself. Questions of physiology, embryology, nutrition and general medicine, are omitted except only in so far as they are strictly relevant to the subjects under discussion. A knowledge of those is assumed. The book does set out to describe the normal variations in the normal child, variations which cause a great deal of worry to the parents, and which, if improperly managed, may cause a great deal of suffering to children. It sets out to give the doctor as much help as possible in trying to decide whether an individual child is normal or abnormal: it sets out to give him as much guidance as possible in the management of simple behaviour problems, such as any doctor concerned with the care of children ought to be able to deal with himself. The range of topics discussed includes behaviour problems, feeding problems, problems of physical and mental development, and certain problems of preventive pædiatrics. It is intended for all doctors who are concerned with the care of children, especially family doctors and doctors in the Child Welfare Service. It is hoped too that it will help them with their own children.

In planning the book I was constantly faced with the difficulty of deciding what is normal and what is abnormal, and what, therefore, should be included in the book and what excluded. It is almost impossible to define the normal. It is certainly not synonymous with the average. A child may differ very widely from the average child in physical and mental development and yet be perfectly normal. An attempt has been made to include the extreme range of normal variations which may occur. This was a matter of great difficulty, for so little has been written about the subject, and differences of opinion are wide. The preparation of the book has certainly taught me how much we do *not* know about the normal child, and how much awaits investigation.

Behaviour problems are included in the book because every normal child has them. I feel that a child with no behaviour problems would be highly abnormal. The book may well be criticized for including topics which are on the borderline between health and disease, such as cyclical vomiting and motion sickness. They are, however, extremely common, and are unrelated to any known organic disease, and accordingly it was felt that they should find a place in this book. Infections are not discussed, but a section is devoted to the prevention of infection and so to the preservation of health.

Another difficulty experienced was that of repetition. So many different subjects have been discussed in this book that any attempt to give a reasonably comprehensive account of each individual problem has inevitably led to minor repetitions. I felt that this was preferable to an excess of cross references, which are so often irksome to the reader. Many of the repetitions are simply due to the fact that numerous different problems arise from the same basic causes.

It is difficult in a book of this nature to give full credit to all papers which have been read in its preparation. It was felt undesirable to list all the hundreds of articles read. Instead an effort has been made to include at the end of the book only those references which the reader will find of value. Specially recommended reading is printed in heavy type. A few references to articles which are particularly worth reading, but which are not specifically referred to in the text, are given at the end of this list. References to articles which are not otherwise relevant to the subject under discussion are referred to by asterisk, and the reference is given at the foot of the page. Any references which I was unable to read personally are denoted by the words " quoted by," referring to the author who referred to that work in his paper or book. I have made every effort to include in the references those papers which do not accord with my opinion, so that both sides of the question can be read.

In conclusion, I wish to express my gratitude to Professor Wilfred Vining of Leeds, who taught me so much when I was a student, and to Dr. Arnold Gesell, of New Haven, who taught me so much about the normal child while I was in his Department. The section on Developmental Problems is inevitably based largely on Gesell's works —on knowledge which I acquired from him and his staff, and from his numerous books and papers. In the section on Behaviour Problems I have frequently referred to an excellent series of articles in the *Journal of Pediatrics* by Dr. Harry Bakwin, and I wish to thank the Editor for permission to do so.

Professor Vining (Leeds), Professor Capon (Liverpool), Dr. Donald Court (Newcastle-upon-Tyne) and Dr. Doxiadis (Sheffield) have read and criticized the entire script. Dr. Harold Waller (Tunbridge Wells), Dr. John Emery (Sheffield), Dr. John Lorber (Sheffield) and Mr. Robert Zachary, F.R.C.S. (Sheffield) have read parts of it. To all these friends I wish to express my thanks. The opinions expressed in the book, however, are my own, and they do not necessarily accord with those of my friends. This could not be, for many of the subjects are highly controversial, and in the present state of our knowledge, purely matters of opinion, so that on some of the topics there was no agreement between my critics. Readers of the book will probably differ still more, and I should like it to be known that I should welcome their criticisms and suggestions.

I also wish to thank Mr. A. Foster, Medical Artist to the United Sheffield Hospitals for the sketches on pp. 177–191 ; Mr. Larway and A. K. Tunstill of the Photographic Department of the United Sheffield Hospitals, for the clinical photographs ; Messrs. J. & A. Churchill Ltd., for permission to reproduce the illustrations on pages 30 and 37 from the book by Evans and MacKeith on " Infant Feeding and Feeding Difficulties " ; Nea Service Inc., for the right to reproduce the Wetzel Grid ; the Editor of the *British Medical Journal*, for Table 5 ; Dr. H. Stuart of Boston for Table 7 ; Messrs. Allen and Hanburys for the photographs on page 33 ; and Messrs. Charles Dent and Little, Brown & Co., for permission to publish extracts from two poems by Ogden Nash.

R. S. ILLINGWORTH.

CONTENTS

Section 1

FEEDING PROBLEMS

Section 2

PHYSICAL PROBLEMS

Section 3

DEVELOPMENTAL PROBLEMS

Section 4

BEHAVIOUR PROBLEMS

Section I
PROBLEMS OF INFANT FEEDING

CHAPTER 1

BREAST FEEDING OR ARTIFICIAL FEEDING?

Incidence of Breast Feeding

THERE are wide differences in the incidence of breast feeding in this country and abroad. Selber [374] reported that 93·4 per cent. of 1,382 European babies were fully breast fed on discharge from two hospitals in Durban, South Africa. The corresponding figures for coloured and Bantu babies were 97·9 per cent. and 98·6 per cent. Jelliffe [218] wrote that 100 per cent. of 155 mothers from poor Bengali villages were fully breast feeding their babies 1 and 6 months after birth. Only 54 per cent. of 78 women from the upper socio-economic class in Calcutta were breast feeding their babies at 6 months. In 1951, 94·4 per cent. of mothers discharged from the Jessop Hospital for Women at Sheffield were fully breast feeding their infants. In contrast to the above figures, I am told that not more than 2 per cent. of mothers discharged from some maternity units in Canada and the United States are breast feeding their babies. Steps are even taken by some [114] to prevent lactation by administering testosterone cyclo-pentyl-proprionate in cotton seed oil to the mother before the baby is born.

Many years ago Sedgwick and Fleischner,[371, 372, 373] being concerned about the falling incidence of breast feeding, conducted an intensive campaign in Minneapolis in order to prove that women could breast feed their babies if lactation were properly managed. Manual expression of the breast was carried out as a routine until lactation was established. The result was that 96 per cent. of 2,847 women were fully breast feeding their babies at the end of the second month, and 84 per cent. of 2,355 women at the end of the sixth month ; 1,000 consecutive babies were discharged from maternity units fully breast fed. Similar experiments were carried out elsewhere.[348, 350]

There is little doubt that if women really want to breast-feed their babies, and if lactation is properly managed, the great majority of babies will be fully breast fed for the first 3 or 4 months until a weaning diet is introduced. In the sections to follow I shall discuss the most important problems of breast feeding.

Possible Advantages of Breast Feeding

The Incidence of Infection

By far the most important advantage of breast feeding is the very much lower incidence of infections in babies fed on the breast than in those who are bottle fed. There have been numerous papers on the subject. The most frequently quoted paper is that of Grulee,[171] concerning the morbidity and mortality in 26,061 babies under the care of the Infant Welfare Society of Chicago between 1924 and 1929. The mortality in the breast-fed infants was 1·54 per 1,000 as compared with 84·36 per 1,000 artificially-fed babies. The incidence of infections in the breast-fed babies was 37·4 per cent. as compared with 63·6 per cent. in the artificially fed ; 5·2 per cent. of the breast-fed babies and 16 per cent. of the artificially-fed ones had gastro-intestinal disorders. Robinson [355] studied the morbidity and mortality of 2,295 babies who were entirely or partly artificially fed, comparing it with that of 2,412 babies who were fully breast fed. The mortality from infections was 30 per 1,000 in the 2,295 infants who were being artificially fed at the time of the onset of the fatal illness, as compared with 3·3 per 1,000 in the 2,412 infants who were being breast fed ; 17·9 per cent. of the breast-fed babies had some illness in the first seven months, compared with 40·7 per cent. of the artificially-fed babies. There was a three times greater incidence of otitis media in the artificially-fed babies, and there was a higher incidence of measles and whooping cough. The overall mortality was two and a half times greater in those artificially fed. When breast-fed babies became ill, the duration and severity of the illness was less than that of those artificially fed. Robinson thus gave convincing proof that the morbidity and mortality of artificially-fed babies is much higher than that of breast-fed ones. Stevenson [401] drew attention to the fact that in babies artificially fed for the first 6 months there is a higher incidence of respiratory infections (colds, bronchitis, pneumonia) than in breast-fed babies, not only in the first 6 months but also in the second 6 months of life. It seemed as if the breast-fed baby obtained something in the first 6 months which provided him with a greater resistance to infection in the second 6 months, when he was on ordinary mixed feeds.

Joensen,[219] in his 445-page monograph on breast feeding, found that fully breast-fed babies had considerably fewer colds and attacks of bronchitis or pneumonia than artificially-fed babies, and, when they did get a cold, they were less likely to develop bronchitis after it ; 1·87 per cent. of those who were artificially fed from birth developed pneumonia, as compared with 0·15 per cent. of those fully breast fed for 6 months. In addition, those fully breast fed in the first 6 months were less liable to acquire measles, influenza, acute tonsillitis or unexplained fever in either the first or second 6 months, and less rubella, chickenpox or otitis media in the first 6 months. Several others[116, 383] found a similarly high incidence of respiratory infection in artificially-fed babies as compared with those breast fed. Stevenson thought that one factor might be the high vitamin A and C intake of the breast-fed child. The breast-fed baby at 6 months obtains about 3,250 International Units of vitamin A from the mother, as compared with the commonly recommended dose of 1,500 units for the bottle-fed baby, and 55 mg. of ascorbic acid as compared with the commonly recommended dose of 30 mg. There is, however, no evidence that this is the factor concerned.

Numerous other papers have shown that there is a very much higher incidence of gastro-enteritis in artificially-fed babies than in those breast fed, and that the mortality of those who acquire the infection is much higher if they are artificially fed. Much of this difference can be ascribed to errors in the feeding technique. Unless the food, bottles, teat and everything else necessary for the preparation of feeds are handled with full aseptic precautions, infection of the baby may occur. It is, in fact, impossible to ensure in most homes that feeds are handled with proper care. It is certainly true that, if the feeds were prepared in the way recommended by the American Academy of Pediatricians,[14] the incidence of gastro-enteritis in artificially-fed babies would be greatly reduced. Such surgical asepsis can and should be achieved in every hospital handling babies, but it is common knowledge that in many hospitals the standard falls a great deal short of this. Gordon and Levine[161] advocated modified cow's milk for premature babies, largely on the grounds that they gain weight faster than on human milk. In a very well equipped hospital with an adequate and properly trained staff that may be true, but it would not be true for many other hospitals. The results of the application of such a recommendation might well be disastrous. In Egypt during the War[402] severe malaria spread northwards from the Sudan and affected large numbers of the natives. The babies mostly escaped the malaria, perhaps because of the prevalent practice of wrapping them up entirely from head to foot at night. So many mothers became seriously ill that, with American help, suitable artificial feeds were given from water-buffalo milk, every effort being made to teach the people clean methods of handling food. The babies were given proper supplies of vitamins. Almost every one of the babies died. The deaths were not due to unrecognized malaria, for the same thing happened in non-malarious districts.

The explanation for the lower incidence of gastro-enteritis in breast-fed babies may lie in two observations. The intestinal flora of a fully breast-fed infant is characterized by the prevalence of *Lacto-*

bacillus bifidus, in contrast to the mixed flora of infants fed on cow's milk. György [177] found that a mutant of *Lactobacillus bifidus* required for its propagation a specific growth factor, containing glucosamine, fructose and galactose, present in large quantities in human milk, and in still larger quantities in colostrum. Cow's milk has only a thirtieth to a hundredth of the activity of human milk. He suggested that the increased resistance to gastro-enteritis may be related to this factor in its effect on the bacterial flora of the bowel.

The stools of the fully breast-fed infant are more acid than those of the baby fed on cow's milk, partly as a result of the intestinal flora described above, and Ross and Dawes [360] showed that the specific types of *Esch. coli* which are related to infantile gastro-enteritis will not multiply at the *p*H of the breast-fed infants' stools. Even a single complementary feed of cow's milk caused an immediate rise of the *p*H of the stool, with the result that the specific types of *Esch. coli* would be enabled to multiply.

By far the safest way of feeding a baby, particularly if the social circumstances, hospital arrangements or sanitary conditions are poor, is direct from the mother's breast.

Convenience

There can be little doubt that in most ways breast feeding is far easier for the mother. There is no equipment to sterilize and there are no feeds to mix and measure. It is an advantage to mother and child that the quantity of milk taken by the breast-fed baby cannot be determined except by test feeds. This relieves the mother of much anxiety caused by the day-to-day variations in the child's appetite. When the mother visits friends or travels, it is much easier for her to feed the baby on the breast than to take all the necessary equipment for artificial feeds. When the baby demands feeds at night, as he usually does in the first 10 weeks, it is a great deal easier for her to feed the baby on the breast than to prepare an artificial feed. Few mothers have a refrigerator in which to keep the day's feeds ready made up. In my opinion too many mothers with organic diseases, such as rheumatic carditis, are advised to bottle feed their babies on the grounds that it will be easier for them. In fact artificial feeding causes much more work than breast feeding.

Psychological Factors

Quite a number of papers [89, 107, 191, 300, 313, 330, 333, 375] have set out to determine whether there is any relationship between the duration of breast feeding and later behaviour. Some of these papers work back from psychiatric disorders in later childhood to the mother's version of the duration of breast feeding. In general these papers suggest that the breast-fed baby fares better in later childhood than the bottle-fed baby, but the fallacies in all of the papers are numerous. One such fallacy is the fact that the mother who breast feeds her baby may be a different kind of mother, with different attitudes to life, from the mother who prefers to feed her baby on the bottle. In that case the child would be influenced not only by the duration of breast feeding but by the attitude of the mother. Newton,[313] setting out to determine whether there was a relationship between infant-feeding experience and later behaviour, found that 67 per cent. of the fully breast fed group were "especially sought after as playmates," "accept adult suggestions," "take responsibility well," "never like to show off or act silly." On studying the table in the paper it was found that there were only 3 children in the group. Two out of three was evidently thought to be synonymous with 67 per cent. Rasmussen [344] went further and claimed that fitness for military service in 6,744 men at the age of twenty in Thuringia and Saxony was directly related to the duration of breast feeding!

Hoefer and Hardy [195] examined 383 children aged 7–13 years and investigated the duration of breast feeding. They found that those who had been artificially fed were inferior physically and mentally to the breast-fed ones. They had proved more susceptible to childhood diseases and had been later in walking and talking. (Those breast fed for an excessive length of time—over 10 months—had not fared so well.) It is unfortunate that the study was a retrospective one. Rogerson and Rogerson [358] in a careful paper attempted to relate feeding difficulties and other experiences in infancy to the psychological status at school age. The study was a follow-up one, not a retrospective one like most of the other papers mentioned above. They found that a higher proportion of the breast-fed babies had good physical and mental health in later childhood. They thought that there was a significant difference in the school achievement of the breast-fed babies compared with that of the artificially-fed babies who had experienced various feeding difficulties. The breast-fed babies were almost consistently superior. Psycho-analysts see a deep sexual significance in breast feeding. Readers who are interested should read the papers by Turner [417] and Markey.[269]

Orlansky [322] rightly shows that there is in fact very little evidence for the statements that breast feeding is of psychological value to the baby. The fact that evidence so far adduced is largely fallacious, however, does not preclude the possibility that breast feeding is of value to the child from the psychological standpoint. It may well be that the baby gains something from the closeness to his mother. He may certainly gain from the psychological effect which breast feeding has on the mother. When one watches a proud mother feeding her baby, one can hardly fail to notice the evident satisfaction which both are obtaining from the act. One does not obtain the same impression when watching a mother feeding her baby on the bottle. The mother has a sense of achievement when fully feeding her baby. She knows that he is utterly dependent on her and that no one else can replace her. This can hardly fail to strengthen the bond between mother and child and increase the mother's affection for him. If it does, the baby will certainly benefit. Her success, furthermore, gives her confidence which stands her in good stead when other problems arise.

Economic Factors

There can be no doubt that breast feeding is cheaper for the mother. She has no equipment to buy. The milk costs her nothing.

Chemical Differences and Digestibility

There are many chemical differences between human and cow's milk, but this is not the place to discuss them in detail. They have been well reviewed by Jeans.[217] There are differences in the protein and amino acid content, in the composition of milk fat, in nitrogen retention, in the calcium and phosphorus content, in the nature and degree of absorption of the carbohydrates, and in the vitamin content. There is little evidence, however, that the differences are in any way such that on these grounds alone human milk must be recommended in place of cow's milk. The increased calcium and phosphorus content of cow's milk does not seem to benefit the child in any way, though it is true that the artificially-fed baby stores more calcium and nitrogen than the breast-fed baby.

It is not easy to adduce evidence that breast milk is more easily digested than a properly constituted artificial feed. The digestibility depends to a large extent on the size of the curd. Breast milk produces a very fine curd in the stomach, whereas undiluted cow's milk produces a large tough one. But cow's milk is modified by boiling, drying or adding such substances as lactic acid, and the curd so produced is much smaller than that of untreated cow's milk and so is easily digested. Many pædiatricians, nevertheless, feel that an ill baby thrives better on breast milk than on cow's milk. An ill child who has been almost completely weaned may refuse anything else but breast milk, reverting to the ordinary mixed feeds when better.

Perianal Dermatitis

In fully breast-fed babies perianal dermatitis is less frequently seen than in babies fed on cow's milk. Pratt and Read [338] found that the lower the *p*H of the stool and the perianal skin, the lower was the incidence of perianal dermatitis. They found that it was from three to five times more common in white babies fed on evaporated cow's milk and maltose dextrin formulas than it was in those fully breast fed.

Other Possible Advantages

Grulee and his co-workers [171] found that the incidence of infantile eczema was seven times greater in artificially-fed babies than in those fed on the breast. Joensen [219] did not confirm this in his study. Some have thought that breast feeding in the early days of the puerperium favours the involution of the uterus. Hammond [180] showed that this is the case in rabbits, but there is little evidence that it applies to human beings. It is true, however, that when a new-born baby sucks at the breast multiparæ may feel cramps in the abdomen due to contractions of the uterus. These contractions are presumably due to reflex liberation of the oxytocic principle of the pituitary body as a result of the sucking. There is a greater incidence of rickets in bottle-fed babies, but this can be prevented by adequate administration of vitamin D.

Possible Disadvantages of Breast Feeding

I have not found papers which show that there are any disadvantages in breast feeding, with the exception of those referring to the premature baby, which have already been discussed. A minor disadvantage is the utter dependence of the baby on the mother. The mother is apt to feel worried if she is delayed for any reason when shopping, because she fears that her baby will be hungry and that no one else can feed him. She may also feel worried about the feeding of the baby if she acquires some acute infection which would make breast feeding unwise. In such a case, however, lactation can be maintained by manual expression of the milk.

The looseness of the stools of the breast-fed baby is troublesome for the mother. The much firmer stools of the baby fed on cow's milk give the mother less work.

Conclusion

There is no doubt that breast milk is safer for the child. The breast-fed baby is less likely to acquire infections than the artificially-fed baby, and if he acquires them his chance of survival is better. Breast feeding is easier and cheaper for the mother. It may have advantages from the psychological point of view. There are no disadvantages of importance.

CHAPTER 2

THE FEEDING SCHEDULE

" The hours of suckling it I do not fix,
Nature in that must guide the nursing sex.
When by its cries it calls you, do not spare
Your labour, nor be loath your breasts to bare."
St. Marthe (1584). " Pediatrophia."

There are still many advocates of a rigid feeding schedule in this country. Many books concerning infant and child care advocate absolute rigidity. Liddiard[255] says that the baby must be fed with absolute regularity and that no night feed should ever be given. In support of her thesis she quotes in all seriousness this statement in a textbook of Fairbairn's : " The careless, shiftless and ignorant mother, whose child is brought up without method, and given the breast whenever he cries for it, is injuring both the health and character of her child. Not only is he likely to have disturbed digestion and irregularity in the character of his bowels, but he is acquiring the slipshod ways of his parents, and without discipline or self-control, he grows up self-willed and unable to adapt himself to our customs, and is neither physically nor morally a credit to the race."

There are many pædiatricians in this country who feel that there should be elasticity in the feeding schedule. There are so many books, however, which still advocate rigidity that it was thought desirable to discuss the points for and against rigidity and elasticity in the schedule.

The problem can be conveniently discussed under the following headings.

Habit Formation

The advocates of a rigid feeding schedule insist that rigidly fixed feeding times are essential for good habit formation. It is argued, for instance, that a baby must not be given feeds at night in the early weeks of infancy because this will lead to bad habits. He must be " trained " not to expect night feeds. To the best of my knowledge, however, there is no evidence that a rigid feeding schedule does in fact lead to good habits or that a self-demand schedule leads to bad ones. It has been shown that babies fed on a self-demand schedule early develop a regular rhythm of their own. Aldrich,[12] after an extensive study of babies in Rochester (Minnesota), found that " self-regulation leads to feeding habits of great regularity in 98 per cent. of babies by the end of the first month." Elsewhere[11] he gave a statistical analysis of the feeding schedule of 668 babies who were allowed to take food when they were hungry. By 1 month of age the great majority had chosen a regular rhythm ; 61 per cent. of them had three-hourly feeds, and 26 per cent. four-hourly feeds. Less than 1 per cent. of the 668 babies presented any feeding problems at the age of 1 year. It is certainly my experience that the great majority of babies fed on a self-demand schedule have adopted a regular rhythm by about 1 month of age—many of them much earlier. Nearly all babies who are fed in the night when hungry drop the night feed by the age of 10 weeks. In my experience it is very exceptional for a baby to demand night feeds after 12 weeks, and if he does some other error of management is usually responsible. *There is no evidence that a self-demand schedule leads to bad habits. Night feeds should be given when the baby wants them, and they do not lead to trouble later. Babies stop demanding night feeds when they are ready to do so, usually by* 10 *weeks of life, and often much earlier.*

Neither is there evidence that self-demand feeding leads to irregularity of the bowels. Irregularity of the bowels, meaning that stools are passed at irregular times, is commonly found in babies irrespective of the feeding schedule, and in any case it is harmless and unimportant.

Psychological Factors in the Child

Gesell [144] wrote : "Superficially it might appear that the self-demand schedule would encourage whims and instability in the child. Exactly the opposite is true. For by individualization of feeding the infant is most directly and completely satisfied. He is satisfied vegetatively and emotionally. He escapes periods of want, anxiety and distress. The promptness and certainty of satisfaction cumulatively experienced . . . will nourish that sense of security which is essential to mental health." Weinfeld [445] wrote : "My personal experience leads me to the conclusion that if the infant has been gratified during his newborn period, through a reasonable application of the self-demand regimen, he can more easily learn to make the adjustments which society demands in later life."

It is, of course, extremely difficult to prove that any one factor in the management of an infant has a significant effect on the child's emotional development in later years, because so many other factors arise in the environment long after the original factor has disappeared. There can be little doubt that a self-demand schedule reduces the amount of crying. There is every reason why it should, for one of the chief causes of crying is hunger. It is obvious by the age of 2 or 3 years that any factor which causes a feeling of insecurity in a child, any persistent failure to satisfy his everyday needs, does lead to serious emotional disturbances. It seems reasonable to suppose that a similar failure to satisfy a baby's basic needs would also have a bad effect on his emotional development. Several workers have attempted to prove this, but the studies are mostly retrospective ones, from later childhood back to the feeding history, and they cannot be said to prove anything. There is, therefore, no satisfactory evidence that elasticity in infant feeding has a beneficial psychological effect on the child which will affect him in later years. It would be exceedingly difficult to prove this one way or the other. But the fact that there is no such evidence does not prove that it has no such effect.

Psychological Factors in the Mother

A rigid schedule may worry the mother through causing the baby to cry a great deal because of hunger. There are many who say that a young baby should never be fed in the night because it will cause bad habits. The advice almost inevitably means that the baby will cry for prolonged periods in the night, keeping the mother and father awake and making them tired and irritable. In the morning the baby may be tired as a result of his disturbed night, and the mother is worried because he does not suck well. In a maternity unit in which the baby is kept with the mother day and night, as he should be, a rigid schedule would hardly be practicable, because a good mother would find it difficult to do nothing when her baby is crying for food.

A self-demand schedule may cause the mother some anxiety. She may fear that she will not be able to tell when he is hungry. Bakwin[30] pointed out that there are many mothers to whom the task of individualizing child rearing is a source of great anxiety. Women with a very orderly nature may find a self-demand schedule tiresome, much preferring precise instructions for feeding, to which they will rigidly adhere. It would certainly be unwise to press such mothers to adopt a self-demand feeding schedule. In my experience this difficulty is not often seen.

The Convenience of the Mother

A favourite argument against a self-demand schedule is the suggestion that the mother will find it very difficult because she will never know when the baby is going to be hungry. Wanning[439] suggests that " the psychiatrists are sending a bevy of mothers into a flurry of warming bottles, only to have them go cold again, ignoring their other children to wait on the cry of the youngest, to say nothing of having them find themselves in a constant state of indecision." This is not true, for the vast majority of babies fed on a self-demand schedule get into a regular rhythm of their own. It is the responsibility of the pædiatrician, when explaining the feeding technique to the mother, to explain to her how she can tell when the child is hungry and wants feeding. In my experience mothers do not find that a self-demand schedule causes any difficulty in this way. It is true that some mothers may interpret the self-demand schedule too literally and carry it too far. Weinfeld [445] was right when he wrote that a self-demand method can be employed just as inflexibly as were the rigid schedules. It is wrong to make a mother feel that she must feed a baby the moment that he cries, dropping everything that she is doing, or that it is always wrong to awaken a baby for a feed. If there is a good reason, such as the parents' bedtime, for awakening a child for a feed, then he should be awakened. That is a different matter from awakening him at a fixed time for every feed if he is asleep. It is one matter to leave a baby crying for half an hour occasionally for food and another to leave him crying for food for prolonged periods every day. As long as a self-demand schedule is not applied too rigidly it is not inconvenient for the mother.

Another argument brought forward against demand feeding is the idea that a mother will be exhausted by the frequent demands for food. It is true that in the new-born period, especially between the fourth and the eighth day, there may be very frequent demands for food—as many as twelve in the 24 hours. This may be advantageous to the mother in that it helps to empty her breast and to reduce over-distension. In any case, if the baby were not fed as frequently as this when he wants food, he would cry and keep the mother awake. After the new-born period the demands are much less frequent, and may indeed be less frequent than in most rigid schedules.

The feeding of twins on a self-demand schedule is very difficult. This question is discussed on p. 23.

Deciding when the Baby is Hungry

This presents no difficulty on a rigid schedule, because the baby is given food whether he wants it or not, and if he is hungry before the allotted time he cannot have it. There is no doubt that some mothers, and particularly those of low intelligence, do make mistakes when feeding babies on the demand schedule. I have seen babies who were being fed almost every half hour because the mother interpreted every cry as a cry for food. Some mothers do not seem to know that babies cry because they want to be picked up and loved. After about 3 months they are apt to cry because of boredom. They want to see what is going on and they want to be propped up instead of being kept lying down. One of the commonest sources of trouble is the so-called "three-months' colic," which causes much crying in the evenings in the first 3 months of life (see p. 60). I have seen many of these children who were being given almost continuous feeds in the evening as a result of the crying. The mothers quite naturally interpreted the baby's crying, which failed to respond to picking him up, as a sign of hunger. Sucking does seem to give some temporary relief to the colic, and their beliefs were thereby apparently confirmed. I was asked to see an 8-month-old child on account of a feeding problem. He was being fed almost two-hourly because his parents interpreted every cry as a cry for food. They failed to realize that a child cries for company, toys and other things. They had been told never to pick him up if he cried because if they did they would "spoil" him.

Another mistake which can be made in a self-demand schedule is to fail to realize that a baby is ill and for that reason not demanding feeds. A chronically starved or cold baby may become dangerously lethargic and fail to demand feeds. A less severely underfed baby is likely to demand very frequent feeds because he is never properly satisfied. A mentally defective child may present difficulties because he may show little interest in food and fail to demand feeds. A baby with inertia in the first few days of life may fail to demand feeds. Some particularly placid babies may fail to demand as many feeds as they really need for an average weight gain.

These mistakes are due to one of two things : failure of the doctor to explain the demand schedule, or to a low level of intelligence in the parents. It is essential for the doctor, in recommending a mother to feed her baby when he wants it, to explain that there are other causes of crying than hunger. She should understand that a baby commonly cries to be loved and picked up. The crying stops and the child remains contented as long as he is in his mother's arms. The crying of a hungry baby is certainly not stopped for long by picking him up. He cries even though he is in his mother's arms. The crying of a child with colic is not stopped by picking him up—at least, not for long. The peculiarly high-pitched scream is characteristic of pain. He becomes red in the face, frowns, screams and draws his legs up with spasms of pain. Proper supervision is just as necessary when a baby is fed on a self-demand schedule as when he is fed on a rigid one. The difficulty of the starved baby failing to demand feeds is avoided by such supervision.

There is little place for self-demand feeding after about 3 months. The demands are then regular and the baby's mealtimes are readily made to fit in with the mother's convenience. There is no excuse for feeding a baby at the age of 8 months every 2 hours, for no normal baby demands feeds so frequently at that age. This sort of mistake is readily avoided by proper supervision.

The Effect on Lactation

I have been unable to find any work on the effect of the feeding schedule on the establishment of lactation. At the Jessop Hospital for Women at Sheffield, therefore, a controlled experiment was carried out,[207] 106 babies being fed on a rigid feeding schedule (six feeds per 24 hours) and 131 on a self-demand schedule. The following is a summary of the findings: (i) Many of the "demand" babies took very frequent feeds between the fourth and the eighth days. On the fifth day 36 babies (28·6 per cent.) took eight feeds or more in the 24 hours, 12 of them (9·5 per cent. of the total) wanting nine feeds or more. (ii) The demand babies gained weight more rapidly than those on a rigid schedule. (iii) There was a strong positive correlation between the number of feeds taken in the 24 hours and the amount of milk taken from the breast, as shown by test feeds, and with the weight gain. (iv) There were twice as many cases of soreness of the nipples and overdistension of the breast on the rigid schedule as on the demand schedule; 29 of 106 mothers (27·4 per cent.) feeding their babies on a rigid schedule developed soreness of the nipples as compared with 16 of 124 mothers (12·9 per cent.) who were feeding them on a demand schedule; 36 of 106 mothers (34 per cent.) who were feeding their babies on a rigid schedule had overdistension of the breasts, compared with 21 of 124 mothers (16·9 per cent.) who were feeding them on a demand schedule. (v) A significantly greater number of babies fed on a demand schedule were fully breast fed on discharge from hospital and at 1 month of age; 94·4 per cent. of the demand babies were fully breast fed on discharge, and 80·3 per cent. at 1 month, compared with 88·1 per cent. of the rigidly-fed babies on discharge and 64·5 per cent. at 1 month. These figures indicate that a self-demand schedule is better than a rigid one for the establishment of lactation. The two factors responsible for this are probably the more efficient emptying of the breast when a demand schedule is used, as a result of more frequent feeds, and the lower incidence of soreness of the nipples because the baby is less ravenous when fed. Another factor may be the fact that a mother who feeds her baby when he wants it worries less about her baby, because he cries less than when a rigid schedule is used.

It might be thought that the irregularity of the feeds would cause difficulty in upsetting the breast rhythm. In fact our experience showed that this does not happen. In any case, babies fed on a demand schedule acquire a fairly fixed rhythm of their own by about 3 or 4 weeks of age, so that the feeding times are by then fairly regular. Every mother ought to be shown how to express milk from the breast, and if at any time some discomfort should be experienced as a result of overdistension, because the baby has not demanded food for a particularly long time, she can relieve the discomfort readily by expressing milk. This is very liable to happen when the baby first misses the night feed and the breast therefore remains unemptied for an unaccustomed time.

A real difficulty does sometimes arise on a self-demand schedule. An occasional baby, as young as 2 months of age, may only demand three feeds in the 24 hours. The baby thrives and gains weight satisfactorily. The mother's breast, however, is left unemptied for too long and so lactation is endangered. This difficulty is easily dealt with either by encouraging the baby to take more frequent feeds or by manual expression of milk half-way between the feeds. I have seen artificially-fed babies fail to gain sufficient weight because they were only demanding three feeds a day.

Individual Variations in Babies

There is no doubt that a rigid schedule suits many babies well during the day, though few young babies are willing to do without a feed in the night. There are many babies, however, whom a rigid schedule does not suit, and it is indeed to be expected, for babies are individuals as much as are adults. Hunger is largely associated with the emptying of the stomach, and babies differ just as much as adults in their stomach-emptying time. It has been shown that when cow's milk is given the stomach empties less quickly than when the baby is fed on human milk. Furthermore, there are differences in the hunger of babies. There are little eaters and big eaters. To a certain extent the baby is affected by the temperature and humidity. In hot, humid weather it is reasonable to expect a baby to want a feed sooner than in cold weather. Babies have periods of activity and periods of sleep, and hunger is likely to occur sooner in an active play period than in a period of sleep. Much depends on the personality of the child, for the placid child is likely to demand fewer feeds than the active one. All these variations between babies make a self-demand schedule a desirable one, for rigid schedules take no account of individual variations.

Many babies present no difficulty during the establishment of lactation. Others are irritable, cry a great deal, refuse to suck properly, or suck for a minute or two, bite at the breast and then withdraw and cry. Such babies are very difficult to manage. A self-demand schedule is most desirable for these babies, because with such a schedule they are less likely to be intractable when offered the breast. If kept waiting a long time they are particularly liable to be difficult.

Duration of Crying

It would be reasonable to suppose that there would be less crying in babies fed on a self-demand schedule than in those on a rigid schedule. There is, however, no statistical evidence for this, for the simple reason that it is a difficult, laborious task to record accurately the amount of crying which babies do. It has already been explained that a rigid schedule does suit many babies, because it happens to coincide with their needs. There are many babies, however, who are not suited by such a régime. I have seen scores of babies who were not suited by a rigid schedule and who cried excessively as a result. The crying was greatly reduced when some elasticity was allowed. Refusal of a night feed because of the fear of habit formation inevitably leads to prolonged crying. Not only does this worry the mother but it tires her and her husband. Both worry and fatigue have a bad effect on the mother's lactation. The baby, furthermore, is tired by prolonged crying and lack of sleep and sucks less well when he is eventually offered the breast. In addition, crying leads to air swallowing and even vomiting, and the baby then approaches the breast when already distended with wind. He therefore empties the breast less well. A self-demand schedule avoids this difficulty. The baby is given a night feed and immediately falls asleep when it is completed, and is likely to sleep soundly until the next feed time. At the Jessop Hospital for Women at Sheffield, where self-demand feeding was gradually introduced, visitors have remarked about the quietness of the hospital, because there is so little crying.

Compensation for Undue Loss of Weight or Slow Initial Weight Gain

When a baby has lost weight excessively in the newborn period, or when weight progress has been slow, owing to the milk coming in slowly, babies may show a compensatory increase of appetite and demand very frequent feeds until they have caught up to the expected weight. Their weight gain is unusually great during this period. I saw a child whose birth weight was 9 lb., who lost $1\frac{1}{2}$ lb. owing to irritability and difficulty in sucking. When the baby settled down as a result of tactful handling, ten to twelve feeds per day were demanded, and there was a weight gain of 15 oz. a week until the expected weight was reached, when the frequency of feeds and the weight gain fell to the average figure. The same compensatory increase of appetite occurs in babies in the convalescent stage of an infection, and even at 6 months of age a night feed may again be demanded for a few days after an infection, until the lost ground has been made up. These cases are not exceptional. A rigid schedule does not allow for such changes. A self-demand schedule does and so avoids a great deal of unnecessary crying.

Hospital Routine

It is commonly said that a rigid routine is necessary in hospital, in order that the ward work can be properly attended to. In the Jessop Hospital at Sheffield self-demand feeding gradually evolved over a period of about a year, replacing a completely rigid routine in which not even night feeds were allowed. The change coincided with a change from a partial association of mother and infant to the full one, in which the baby is not removed from the mother's room for any purpose such as bathing or napkin changing. There was a serious shortage of nurses throughout the period. The nursing staff had been suspicious of suggestions that some elasticity in the schedule should be allowed. They became unanimously enthusiastic for a self-demand schedule, so much so that, when a controlled experiment was started, necessitating babies in one ward being placed on a rigid schedule, there was considerable opposition to the use of a rigid schedule and difficulties arose in the conduction of the experiment. The chief point made by some of the sisters was that, whereas previously the shortage of nurses made proper supervision of feeding impossible when thirty babies had to be fed at the same time, much better supervision was now possible because the babies were being fed at different times when they needed it. They noted the fact that there was less crying, that the mothers were happier and less worried about their babies, and that the nurses themselves were less irritable because they were able to cope with the work better.

Conclusion

On almost all counts a self-demand schedule is preferable to a rigid one. It must be Nature's method, for Nature could hardly have intended that feeding should be strictly regular. A considerable proportion of mothers have adopted the common-sense attitude and feed their babies when they want food, against the advice of their doctors. It does not lead to bad habit formation. Though it is impossible to prove that failure to satisfy the basic needs of infancy, such as hunger, may lead to some psychological disturbance later, it is reasonable to suppose that it may have such an effect. An elastic schedule presents psychological advantages to the mother. It is not inconvenient to her, because babies fed on a demand schedule get into a regular rhythm by 3 or 4 weeks of age. It may cause trouble by the mother's failure to interpret the causes of crying, but this difficulty is avoided by proper discussion with her and proper supervision. A self-demand schedule caters for the individual; a rigid schedule works well for many babies but not for others, and if it does not cater for them it causes a great deal of crying. An elastic schedule allows for a compensatory increase of appetite after a period of defective weight gain. It is a help, not a hindrance, in hospital routine, in allowing better supervision of feeds. Experimentally it has been shown that it halves the incidence of sore nipples and overdistension of the breast in the mother, increases the incidence of full breast feeding and increases the weight gain in the child. It must be admitted that a woman of very low intelligence is less likely to make mistakes with a rigid schedule. Certain orderly and over-anxious types of women find a rigid schedule easier. Otherwise there are no valid arguments against a self-demand schedule.

CHAPTER 3

SOME BREAST FEEDING PROBLEMS

Should Prelacteal Fluid or Foods be given?

A STUDY of the literature shows that there are many papers on the subject of prelacteal feeds (feeds given before the breast milk comes in). Most of them are concerned with the prevention of dehydration fever or the reduction of weight loss rather than with the effect of prelacteal feeds on the establishment of lactation. The prevalent use of prelacteal fluids and feeds is due to a fear that without them dehydration fever will occur, that the baby will starve, and that the normal weight loss in the first 2 or 3 days of life is harmful to the child. There is little foundation for any of these fears, which are based more on impression than on fact. Of these the most doubtful is the prevention of dehydration fever. Unfortunately it is not always easy to make a really confident diagnosis of this condition. Some babies seem to have an elevation of temperature on the first and second day as a result, presumably, of the effects of delivery, and perhaps cerebral œdema. Thereafter it is not easy to eliminate the possibility of an infection. Overclothing or overheating will cause a rise of temperature, and this cause would always have to be eliminated in any investigation. Some workers have tried to relate the giving of prelacteal fluid to the incidence of dehydration fever, mostly without giving a satisfactory definition of such fever. Bruce [70] found that the incidence of dehydration fever was not increased by withholding fluid in the first 2 days. Kaliski [225] found the opposite, as did Rodda and Stoesser.[357] One feels that the answer lies in the fact that in institutions in which prelacteal fluids are not given, and in which there is a high standard of observation, dehydration fever is still very uncommon.

The reduction of the normal weight loss has occupied the attention of several workers. Kugelmass and his co-workers [243] expressed strong feelings on the matter. They wrote that the loss of weight in the new-born period "is a period of semi-starvation . . . that is too stupefying to be ignored, too debilitating to be physiological, too prolonged to be a sacred law of Nature." They found that in animals there is no comparable weight loss. They recommended that a mixture containing gelatine, dextrose and salt should be given two-hourly in the 24 hours after birth, and claimed that this reduced the weight loss to an average figure of 1·7 per cent. as compared with 7 per cent. in controls. Frank [132] wrote that in the Salvation Army Hostel in Chicago they went so far as to inject all the new-borns with saline in order to reduce weight loss. Krost and Epstein [240] gave 5 per cent. dextrimaltose and 0·5 per cent. sodium citrate and made the babies œdematous as a result. On the other hand, Schorer and Laffoon [369] found that neither expressed breast milk from other mothers nor cow's milk prevented weight loss, though it did reduce the incidence of breast feeding. Kaliski [225] and Rodda and Stoesser [357] made similar observations. Sanford [368] said that a third of normal new-born babies will lose 5–8 per cent. of their body weight whatever feed is given them, but in the others the weight loss is reduced by complementary feeds. He too, however, found that complementary feeds reduced the incidence of breast feeding. It has been suggested that the giving of cow's milk for 2 or 3 days after birth, followed by a period on the breast, and then cow's milk when the child is older, might cause allergic manifestations to develop in the weaning period. Parmelee [326] thought that the giving of fluid before milk comes in enables the baby to suck more vigorously. The evidence for this was unsatisfactory.

Withholding of fluid in the first 2 or 3 days, if breast milk is unusually slow in coming in, is found to cause an increased weight loss, but this does no real harm to the baby. It is a common practice to withhold fluid from premature babies for the first 2 or 3 days. Hansen [181] showed that this results in a rise of serum electrolytes and of blood urea nitrogen, but the babies seemed to be unharmed. Campbell [81] noted the acidosis which may result from such starvation, and felt that babies should not be denied fluid for more than 48 hours. The same arguments apply to full-term babies. It is certain that in hot weather babies denied fluid in this way may become dehydrated, and acetone may be smelt in the breath.

It seems reasonable to suggest that there is no ground for dogmatism on the question of prelacteal fluid, and that no rigid rule should be laid down. The giving of fluid other than water may interfere with the establishment of lactation, particularly if manual expression of the breast is not carried out, and it should be avoided before the fifth day, unless there is virtual agalactia. Such fluids as those used by Kugelmass and his co-workers [243] should be avoided. Saline should not be given, because the kidney is immature, and has difficulty in excreting the sodium ion, so that there is a risk of œdema. Excessive weight loss (i.e. over 10 per cent. of the body weight) worries the mother, and should be prevented in hot weather by giving boiled water if the milk has not come in. If acetone is detected in the breath, or if "dehydration fever" occurs, fluid should certainly be given. Otherwise there is no particular need to give additional fluid in the first 2 or 3 days. It should always be remembered that the fluid given may introduce infection into the baby, unless full aseptic precautions are observed.

The Duration of the Breast Feed

A great deal of trouble is caused by rigid instructions about the duration of the breast feed. It is a common practice to advise mothers to feed the baby, of whatever age, for exactly 10 minutes on the breast. This sort of rigidity of ideas fails to take into account the individual variations in the speed of sucking, the increasing speed of sucking with increasing age, the variations in the speed of flow of milk from breasts, the quantity of milk in the breast or the degree of hunger and thirst shown by the baby. There is a great difference in the speed of sucking not only from baby to baby but in the same baby from feed to feed and from week to week. There are good suckers and poor suckers. The older the baby becomes the more rapidly he sucks. In some mothers the milk, particularly in the early morning feed, when the breast is a little distended, squirts or pours out so fast that the baby has to gulp it down as quickly as he can, and often chokes in the process. When the mother has a depressed nipple or there is some mechanical difficulty in the baby, it may take an unusually long time for the baby to obtain the milk. It often happens that a baby sucks for 10 minutes at one breast but falls asleep after about 3 minutes on the second. No rigid rules can take all these factors into account.

I have often been asked to see babies who were in trouble because the mother had been instructed to feed them for not more than 5 minutes on each breast. It is true that a mature baby of, say, 3 months can get all the milk there is in 5 minutes or less on each breast, but the younger baby of 2 or 3 weeks cannot usually do it and so is left hungry and unsatisfied, while the breast is left incompletely emptied. Lactation then fails. Many other babies get into trouble because the mother has been instructed to feed them for exactly 10 minutes on each breast. In the new-born period this may be insufficient. In the first place, it is essential to distinguish the time spent by the baby in actually sucking from the time spent on the breast. A good example of this distinction is given by the irritable baby in the new-born period. He comes up to the breast, then screams and kicks, perhaps sucks for a few seconds and then withdraws and screams again. The baby with inertia may spend quite a long time in breast play, licking the nipple and not sucking at all. A mother who has been instructed to feed the baby for exactly 10 minutes on each breast may make the mistake of including all the time spent in crying or breast play in the feeding period, and as a result the feed is stopped before the baby is satisfied. The irritable baby may take nearly an hour at each feed—thoroughly exhausting the mother in the process—but only a fraction of that time is spent in actual sucking. Even when the new-born baby is sucking well he may need more than 10 minutes on each breast, but I have not seen a baby, in the presence of an adequate supply of milk, require more than 15 minutes on each breast, and I therefore believe that that should be the limit. The baby who spends longer is probably using the breast as a pacifier.

The mother who has been instructed to feed a baby for exactly 10 minutes on each breast frequently gets into another difficulty. When the baby is mature he frequently obtains all there is in about 5 minutes or less at each breast, and the mother then tries to compel him to keep sucking. If she succeeds, he swallows air as a result of sucking on an empty breast, and so has colic and perhaps vomiting. In addition there is a risk that he will make the nipples sore, while he becomes tired with sucking on the first breast and falls asleep as soon as he is placed on the second. I agree with Richardson,[349] who wrote : " My own position is strongly against any arbitrary time limitations, which I believe to be the cause of many unnecessary weanings. I have never seen anyone with patience or perseverance enough to overfeed a baby." Discussing test feeds, he wrote : " I rely on the baby himself to indicate to me and his mother when he has had enough."

Many advocate severe restriction of the duration of the feed in the first 2 or 3 days, until the milk has come in, on the grounds that more prolonged sucking will cause soreness of the nipple. They suggest that on the first day the feeds should be limited to 2 or 3 minutes per breast two or three times in the 24 hours, and to 5 minutes per breast 6-hourly on the second day. A controlled study at the Jessop Hospital, Sheffield, in which some mothers fed their babies on the first 2 or 3 days as often and as long as they wanted, while others kept to the rigid schedule described above, indicated that the elastic method did not increase the incidence of soreness of the nipple.

The baby himself is the best guide to the duration of the feed. He is allowed to suck on the first breast until his speed of sucking slows down. He is then transferred to the second breast and allowed to suck until he falls asleep (if a young baby), or until he stops sucking and withdraws, if older. He should not have longer than 15 minutes per breast. By the age of 3 or 4 months he is unlikely to take more than 5 minutes per breast.

The Duration of Breast Feeding

It is said that Plotinus, when 8 years old and having lessons with his tutor, would run to his nurse and clamour for the breast. In China, New Guinea and among many primitive peoples it is common for a child to be breast fed till 2 or 3 years old.

No rigid rules can be laid down about the age at which weaning should begin or at which breast feeding should be completely stopped, except in the case of disease, such as pulmonary tuberculosis, or of a new pregnancy. Babies often make the decision for the mother. At any age from four months onwards a baby may suddenly and without any apparent reason refuse the breast. Robinson [355] thought that breast refusal only occurs in babies fed on a rigid schedule, but I do not think that that is true. It is usually the mother who has to decide when to give the baby some food other than breast milk. If there is a fully adequate supply of milk, weaning is likely to begin later than if there is a slight insufficiency. Normally, however, one decides by the maturity and size of the baby. Most full-term babies are equipped to take thick feeds * at 3 or 4 months, particularly if they are placed well back on the tongue. Before that date the baby's tongue is apt to eject the food instead of taking it back into the throat. When a baby is showing any sign of excessive weight, weaning is indicated, for some babies with excessive appetites may take a very large amount of milk, which is undesirable. I have seen two fully breast-fed babies who weighed over 32 lb. at the age of 9 and 10 months respectively. Assuming that they were taking $2\frac{1}{2}$ oz. per pound per day, they would be taking 4 pints of milk from the mother per day, which is far too much. In general, therefore, when a baby weighs 16 lb. or reaches 4 or 5 months of age, whichever is sooner, there is a good reason for beginning to wean. A 16-lb. baby would probably take 2 pints of milk per day from the mother, and more should not be allowed, for the mother's sake as well as in the interests of the baby. On the other hand, if a baby is determined not to have anything else but the breast milk, it would be undesirable to force the issue. It is common for a baby to insist on a breast feed at the last feed of the day for some weeks after weaning has otherwise been completed. This is harmless, but when the baby aged 6–12 months insists on breast feeds throughout the day, and refuses everything else, his nutrition may suffer and a firmer line has to be taken.

Weaning of difficult babies is achieved among the Mundugumor natives by applying bitter sap to the nipples, and in Manus by wrapping the nipples in human hair.[281, 282] Some Zulus paint the nipples with aloes or mustard. I cannot recommend such drastic measures in this country, but it should be remembered that the longer weaning is postponed the more difficult it is apt to become, for the child is passing further and further into the period of resistance. Generally speaking, if weaning has begun at 4 or 5 months of age, the last breast feed is likely to be relinquished by the age of 8 or 9 months.

The choice of the particular feed at which thickened food should be introduced is a matter for the mother's convenience.

The question of when to replace thickened feeds by solids is an easy

* By thick feeds I mean fruit or vegetable purée, soup, jelly, squashed banana, lightly boiled egg, grated cheese, etc.—substances which do not have to be chewed.

one. A child is given solids when he can chew, which is usually at about 6 months of age. There is no need to wait for teeth to come through.

The question of when the late evening feed should be dropped is an individual matter which can only be decided by a process of trial and error. If he is not given the feed and he awakens crying for food at 2 or 3 a.m., it means that he is not ready to do without a feed in the late evening. Tests at intervals will enable the mother to determine when the late evening feed can be discarded. Sometimes the baby decides for the mother by refusing to take an evening feed.

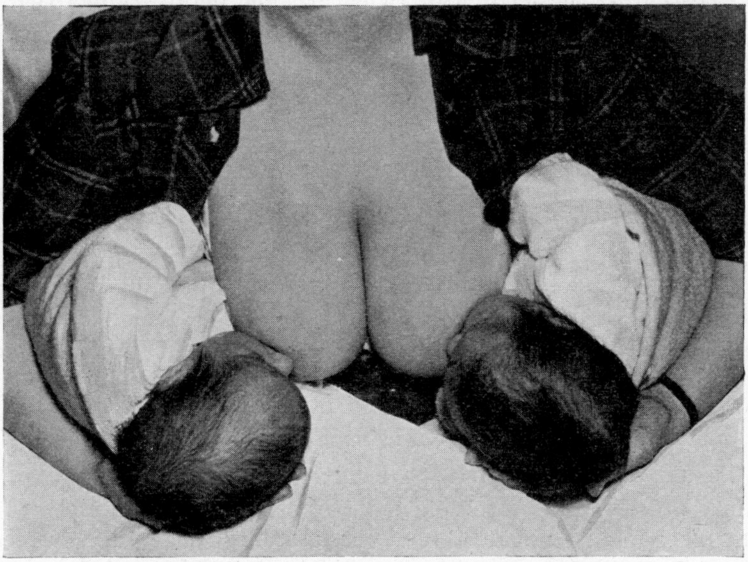

FIG. 1. Twins being fed simultaneously on breast.

The Feeding of Twins

The easiest and the quickest way to feed twins on the breast is to feed them simultaneously, one on each breast (Fig. 1). The babies' legs are behind the mother, and each head is supported by the mother's hands with the help of a pillow or cushion. If one twin feeds on the right breast at one feed he feeds on the left at the other. Some mothers are reluctant to do this, for it is not very comfortable, but it does save time and it avoids the difficulty of keeping one baby crying for food while the other is being fed. It is not possible if the twins demand feeds at different times and refuse to suck when they are both put to the breast at the same time.

A self-demand schedule is obviously difficult with twins, because they are apt to want feeding at different times. A record of twins fed on demand was given by Trainham and co-workers.[416] It was evident that such a schedule presented considerable difficulties and a more or less rigid schedule, allowing such elasticity as is convenient, should be advised.

Every effort should be made to enable the mother to produce sufficient milk for both. It would seem desirable to practise manual expression as a routine after feeds from the third day until lactation is well established in order to stimulate the supply of sufficient milk. If in spite of this there is not enough the procedure to be adopted depends on the quantity of milk available. Charlotte Naish,[305] who discusses the question of the feeding of twins in some detail, thinks that it is wrong to give the babies a breast feed followed by a complete artificial feed, because they are liable to suck badly on the breast if that is done. On the other hand, it would be difficult for a mother to feed both babies on the breast simultaneously and then give them complementary feeds, for the process would be too time-consuming unless she had domestic help.

Drugs in Milk

I have reviewed the excretion of drugs in milk elsewhere.[210] Probably the only substances which are found in a higher concentration in milk than in the blood or urine are thiouracil[459] and radioactive iodine.[259a] In one patient the concentration of thiouracil in the milk was twelve times that in the blood. Bromides and iodides may cause a rash in the baby when taken by the mother : bromides in addition may make the baby drowsy. I have seen three babies who were unduly drowsy while receiving milk from their epileptic mothers who were receiving phenobarbitone. Experimental changing of the feed and return to the breast milk proved that their drowsiness was due to the phenobarbitone in the mothers' milk. Phenytoin passes into the breast milk and may cause methæmoglobinæmia and cyanosis in the baby.[129]

Alcohol, if taken in excess by the mother, may affect the baby. Bisdom [47] described an 8-day-old baby who was intoxicated by the alcohol received through the milk of his mother, who had drunk a whole bottle of port in one day. The baby was in a deep unrousable sleep, with a poor pulse and no reaction to pain. Alcohol was demonstrated in the baby's blood. Nicotine may pass into the breast milk, and is said to have rendered babies restless, and to have caused diarrhœa, vomiting and tachycardia in babies. Ergot may cause symptoms of ergotism in babies. When a mother ate large quantities of carrots while breast-feeding, her baby became yellow as a result of carotinæmia.

Dicoumarin, tromexan and allied substances pass through into the milk [90] and may affect the baby at a time when the prothrombin is low. They are said to be an occasional cause of liver damage in the baby. I have seen a considerable number of mothers breast-feeding their babies while receiving tromexan, and have never yet seen any adverse effect in the baby.

No other drugs have been proved to have an adverse effect on the baby. There is a difference of opinion as to whether the emodin-containing drugs—rhubarb, cascara, senna and aloes affect the breast milk, but it is the impression of many that they do, and may cause diarrhœa and colic in the baby.

There is no evidence that caffein, sulphonamides, mandelic acid, salicylates, quinine, penicillin or other antibiotics pass into the milk in sufficient quantity to affect the baby.

Other Substances in Breast Milk

Protein substances may pass into the breast milk, and have been said to cause allergic manifestations in the baby. Amongst these is egg white.[115, 376, 376a] Rhesus antibodies are found in breast milk, but have no adverse effect on the baby.[85, 421]

If a mother eats a considerable number of oranges or some unripe fruit it is possible that the baby may have colic as a result. It is customary to warn nursing mothers not to eat onions, pickles or turnip, on the ground that they may affect the baby. In a study of three months' colic, I could find no relation between food taken by the mother and the development of colic in the baby. The evidence for this is uncertain. It is not known whether foodstuffs taken by the mother have an adverse effect on the taste of the milk. It is known, however, that many plants and foods give undesirable flavours to cow's milk.[332] The onion–garlic group affects the milk by allyl sulphide. Essential oils, aromatic esters and aldehydes taken in feeds cause an unpleasant taste in cow's milk.

There have been several papers concerning the toxic effect of the milk of a mother suffering from beriberi.[127] The toxic substance is thought to be methylglyoxal and other intermediary metabolites. A baby suffering from galactosæmia will not tolerate milk.

Human milk is by no means sterile. It may contain staphylococci and other organisms, but there is no evidence that they have a bad effect on the baby.

A few babies have colic and irritability when breast fed at the time of a menstrual period. The cause of this is unknown. The literature was reviewed by Grulee and Caldwell,[170] but no definite conclusion as to the ætiology of the colic was reached. It is commonly supposed that there is a temporary falling off of the milk supply at the time of the period, but there is a disagreement about this, some having found the reverse to be true.

Plantenga and Filippo [336] claimed that they found certain chemical changes in the breast milk about 24 hours before the onset of the menses in mothers whose babies had colic. The changes included a fall in the lactose content and an elevation in the chloride content of the milk. There were no changes in the milk of mothers whose children were symptom free.

In the present state of our knowledge we can only say that the cause of colic at the time of the menstrual period is unknown. I even doubt whether it really exists.

CHAPTER 4

BREAST AND NIPPLE DIFFICULTIES

Overdistension of the Breast

Definition and Ætiology

According to Waller,[434] who has given a full account of overdistension of the breast, about seven of every ten primiparæ have some degree of " overdistension " (usually termed by him " overload "). In one out of five primiparæ the overdistension is marked. He classified the breasts of lactating women into four categories : (1) Normal. There is hardly any rise of tension and the outflow is free. (2) Overload. There is a moderate overfilling with a rise of tension. (3) Engorgement. A greater degree of overfilling, often with some œdema of the nipple and of the skin over the breast. (4) Engorgement with obstruction. This is the extreme type without any outflow. The breasts are considerably enlarged. The margins stand out as a sharp ridge from the chest wall. The skin is tightly stretched and glistening, while the veins are congested. There is pitting œdema over the breast and the nipple is œdematous. There is extreme tenderness to the touch and considerable pain. I prefer to term these cases of overdistension mild, moderate or severe.

The cause and nature of overdistension of the breast is not clear. Waller thought that a relevant factor is the elasticity of the skin. If the skin is rigid and inelastic it will not permit enlargement of the breast, and pain and engorgement are apt to occur. It seems likely that another basic trouble is inadequate emptying of the breast after the milk has begun to come in. This may be due to the baby having difficulty in obtaining the milk because of depression of the nipple, or because he is lethargic, irritable or sucking badly. The difficulty may be caused by the doctor or nurse, in preventing the child sucking or only allowing him to suck at infrequent intervals. In more severe cases the breast tissue is hard and the nipple fails to protract, so that the baby cannot get his jaws far enough behind it to get the milk. The doctor or nurse may fail to try to express milk if the baby does not relieve the distension. The distension may then increase, so that eventually the distension of the alveoli obstructs the venous return. It then becomes much more difficult or impossible for the baby to obtain the milk or for the attendant to express it, for the ducts in turn become obstructed by venous obstruction and œdema of the breast tissue develops. Newton and Newton [312] attempted to demonstrate the mechanism experimentally. They weighed babies before and after feeds. Ten minutes after their feeds they used an electric breast pump for 5 minutes on each breast. A subcutaneous injection of 0·3 ml. of pitocin was given, and a minute later the breast pump was used again for a further 5 minutes. They worked out the total quantity of milk produced and found that the quantity was directly related to the degree of engorgement. They thought that the retention of milk in the alveoli, which if severe leads to vascular obstruction, may be due to a failure of the " let-down reflex," or to failure to allow the baby to suck enough.

The Results of Overdistension

Overdistension of the breast causes pain to the mother, and so leads to insomnia and worry. Both pain and worry have an adverse effect on the supply of milk, and pain, by interfering with the let-down reflex, aggravates the overdistension. Severe or prolonged overdistension presents a considerable danger to lactation, for involution sets in and the milk supply then fails. Waller [434] thought that unrelieved overdistension is probably the commonest cause of failure in the milk supply.

With the less severe degrees of overdistension, the prognosis for lactation is good, provided that the overdistension is relieved. It was shown in the Jessop Hospital for Women at Sheffield that, when all cases of overdistension, mild and severe, were grouped together, the prognosis for lactation was in fact better than if no overdistension at all occurred. Table I shows the incidence of breast feeding in mothers who were feeding their babies on either a rigid or a demand schedule.

TABLE I

Relation of Overdistension of the Breast to Incidence of Breast Feeding

	Incidence of Full Breast Feeding			
	On Discharge		At One Month	
No Overdistension	Number	Per cent.	Number	Per cent.
Rigid schedule	54/64	84·4	33/59	55·9
Demand schedule	95/102	93·1	81/101	80·2
All cases	149/166	89·8	114/160	71·3
Overdistension				
Rigid schedule	34/36	94·4	29/36	80·5
Demand schedule	21/21	100	18/21	85·7
All cases	55/57	96·5	47/57	82·5

It will be seen that, whereas 80·5 per cent. of mothers who had overdistension on a rigid schedule were fully breast feeding at 1 month, only 55·9 per cent. of those who did not have overdistension were breast feeding their babies at that age. It seems that overdistension suggests that the milk supply is abundant and that, if it is properly treated, the outlook for breast feeding is therefore good rather than bad. There is no doubt, however, that if overdistension is severe, so that expression of milk is impossible, lactation is in great danger of failing.

Overdistension is apt to lead to infection and breast abscess as a result of stasis. A further danger of moderate or severe overdistension is the fact that the baby cannot obtain the milk, partly because he cannot get his jaws behind the nipple, owing to the hardness of the breast, and partly because the outflow is obstructed by the venous engorgement. If, therefore, he is allowed to suck, he inevitably makes the nipple sore, and in addition he swallows air, gets colic, may vomit and fails to gain weight.

For many reasons, therefore, overdistension must be adequately and promptly treated.

The Treatment

In mild cases no treatment is necessary, though a self-demand schedule is advisable, because a baby on this schedule is likely to have more frequent feeds than a baby on a rigid one. If necessary he should be encouraged to take frequent feeds in order to help to empty the breast. If there is some discomfort from overdistension between the feeds, the milk should be expressed by hand.

The technique of manual expression is as follows. Expression of milk is achieved by two movements (Fig. 2). The first is compression of the whole breast between the two hands, starting at the margin of the breast tissue and continuing down as far as the areola. Firm pressure is maintained throughout the movement, which is repeated ten or twelve times. The aim of this movement is to impel milk from the smaller into the larger ducts and lacteal sinuses. The second movement is designed to empty the sinuses. The breast tissue just behind the areola is pinched sharply and repeatedly between the thumb and forefinger of one hand while the breast is held firmly fixed by the other. The direction of this force is backward towards the centre of the breast rather than towards the base of the nipple.

A common mistake is to move the finger and thumb over the surface of the skin, thus rubbing the skin. The finger and thumb remain over the same piece of skin and should not move over it. The other common mistake is to move the skin over the breast tissue instead of compressing the sinuses. It should be possible to make the milk squirt out when the movement is properly performed. Unless overdistension is severe it causes no discomfort to the mother.

In moderate cases of overdistension the baby should be encouraged to take frequent feeds, provided that he can obtain the milk. If there is any œdema he should not be allowed to suck. If he cannot obtain the milk and the overdistension is only moderate, some milk should

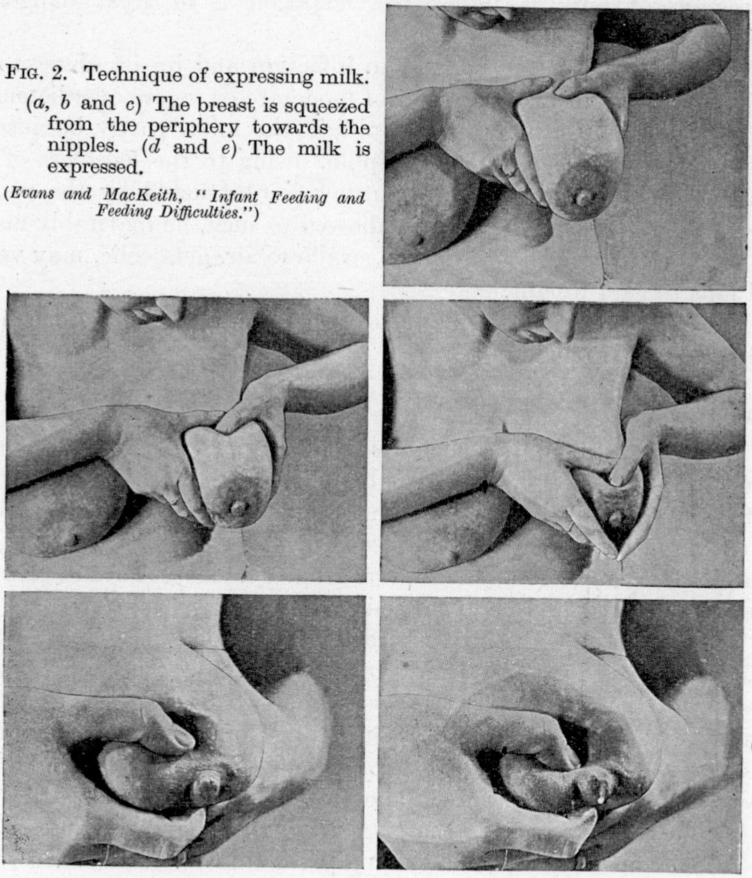

FIG. 2. Technique of expressing milk. (*a*, *b* and *c*) The breast is squeezed from the periphery towards the nipples. (*d* and *e*) The milk is expressed.

(*Evans and MacKeith, "Infant Feeding and Feeding Difficulties."*)

(*a*) (*b*) (*c*) (*d*) (*e*)

be expressed by hand and then the baby should be allowed to suck. Any excess of milk after his feed is removed by hand.

In some women the breast fills so rapidly that manual expression of milk is insufficient to prevent overdistension. Almost as soon as the milk has been expressed the breast fills up again and discomfort is experienced. In such cases it is essential to give stilbœstrol, in doses of 10 mg. four-hourly by mouth day and night, until the pain is relieved. Usually three or four doses are sufficient.

In a critical review [189] of the action of diethylstilbœstrol, it was shown that its mode of action is not clear. It seemed to do little to prevent the secretion of milk when given routinely to 153 patients for 4 to 10 days post-partum in a daily dose of 5 to 25 mg. ; 13 of 83 "non-lactators" needed breast binders for overdistension, and 70 supplied enough milk for their babies in spite of it. Nevertheless 90 per cent. of the lactating women avoided engorgement of the breast, and in those who did develop overdistension, pain was prevented. These confusing findings at least indicate that stilbœstrol is worth giving, even though it is not altogether successful, and we do not know how it works.

In moderate cases a mechanical device called the "Humalactor," made by Messrs. Gascoignes of Reading, has proved useful.

In severe cases it is probably better not to attempt to express milk. Any attempt to do so causes very severe pain and no milk, or practically no milk, is obtained. The baby is not allowed to suck but is maintained by expressed milk from other mothers or by artificial feeds. Stilbœstrol is administered and the breast is firmly supported. As soon as possible milk is expressed by hand, and as soon as all œdema has gone the child is allowed to suck. Manual expression is continued after feeds until lactation is fully established, and milk is expressed between feeds if there is any discomfort from overdistension.

On no account are hot fomentations applied to the breast.

Prevention

Waller [434] showed that daily manual expression of colostrum in the last 3 months of pregnancy reduced the incidence of "overload." His results were as follows :

Overload	Manual Expression (per cent.)	Controls (per cent.)
None	63	23
Mild	12	21
Moderate	20	37
Severe	5	19

It seems as if the daily expression of colostrum during pregnancy makes the outflow easier after the baby has been born. Every mother ought to know how to express milk, and if she has learnt to express colostrum before the birth of the baby, it will be easy for her to deal with mild overdistension by expressing the breast. The value of self-demand feeding in reducing the incidence of overdistension has already been mentioned. Newton and Newton [312] thought that there was less overdistension if babies were kept with their mothers instead of being placed in a nursery, and if they were fed on a self-demand schedule. It is not yet known whether self-demand feeding in the first 2 days of life affects the incidence of overdistension or not. It is certainly a bad thing to prevent a baby sucking after the second day, for that is liable to lead to overdistension of the breast. Both breasts must be used at each feed, for otherwise the breasts will be improperly emptied and overdistension may occur.

Local Overdistension

This is not uncommon. A segment of the breast is painful and distended, the rest of the breast tissue being unaffected. It may occur at any time during lactation. It may be due to the mother lying in a particular position, or to an abnormal opening of a duct, or to the need of a better-fitting breast support. The absence of fever and malaise distinguishes it from mastitis, which it otherwise closely resembles. Treatment is that of the cause, together with manual expression of the affected part.

Soreness of the Nipples

Soreness of the nipples is very common. The incidence of soreness varies from hospital to hospital, depending largely on the management of the breasts. Probably about three out of every ten women have some soreness of the nipples. Some have given a higher incidence.

Ætiology

Gunther [172] wrote an excellent review of the subject and described experimental work into its ætiology. She describes two forms of sore nipples : (1) The erosive or petechial. In this form there is swelling of the papillæ, usually at the centre of the nipple. There may be small, almost translucent, œdematous areas, and later petechiæ. In some there are petechiæ without œdema. In severe cases the petechiæ merge to form a red crescent transversely across the nipple. Sometimes the superficial layers of epithelium are eroded as a ruptured blister. This form is most common in the first few days and rarely begins after the first week. (2) The ulcerative or fissured type. In this form there is an ulcer, usually at the side of the nipple. It is not seen before the fifth day. In some cases of soreness of the nipple there is no visible lesion.

There are many causes of soreness of the nipples. Gunther thinks that the cause of the erosive or petechial form is negative pressure caused by the baby's suction ; hence the observation that the greatest pain is felt in the first few sucks. The larger the baby in general the greater was the suction. The older infant may approximate his jaws so closely round the areola that he creates a vacuum and, unless a

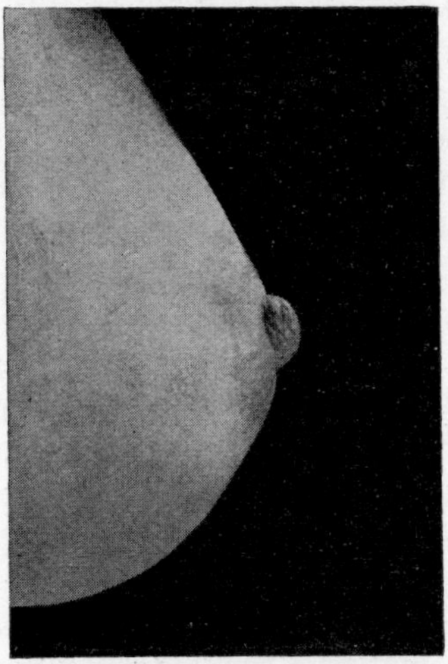

(*a*)

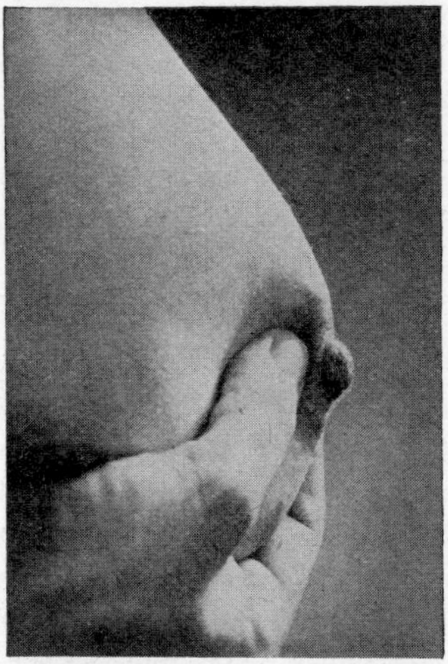

(*b*)

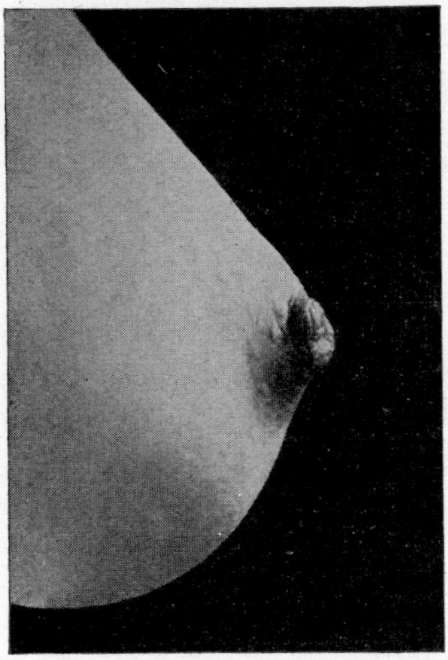

(*c*)

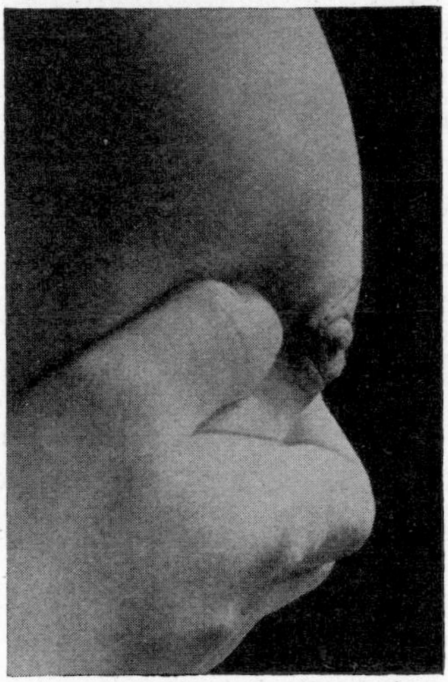

(*d*)

FIG. 3

(*a*) Normal nipple.
(*b*) Normal nipple projecting from breast when areola is pinched.
(*c*) A nipple which will retract when areola is pinched.
(*d*) Nipple retracting when areola is pinched.

(*Photographs by courtesy of Allen and Hanburys.*)

finger is inserted into the corner of his mouth to release the vacuum when he withdraws from the breast, it may hurt the mother. Gunther thought that the ulcerative type is due to mechanical trauma at a time when there has been a sudden withdrawal of œstrogen.

Abramson[1] thought that mechanical trauma from clothes or gauze was an important factor, together with thinness or soddenness of the epithelium and defective hygiene. He devised a plastic breast shield (not a nipple shield) which fitted comfortably over the whole breast and was kept in place by a brassiere between feeds. It was removed at feed time and restored immediately after. Using this method only 2·4 per cent. of 1,000 patients developed soreness of the nipple.

Waller[434, 435] thought that defective protraction of the nipple was an important factor. It may be due to a persistence of the original invagination of the mammary dimple which has failed to become detached when it became everted. When the examiner's fingers pinch the areola in such cases behind the base of the nipple, the nipple is pulled in instead of extended, as it should be (Fig. 3). The nipple is anchored to the underlying tissues instead of being loosely attached to the breast and, when later the child sucks, it reacts by retracting towards the breast instead of projecting into the mouth. Such a nipple lies during suckling in the front of the baby's mouth instead of well back against the palate, and suction falls on its surface instead of on the areola. The nipple is therefore damaged. (It is felt by some that the practice of applying finger pressure behind the areola so that the breast tissue is kept away from the baby's nose during suckling may lead to a similarly abnormal position of the nipple in relation to the baby's palate, and so to soreness of the nipple.) Waller said that about a third of primiparæ have sufficient defect of the nipple to threaten difficulty in the puerperium.

This work was confirmed by Ogden and MacKeith[318] and Gunther.[174] The former found that many nipples which on superficial scrutiny appear to stand out well from the breast prove to protrude inadequately when tested by pressure between finger and thumb at the areolar margin ; 20 per cent. of primiparæ had normal-looking nipples which proved to be nonprotractile in this way. Of 234 mothers studied, 52 (22 per cent.) required treatment, and of those only 2 had visibly malformed nipples ; 49 of the 52 were cured by antenatal care with the Waller glass or plastic nipple shield. It was not thought advisable for the mother to try to pull the nipple out herself.

Waller thought that the other major cause of soreness of the nipple is sucking when the nipple is œdematous as a result of overdistension of the breast. The baby is unable to get his jaws behind the nipple because it fails to protract into his mouth. If the baby sucks, soreness of the nipple is an inevitable result.

Soreness of the nipple may be due to the baby sucking too long on the breast. It was shown on p. 21 that restriction of time on the breast in the first 2 or 3 days did not seem to reduce the incidence of soreness of the nipple, but it seems likely that if a baby sucks on the breast after obtaining the milk he may cause soreness.

Newton [314] studied the effect of various methods of nipple care in relation to soreness. Four methods were used in 287 women. Some washed the nipple with soap and water before each feed ; others applied 70 per cent. alcohol to the nipples ; others washed them in water ; others applied an ointment containing vitamin A and D. The mothers using soap and water and alcohol had the highest incidence of soreness. It was thought that the soap washed off the protective greasy covering. It was thought that lanoline, perhaps with added vitamin A or D, reduced the incidence of soreness. She warned against the use of the compound tincture of benzoin, because of its alcohol content.

The rôle of the feeding schedule after the first 2 or 3 days has already been discussed. It was found that the incidence of soreness of the nipples was twice as great when a baby was fed on a rigid schedule as when fed on a self-demand one. Newton did not find that limitation of the duration or number of feeds in the first 2 days was of value. She felt that a baby should suck when he wants and as much as he wants till he is satisfied. During the course of a study of sore nipples at the Jessop Hospital at Sheffield, we found that the average number of feeds given to babies on a self-demand schedule from birth was only 2·2 in the first day—whereas we had given 3 feeds in the first day to babies fed on a rigid schedule. In other words, a self-demand feeding schedule did not increase the number of feeds in the first 3 days. Walser [438] said : "In many cases the mounting incidence of cracked and sore nipples is not because the nipple has little rest between feedings, but because in many cases the baby is kept in the nursery too long after birth and brought in so infrequently that a starving, ravenous baby results and the mother's breast is damaged by the child's own efforts." Margaret Mead noted that among primitive tribes in the Pacific, amongst whom the practice was to feed babies on the breast at extremely frequent intervals, soreness of the nipples was practically unknown, for "the satisfied infant did not draw so ravenously."

Some books still recommend that the nipple should be scrubbed in the ante-natal period with a scrubbing brush, and that it should be hardened with spirit. Both these methods are much more likely to damage the nipple than to protect it. Hard skin cracks a great deal more easily than soft skin.

Waller and others have drawn attention to the danger of trying to remove dried secretions from the nipple without soaking them off. Soreness of the nipples may result from the abrasions caused.

Poor hygiene is an important cause of soreness of the nipples. I have seen women who were in the habit of " cleaning " the nipple before feeding a baby by spitting on to the hand and then rubbing the hand over the nipple. Failure to keep the nipples clean before and after the feeds may lead to soreness.

Psychological factors play an important part in complaints of soreness of the nipples. They should always be suspected when careful examination of a nipple with a lens fails to show any abrasion or abnormality, or when the pain complained of is out of all proportion to the extent of the lesion found. Worry about previous genuine soreness may well lead to soreness in another pregnancy. Often, too, there is an underlying revulsion to breast feeding, and if that is the case it is usually better that the baby should be artificially fed.

The Dangers of Soreness of the Nipple

The dangers of soreness of the nipple are several. It causes a great deal of pain to the mother, and pain alone has an adverse effect on the supply of milk—partly by inhibiting the draught reflex. In addition it causes worry and insomnia, and both have an adverse effect on lactation. If the baby is wrongly allowed to continue to suck after soreness has developed, the pain increases and failure of lactation is likely to result. Many babies are taken off the breast on account of improperly treated soreness of the nipples, the mother having felt that she " could not carry on any longer " with breast feeding because it was so painful. There is a danger that the staphylococcus, which has probably gained entry at the site of the abrasion on the nipple, will cause mastitis and abscess. Sometimes the nipple bleeds when the baby sucks, and the baby is then found to have melæna.

Prevention and Treatment

When a nipple is found to be insufficiently protractile, the mother is supplied with the Waller plastic * or glass nipple shield. The shields are applied so that the nipple lies in the centre of the opening. They are held in position by a well-fitting brassiere, which should have a diaphragm. It is advisable for comfort to replace narrow shoulder straps with wider ribbon so that extra uplift can be given without making the shoulder sore.[318] They should be worn from the twentieth week, or earlier in severe cases.

Waller compared the incidence of soreness of the nipples in women who expressed colostrum in the last 3 months of pregnancy with that of controls. Soreness developed in 12 per cent. of the mothers who expressed colostrum, and 24 per cent. of those who did not.

If the nipple in the ante-natal period is hard it may be softened with

* The Woolwich Breast Shield (Allen and Hanburys).

lanoline. Other preventive measures are implicit in the remarks made above.

As soon as any soreness develops and any lesion can be seen on careful examination the baby should be taken off the affected breast. The milk is expressed at the usual feed intervals and given to the baby.

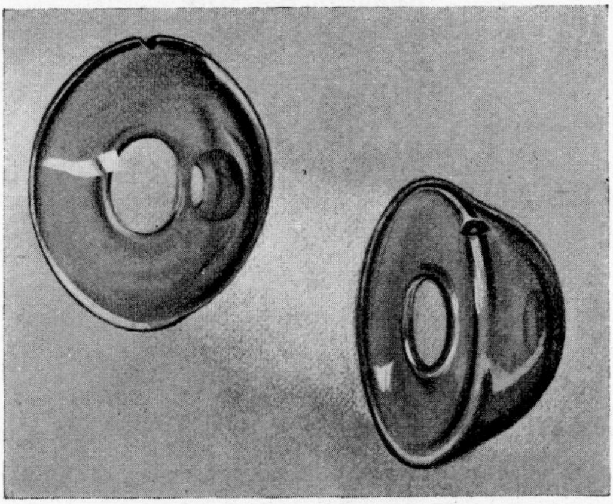

(*a*)

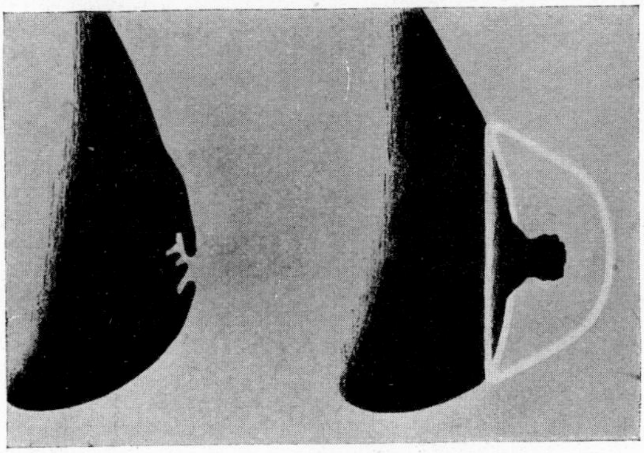

(*b*)

FIG. 4.

(*a*) Glass shields. (*b*) The shield in use.

(Evans and MacKeith, "Infant Feeding and Feeding Difficulties.")

Penicillin cream should be applied four times a day. As soon as the nipple has healed the baby is returned to the breast.

A sore nipple will heal more quickly if it is exposed to the air, and particularly to sunlight. A breast binder or brassiere is better avoided.

If there is frequently recurring soreness of the nipples, continued expression may be needed, the milk being given to the baby. I have not had experience of the use of nipple shields in such cases.

Too Large a Nipple

One occasionally sees nipples which are so large that the baby cannot get his jaw sufficiently far back to obtain the milk. In such cases the milk has to be expressed by hand and given to the baby in a bottle.

Blood in the Milk

When a nipple is deeply cracked, blood may be found in the milk. Occasionally, however, one sees blood in the milk when there is no visible crack or fissure. This may be due to a duct papilloma, and the woman should be carefully studied and followed up by the gynæcologist on that account. There is no doubt that in some mothers there is no discoverable cause for the bleeding, but one presumes that there must be an anatomical cause. Haagensen* regarded it as " an expression of the intensity of the epithelial proliferation in the rapidly growing breast " rather than as a manifestation of disease. For psychological reasons it may be better to take the baby off the breast and suppress lactation by stilbœstrol (10 mg. four-hourly for 5 days or so).

* Haagensen C. D. (1956). " Diseases of the Breast," Philadelphia. Saunders.

CHAPTER 5

INSUFFICIENCY OF MILK

THE high incidence of artificial feeding in this country and elsewhere is an indication of the importance of the problem of insufficiency of milk and the failure of lactation. Insufficiency of milk may arise as a result of defects in the mother, child or her attendants, and it may lead to complete failure of breast feeding.

Ætiology

Inadequate Emptying of the Breast. The amount of milk produced by a mother depends largely on the demand. There is a delicate regulating mechanism which enables a woman to feed a large baby just as adequately as a small one. If the breast for any reason is not fully emptied, then the supply of milk falls off. Conversely, if the breast is fully emptied by manual expression after feeds (assuming that there is some milk to express), more milk will be secreted. A woman had persistent trouble with sore nipples, and so fed her baby entirely on expressed milk[267]; she was so efficient in expressing that in two lactation periods she sold a surplus of 30,000 ounces of milk for 3,717 dollars. Another woman sold 20,000 surplus ounces in one lactation period for 2,020 dollars. A wet nurse is known to have produced 5,770 ml. of milk in one day—and was able to maintain seven babies at a time with the quantity produced.

Von Sydow[430] found that routine expression of milk in a Gothenberg Hospital led to 20 litres of milk being available every day for the milk bank. He found that if a mother was secreting 300 ml. of milk or more by the sixth day, she had almost a hundred per cent. chance of fully breast feeding if she was healthy, had normal nipples, and if the baby were sucking well, and she did not belong to a particularly low social class. Even with a secretion of 200 ml. she would have a ninety per cent. chance of fully breast feeding.

One of the most important causes of inadequate emptying of the breast is overdistension during the first few days of the puerperium (p. 28). In a moderate or severe case the baby is unable to get the milk, and in a severe case it is almost impossible to express the milk by hand. Involution sets in as a result and lactation fails, or at least the supply of milk is inadequate for the baby's needs. Every farmer knows that if a cow is allowed to go unmilked the milk production falls off. Waller [434, 435] thought that high milk tension, which may lead to inadequate emptying of the breast, is probably the main factor leading to insufficiency of milk. He thought that if there is much milk left after a baby has sucked, the emptying of the breast is inadequate unless completed by manual expression, and lactation fails. He recommended that in the period of the establishment of lactation manual expression should be tried after the baby has sucked in order to determine how much milk there is left. If there is much milk there, it should be expressed. From one mother, whose baby was gaining weight well, the residual milk removed in 12 days exceeded what was taken by 55 per cent. From his studies at Woolwich he emphasized that the difficulty in most women is not in producing enough milk but in maintaining the yield.

Inadequate emptying of the breast may be due to a wide variety of causes. The baby may suck badly as a result of a minor degree of birth injury, cerebral irritability, inertia or other causes. The baby may suck less well if he has an intense physiological jaundice. He may be an irritable baby who snarls at the breast, screams as soon as he gets near the breast or after he has sucked for a minute or two, and takes very little even though the milk supply is adequate. There may be a mechanical difficulty in the child, such as a blocked nose, stomatitis or cleft palate, which prevents his sucking well. A mentally defective child is apt to suck very badly and show little interest in food, and so he does not empty the breast well. If the mother's nipples are depressed, any of these difficulties are aggravated and emptying is incomplete.

In my opinion the premature use of complementary feeds is one of the chief reasons for the failure of the milk supply. It is not at all uncommon to hear about babies who were given complementary feeds as soon as the third day of life. If this is done *and the breast is not fully emptied by manual expression,* lactation is very liable to fail. Probably the chief reason, however, for the danger of such complementary feeding is that the baby sucks less well at the breast and so empties it less completely and the supply of milk then fails. It should be quite exceptional to give a complementary feed in the first five days.

Premature complementary feeding is due to a variety of causes. It may be due to undue insistence on a rapid gain of weight, or on recovery of the birth weight by the tenth day. There is no occasion for such anxiety. A baby may be a long way below the birth weight on the tenth day and yet be perfectly well. It is often due to fear that the baby will be harmed by having little milk in the first few days. The baby is not harmed by this provided that, if the weather is hot or the baby becomes feverish or cries a great deal for food, boiled water is given him. One of the chief causes of premature complementary feeding is the test feed. Test feeds are essential under certain circumstances, but routine test feeds are thoroughly harmful in wasting the nurses' time, in causing anxiety to the mother and in leading to premature complementary feeds. *Test feeds show not the amount of milk which the mother is producing but the amount of milk taken by the baby.* Failure to realize this in the case of the irritable baby will almost certainly lead to the giving of complementary feeds. Many are ignorant of the normal rate at which milk comes in. They do not realize that $\frac{3}{4}$ oz. of milk per pound on the fourth day is adequate, and that $1\frac{3}{4}$ oz. per pound is all that most babies get from the mother by the seventh or eighth day.

There is no doubt that the ready availability of tins of dried milk is an important cause of complementary feeding. In countries where such artificial foods are not available the majority of mothers breast feed their babies perfectly satisfactorily.

Inadequate emptying of the breast may be due to the practice of instructing a mother to use only one breast at each feed. If the baby is being fed approximately four-hourly, this means that each breast will only be emptied at approximately eight-hourly intervals. Involution sets in as a result of the small demand for milk. In the same way it may be due to the use of supplementary feeds—complete feeds of cow's milk given in between the breast feeds. Supplementary feeds should never be given except in the weaning period. If they are it means that the breast remains unemptied for prolonged periods. A similar difficulty sometimes arises with babies on a self-demand schedule. An occasional baby on this schedule, even as young as 2 months of age, only demands three feeds a day. Emptying of the breast is inadequate with such a schedule and the supply of milk may fail.

The question of prelacteal feeds is discussed on p. 18. It is uncertain whether they have an adverse effect on the establishment of lactation by reducing the child's hunger and thirst and so reducing the emptying of the breasts.

There are many instances, such as soreness of the nipples and overdistension, in which manual expression of milk is necessary. It is obvious that inefficient expression and therefore improper emptying of the breast may cause a falling off in the supply of milk.

Worry. Worry and anxiety have a bad effect on the supply of milk. This fact is known to farmers. Croft [99] wrote that "anxiety neurosis" is commonly seen in cows. They refuse to let down their milk. A stranger in the cowshed at milking time may cause "neurotic cows" to give almost no milk, although he does nothing more than stand in the doorway of the shed. Thomas Hardy, in "Tess of the D'Urbervilles," described how an animal would let milk down freely for one but not for another. The cause of a morning's unsuccessful milking was said to be disturbance of the herd by the arrival of a new farm hand.

Severe emotional disturbance may stop the supply of milk altogether. Moloney,[300] writing about the people of Okinawa described how bombing stopped the supply of breast milk. Waller * told the story of a woman who was fully and successfully breast feeding her baby suddenly being called to a hospital to see her husband, who was said to have been taken there after a serious accident. When she reached the hospital she saw the patient being wheeled from the theatre with his head and face swathed in bandages. The surgeon expressed his sympathy with her. When she arrived home her husband was waiting for her and cursed her soundly for keeping him waiting for his tea. It had been a case of mistaken identity. The shock, however, was such that the supply of milk completely failed, and it was only after heavy sedation that it returned in a few days. Newton and Newton,[311] discussing the mechanism of the draught or let-down reflex in women, performed experiments to demonstrate the central inhibition of the reflex by distractions of various kinds. The inhibition was overcome by injections of pitocin. The distractions were of a singularly unpleasant kind. While the baby was being fed they either (i) immersed the mother's feet alternately for 10 seconds out of every 30 in ice-cold water ; or (ii) rapidly asked a series of mathematical questions, giving an electric shock of moderate intensity when there was delay in replying or a wrong reply ; or (iii) pulled intermittently at a length of surgical bandage attached to each of the big toes. It seems hardly surprising that each distraction caused a considerable reflex falling off in milk production.

It is very easy to arouse worry and anxiety in a woman who has recently given birth to a baby. She is in a particularly emotional state. She has had a trying and exhausting time for some months, culminating in labour. She knows that a new-born infant has a rather slender hold on life, and the slightest suggestion of an abnormality in the child may cause severe anxiety. A woman may be worried if her baby is separated from her by being kept in a nursery instead of at her side, where she can watch over him. This worry is probably in part the explanation of the observation made by Fields and Rose[128a] and others that there is a higher incidence of breast feeding when babies are kept in their mother's room than when they are kept in a nursery. The mother may hear the crying of a baby in the distance and think that it is her baby who is crying, and she fears that his wants will go unheeded. It is common for the doctor or nurse, in the round of patients, to utter a remark about the baby's head, or poor weight gain, or excessive weight loss, which immediately causes profound worry in the mother,

* Personal communication.

out of all proportion to the abnormality present. Any suggestion that there is not enough milk may cause a great deal of anxiety, and this has a considerable effect on the supply of milk. The mother may in any case worry about the child's appearance, grunting respirations, nævoid staining of the skin above the nose or on the eyelids or other features. She is particularly apt to be distressed by inertia in the baby, or more still by irritability. Sometimes mothers are worried by excessive interference by the nurse in the management of the feeding, especially when the baby is being difficult and irritable. The mother feels that she could do much better if she were left alone. She may have little confidence in the nurse's ability to help her to establish lactation, and worry results.

Routine test feeds are particularly liable to cause worry. They are inherently undesirable because of the mere suggestion which they inevitably carry that the establishment of breast feeding is doubtful and difficult. Babies suck better at some feeds than at others. There are many fallacies in their interpretation. Even though the doctor does not tell her how much the baby has gained in a feed, the mother has ways and means of finding out and worries when she thinks that she has not enough breast milk.

In Palestine test feeds had to be stopped on account of the danger to breast feeding, for the supply of cow's milk was inadequate.[356] It must be admitted that there are differences of opinion about the value of routine test feeds. Harold Waller * said that routine test feeds were on all the 24,000 mothers who passed through the wards of the British Hospital for Mothers and Babies at Woolwich over a 26 year period. He thought that the ability to do these test feeds without disturbing the mother is a test of good nursing.

There are other ways in which the mother is upset. She may be worried because the milk is slow in coming in or because she thinks it normally comes in on the first or second day. She is considerably worried by the pain of overdistension or of a sore nipple. She is anxious if the baby cries excessively, as so often happens on a rigid feeding schedule, or about her ability to manage the child when she gets home. Such worry is more likely if the baby has been kept in a nursery. It is less likely if the mother has had the baby at her side day and night and has become accustomed to handling him, bathing him and changing his napkin. I have many times seen mothers worrying considerably about home, longing to get home and being kept in the hospital because there was an insufficiency of milk. The insufficiency was due to worry, and when the mother's hopes were realized and she got home lactation promptly became adequate. Embarrassment at breast feeding in a ward with others present may

* Personal communication.

inhibit the flow of milk. Excessively frequent weighing leads to anxiety. When the mother gets home she loses the support of a nurse in whom she had confidence and immediately finds all manner of difficulties in the management of her child. She worries and lactation fails.

A doctor may have been unwise in his efforts to convince her of the importance of breast feeding, and have said so much that the woman feels considerable worry about her ability to produce sufficient milk and feels guilty if there are signs of insufficiency.

It is essential to understand the effect of worry on lactation and to realize how numerous are the possible sources of worry for a mother who has recently given birth to a baby, particularly if he is her first-born.

In some East African tribes a woman who is unable to nurse her child loses her man's love ; he turns to another woman.[109]

Fatigue. The mother may have been exhausted by the effects of delivery or by an illness during pregnancy, such as toxæmia. The doctor is apt to think that the patient has a real rest in the maternity hospital. The patient is likely to think otherwise. Rightly or wrongly, hospital routine causes constant interruptions throughout the day, beginning at about 5 a.m. and finishing at about 11.30 p.m. A patient who is a friend of mine kept a record of what she termed an unusually " quiet " day in a maternity hospital, noting the frequency and time of the interruptions in the form of visits from nurses, doctors, cleaners and others. There were thirty-two interruptions before midday, and continual openings and closings of the door of her room after that for one reason or another until the night sister's visit at 11.30 p.m. Some babies cry a great deal more than others and demand food much more frequently than others. The majority of babies demand at least one night feed for the first few weeks (usually 10 weeks), and the mother, even when she gets home, is unable to have a good night's rest. With only one baby at home she is extremely busy during the day. She has to queue for food at the shops. She is likely to have very little help at home and is in a state of constant fatigue for the first 2 or 3 months after delivery. Such fatigue inevitably has a deleterious effect on lactation.

Poverty and Undernutrition. Several workers quoted by Douglas [116] showed that there is a higher incidence of breast feeding in the well-to-do than in the poor. Of the various factors involved nutrition is probably one. Wallace [433] showed that sheep which are malnourished in the last months of pregnancy have a poor milk yield. Several workers [17] showed that working-class women were able to breast feed their babies longer if their diet during pregnancy had been supplemented by additional vitamins and other foodstuffs. There are, however, differences of opinion about this, some workers [432] claiming that even quite severe malnutrition has no effect on lactation or on the quality of milk produced.

Genetic Factors. There is evidence of the importance of genetically determined differences in milk production in cattle and in rats.[220] It is likely that there are similar genetic factors in human beings.

Unknown Factors. In many instances the cause of insufficiency is unknown. It must be emphasized, however, that the cause of insufficiency of the milk supply is likely to be recorded as unknown when in fact it is probably one of the factors mentioned above, such as improper emptying of the breast. Sedgwick [371] said : "I have never seen agalactia and seriously doubt its existence."

I am sure that it is an exaggeration to say that agalactia does not occur, but would agree that it is rare.

The Diagnosis of Insufficiency

The diagnosis is made on the basis of symptoms, the appearance of the child and the result of test feeds. When the deficiency is only slight there may be no sign other than defective weight gain. The child seems to be contented, sleeps well and the stools are normal. When the insufficiency is of moderate degree the baby cries excessively. He is likely to demand very frequent feeds—long after the new-born period, in which frequent demands for food by normal babies are common. He may refuse the breast or suck at the breast for 2 or 3 minutes and then withdraw and cry. He may suck at the breast for a normal time and go to sleep, only to waken up half an hour later and cry. The crying is not stopped by picking him up. He may suffer from flatulence and colic as a result of sucking at an empty breast, with consequent air swallowing. Excessive air swallowing may cause vomiting. Weight gain is defective. He is likely to be constipated. If the deficiency is marked the stools become green and contain mucus without fæcal matter. After a time the child looks undernourished, with a loss of tissue turgor. When severe deficiency of milk continues, the child may lose his appetite and become too languid and exhausted to cry for food at all.

A confident diagnosis of underfeeding should not usually be made without confirmation by test feeds. Such confirmation should certainly be sought if there is the slightest doubt about the diagnosis and if the symptoms are of recent onset. When a test feed is done the baby is weighed before and after every feed for a whole day, so that the total weight gain can be calculated. It is essential that he should be weighed before and after every feed, for the amount of milk produced varies considerably from hour to hour. In general the most productive feed is the first in the morning. The late afternoon or early evening feed tends to be the most deficient. If complementary feeds are needed the knowledge of which feed is most deficient is important, for after these feeds the complements should be given.

It must be admitted that in a busy baby clinic one can often fairly safely assess the amount of milk which the baby is obtaining from the mother by means of the weight gain. Knowing that an average baby after the first 10 days requires approximately $2\frac{1}{2}$ oz. per lb. per day a weight gain of less than half the minimum " normal " weight gain of 6 oz. per week would suggest that the baby is receiving less than half the required quantity of milk from the mother—provided that there is no other cause for the defective weight (see p. 71).

The limitations and fallacies of test feeds must be thoroughly understood. It is particularly important to remember the normal rate at which milk comes in (p. 41). I have seen a child taken off the breast on the second day of life on the grounds that there was not sufficient milk for him. It must be remembered that there are individual variations in the amount of milk needed to satisfy a baby and to give an average weight gain. A test feed may show that the baby is receiving $2\frac{1}{2}$ oz. per lb. per day but that does not prove that the baby would not like to have more. His crying in spite of an intake which is enough for average babies may be due to hunger. The child at all the feeds must be weighed on the same scales, for scales are frequently inaccurate. He must be weighed without clothes. The passage of urine or fæces after a feed just before weighing will affect the figures for that feed. The fact that the test feed shows not the amount of milk which the mother is producing but merely the quantity which the child has obtained from the breast has already been mentioned. A child who is drowsy—perhaps as a result of being over-clothed—will not suck well and test feeds may give an entirely fictitious idea of the amount of milk available. It is obvious that test feeds are much more significant if the breast is fully emptied after every feed, the quantity of milk expressed being added to the quantity taken by the baby. This method alone gives an adequate picture of the quantity of milk produced by the mother.

In considering the diagnosis it must be remembered that any symptoms of insufficiency can also be produced by other conditions. The other causes of defective weight gain, flatulence, colic, vomiting, constipation and irritability are discussed in Chapter 6.

Prevention of Insufficiency

It is clear from what has been said that prevention begins in the ante-natal period, with treatment of depressed nipples and manual expression of colostrum in the last 3 months of pregnancy. Other preventive measures after the birth of the baby are implicit in the remarks concerning the ætiology. Complementary feeds should be avoided as far as possible in the first week (see p. 64), and are practically never necessary in the first 4 days. Preventive treatment includes prompt action in the case of overdistension, and immediate treatment of a sore nipple. Test feeds should never be done as a routine. They should only be done when there is a special indication, in particular suspected insufficiency of milk.

If a woman who had failed to breast feed her first baby was extremely anxious to feed her second one, I feel that the best advice to offer would be that she should express colostrum in the last 3 months of pregnancy. The child should be fed on a self-demand schedule. After the milk had come in, the breast would be emptied routinely after every feed until lactation was fully established. Complementary feeds would be avoided at least until the fifth day. She should have her baby in the room with her.

It may be added that an important preventive measure is the proper teaching of medical students and nurses.

Treatment

In some primitive peoples the baby is killed if the mother is unable to feed it on the breast.[457] In the sixteenth century Phaer [334] recommended powdered earth-worms as a lactagogue. Platt and Gin [337] described a variety of lactagogues in use in China. They included cuttle-fish soup, shrimps' heads cooked in wine, cooked sea slugs, powdered dead silk-worms in old wine, and sweet wine made from glutinous rice with the larvæ of blow-flies collected from fæces. Barats [40] even recommended breast-milk enemas. Zlocisti [468] caused the husband to suck the breast and so empty it. Jacobins caused the mother to suck her own breast by means of a tube attached to a nipple shield. In the Renaissance era a woman who lost her milk was given the udder of a goat to eat.[455] There are numerous examples in the literature of successful breast feeding by women who have not been pregnant.[131, 457] David Livingstone described several instances of grandmothers nursing a child. Wieschhoff [457] wrote that in Java it is the custom for babies to be nursed by their grandmothers if their own mothers are too busy to devote enough time to them. He quoted examples of the same phenomenon in the Maoris, North American Indians, Africans, Indians and South Americans. Margaret Mead [283] referred to the same practice in the New Guinea area. These reports are more than merely interesting. They suggest that it should be possible to get a baby back on to the breast after it has been off for some time. This in fact can be done. Sedgwick [371] described a 4-month-old baby who became fully breast fed after being off the breast for 9 weeks. At first he refused the breast when put to it. Soon he sucked. Milk was expressed after he had sucked and he was supported with complementary feeds. Eventually lactation was fully re-established. Another baby, aged 1 month, who had never been breast fed at all, was put to the breast and was fully breast fed by the age of 2 months. Spence [392] described the complete establishment of lactation in a woman who had not breast fed her baby at all for the first 11 weeks of his life. Probably a great deal more could be done to re-establish lactation in mothers who have taken their babies off the breast as a result of bad advice.

There is no evidence that iodine, thyroid extract, anterior pituitary extract or any other substance acts as a lactagogue. Some substances commonly regarded as lactagogues probably act partly by supplying fluid and food, and partly by their psychological value.

There is no point in forcing fluids. A controlled study on 210 women at the Jessop Hospital at Sheffield [209] showed that mothers who drank a large quantity of fluid (average 107·5 oz. per day) produced if anything rather less milk than those who were left to drink exactly what they wanted (average daily intake 69·1 oz.). There is no evidence that cows produce more milk when given extra water to drink.[302, 320, 321] Olsen [320, 321] gave thirteen nursing mothers widely varying quantities of fluid to drink, and found no correlation between the fluid intake and the quantity of milk produced. Others have made the same observation.

Gunther [173] thought that the flooding of body with water may antagonize the draught reflex. The draught reflex is accompanied by the antidiuretic action of the posterior pituitary gland. If diuresis has been caused, the secretion of antidiuretic substance may be impaired. All that the mother needs to do is to drink when she feels thirsty—as she often will at the moment when the draught reflex occurs.

The importance of avoiding complementary feeds in the first 5 days or so has already been emphasized. It is not necessary to give them before the fifth day, but after that it would be wrong to deny the baby food if he were crying excessively and losing weight. Such crying and loss of weight would worry the mother and be bad for the baby. If test feeds then confirm that the milk supply is inadequate, small complementary feeds should be given, and the breasts are fully expressed after every feed. Richardson regarded this as the most important factor in the very high incidence of breast feeding which he reported in his series (92·1 per cent. of 2,815 babies fully breast fed at 1 month). The complementary feeds are dropped as soon as possible, so that the baby is fully breast fed. If in addition it is found that the baby is having infrequent feeds he should be encouraged to take them more often. One must also see that the baby is being given long enough on each breast.

A controlled study was carried out at the Jessop Hospital,[208] Sheffield, in order to determine whether it was better for the purpose of preserving lactation, to give complementary feeds by spoon, as recommended by Ungar [420] and Naish,[305] instead of by bottle, which is a much quicker method. The experiment showed that nothing whatsoever was gained by using the spoon.

There is very often a temporary falling off of the milk supply when the mother gets up and returns to work. Test feeds will show in which feeds the supply of milk is inadequate, and appropriate complements are then given. In addition, the breasts must be expressed after every feed, and the expressed milk is given to the baby. Again, one must see that the feeds are sufficiently frequent (i.e. not merely three per day) and that the baby is being given long enough on each breast. As soon as possible the complementary feed is dropped.

A good idea of the quantity of breast milk available when a baby is receiving complementary feeds can be obtained by observing how much the baby takes from the bottle. An average baby requires approximately $2\frac{1}{2}$ oz. of milk per pound per day. Supposing that a 10-pound baby is being given a complementary feed after each breast feed, and the mother says that he is taking 18 oz. of properly constituted cow's milk in the 24 hours, it is clear that the baby is probably taking not more than 7 oz. of milk per day from the mother—provided that his weight gain is an average one. (A baby's weight gain may be a great deal more than 6 oz. a week. If so he may be receiving more than the calculated average requirement of $2\frac{1}{2}$ oz. per pound per day). It is most unlikely that there will ever be a sufficient supply of breast milk in such a case, and he should probably be put fully on to the bottle. In general, if it is shown that the mother is not producing as much as half the calculated requirements, in spite of proper emptying of the breast, it is usually wiser to put the baby fully on to artificial feeds. This is an individual matter, and if the mother is anxious to continue partially breast feeding her baby it is her affair, and she should not be discouraged from doing so. It must be remembered, however, that a great deal of time will be consumed by breast feeding the baby at each feed, and then expressing the breasts, and then giving a complementary feed. It takes too long.

When a mother comes to the doctor after the first 2 weeks, and the baby's weight gain is inadequate, the decision as to what to do will depend on how much the baby has gained, provided that there is no other cause for defective weight gain, such as vomiting or an infection. If he is gaining 4 or 5 oz. a week, the introduction of manual expression of the breast after every feed, together with attention to the frequency of the feeds, and to the time on the breast, can usually be relied upon to increase the weight gain to 7 or 8 oz. a week, without giving complementary feeds. The expressed milk is, of course, given to the baby. If the weight gain has been less than 4 oz. a week, in my experience one cannot usually increase the weight gain to the required figure without giving a complementary feed. If the weight gain has been a mere 1 or 2 oz. in the week, one might as well put the baby on to the bottle right away. It should be noted that if a baby has not been seen for 2 or 3 weeks, the weight gain may be deceptive. The fact that he has gained, say, 21 oz. in the last 3 weeks does not by any means prove that the milk supply is adequate : he might have gained 18 oz. in the first 2 weeks and only 3 oz. in the last week.

As for the nature of the complementary feed, it matters little, as long as it is properly constituted. If expressed milk from another mother is available, it should be given (after it has been boiled or pasteurized). Otherwise a dried milk or ordinary cow's milk (diluted and with sugar added) is given. As for the quantity, enough is given to satisfy the baby, and it should not be restricted. If test feeds have shown that the breast milk supply is only defective in one or two feeds in the 24 hours, the complement is given after these feeds only. A supplementary feed, that is a complete feed of cow's milk, is never given except in the weaning period, for if it is given it will mean that the breast will remain unemptied for a prolonged period.

Every effort must be made to avoid worrying the mother, and she should be given as much rest as possible.

The Failure of Lactation

Below is a brief discussion of the causes of the failure of lactation. The problem was discussed in detail by Joensen,[219] working in the Faroe Isles.

Unwillingness of the Mother to Breast Feed her Child

This may be a matter of necessity. The early return to work in industry or elsewhere makes artificial feeding almost inevitable. More often, however, failure is due to a lack of desire to feed the baby on the breast. This may be due to the feeling that breast feeding is too tying. The mother wants to be free to go out to places of entertainment, and to shop without feeling bound to return by a given time to feed her baby. She may have no idea of the importance or value of breast feeding. A friend of mine visited a magnificently equipped American maternity unit and, on seeing a woman feeding her baby on the bottle, asked her why she was not feeding him on the breast. The mother laughed and said, " Well, it never struck me " ! An essential part of ante-natal treatment should be an explanation to the mother of the value of breast feeding and the pleasure and satisfaction which she will derive from it. It is a mistake to dwell too much on the idea that it is a duty for her to breast feed her baby. So much can be said that the mother becomes genuinely worried about being unable to feed him. It has long been an established practice for certain firms to send advertisements of their dried milk products to mothers immediately after the birth of a baby. These are apt to suggest to mothers that artificial feeding is in every way as good as breast feeding, and they tend to discourage lactation.

Some mothers regard breast feeding as an unpleasant or even disgusting procedure. There are presumably deep-seated psychological reasons for this attitude. It is said that husbands may have the same attitude. I think that it is wrong to make determined efforts to persuade such a mother to breast feed her baby. Some mothers feel that it will be embarrassing to feed the baby in front of older children. Sometimes the social conditions are so bad that there is in fact no privacy at all for the mother, and there is good reason for her feeling of embarrassment. Others fear that breast feeding will spoil the figure. There is some truth in it, for the breast tends to be less firm after breast feeding, though this can be largely prevented by ensuring that the breast is properly supported during pregnancy and lactation. Others have the unfounded fear that it will lead to obesity. Some have heard about lactorrhœa, or have experienced it, and fear that their clothes will be soiled by it. Many have had a previous unfortunate experience with an improperly treated sore nipple or breast abscess, and they cannot face a recurrence of the pain which they experienced.

When there is an insufficiency of milk and complementary feeds have to be taken after every breast feed, so much time is consumed in feeding that the mother quite naturally feels that she cannot continue to breast feed the baby.

Of all those causes by far the commonest is a mere lack of desire to breast feed. The mother thinks that it does not matter whether the baby is breast fed or not, and if the slightest difficulty arises or the slightest symptoms of possible insufficiency develop in the baby she takes him right off the breast without consulting any doctor or nurse. She may consult her grandmother or neighbour, and the advice then given is almost invariably that the baby should be put on to the bottle. If the mother has failed to breast feed a previous child she will be all the more ready to feed her second baby on cow's milk.

Lack of Interest in Breast Feeding in the Attendants

This is a major cause of the failure of lactation. Many doctors and nurses are doubtful in their own minds about the value of breast feeding or frankly feel that it has no advantage at all. Many feel that it is " weakening " for the mother, and if she is tired or pale they advise her to put the baby on to the bottle. They fail to realize that this will involve her in a great deal more work. Neale and his co-workers[305A] wrote that "Physicians' advice, more than any other single factor, is still responsible for weaning babies. Physicians still take babies off the breast when there is any difficulty rather than take the trouble to go into the whole difficult question of successful breast feeding." A doctor whose wife has failed to breast feed her babies may react subconsciously by advising his patients against breast feeding. I attended a post-graduate lecture on Infant Feeding in a New York teaching hospital. At the end of the hour's lecture, which was entirely devoted to artificial feeding, a doctor in the audience asked whether the speaker had any views on breast feeding, as he had not mentioned it in his lecture. The speaker said that he had deliberately not mentioned it as he never recommended it. He said that it caused "too many difficulties." Mothers cannot be blamed for making little effort to breast feed their babies when there is widespread disinterestedness in it amongst doctors and nurses.

The basic cause of such disinterestedness is poor teaching in the medical schools. If more time were devoted to practical pædiatrics than to rare diseases of little importance, many more babies would be fed on the breast.

Errors of Diagnosis

By far the commonest mistakes are the diagnosis of insufficiency of milk without carrying out test feeds or properly weighing up the history, and the diagnosis that symptoms such as vomiting or crying are due to the breast milk not suiting the baby. A diagnosis that breast milk does not suit the baby is almost certainly wrong. (The exceptions in the case of beriberi and galactosæmia have already been mentioned.) Attempts to relate symptoms in babies to variations in the chloride or protein content of the mother's milk or changes in other constituents are in no way convincing. The composition of the mother's milk varies from hour to hour and day to day. Slight differences in the method of collecting the sample lead to considerable differences in the chemical analysis, particularly of the fat content. Reinhold[345] described a baby with vomiting and curdy stools, whose symptoms were apparently related to the high fat content of the mother's milk (7·4 per cent.).

I saw a fully breast-fed baby with cheesy constipated stools, and found that the mother was drinking 5 pints of milk a day with the idea of providing nourishing milk for her baby. As soon as her diet was corrected the baby's stools became normal. Wilson[460] conducted a series of analyses of mother's milk obtained for a milk bank. He wrote: "Analyses have shown enormous variations in the fat content, not only as between the milk of one mother and another but in that of the same mother almost from hour to hour in the same period of 24 hours' observation." In one sample he found a fat content of 4·25 per cent., and in another of 12·16 per cent., yet in neither case were the babies in the least upset. Boyd [560] emphasized the great variations in the composition of human milk as a result of emotional and genetic factors and variations in the intake of food. Babies seem to tolerate these differences without trouble, and for practical purposes analysis of the mother's milk on account of feeding difficulties is a waste of time. It is fraught with many serious fallacies. The reason for the child's symptoms should be sought elsewhere.

It is very common to see cases of congenital pyloric stenosis who have been taken off the breast on the grounds that the breast milk was not suiting the baby. There is no excuse for such a diagnosis. Excessive crying is also liable to cause this diagnosis to be made. The causes of this and the other symptoms which frequently lead to this diagnosis are discussed in Chapter 6. Many babies are deliberately taken off the breast because menstruation has recommenced. The reason for this action is the idea that the breast milk of a menstruating woman is poisonous for the baby. There is no foundation for this belief. Many other babies are taken off the breast because of "three-months' colic." The mother or doctor thinks that the colic is due to the breast milk not suiting the baby, or that there is not enough milk for him.

Finger sucking is apt to be regarded as a sign of insufficiency. It is universal in the first 2 or 3 months and means no such thing.

Another diagnosis which is commonly made by doctor, nurse or mother—particularly the latter—is that the breast milk is too watery. *For practical purposes this diagnosis is always wrong.* At least, I have not yet seen such a case. It is easy to understand how the idea arises. The first part of the milk does appear to be watery. The last part of the milk in the breast has the highest fat content, and is therefore much more opaque. I have seen many scores of babies taken off the breast on account of this diagnosis.

Hytten [201] claimed that the fat content of human milk may be so low that the child may be undernourished. I have never seen this phenomenon. This might happen if breast-fed babies were restricted to exactly 2½ oz. per pound per day, but they are not.

The opposite diagnosis is not made so frequently—the suggestion that the breast milk is "too strong" for the baby. *This diagnosis is always wrong.* One has seen babies who on account of vomiting have been placed on half-strength breast milk on the grounds that the breast milk is too strong for them.

It is interesting to note that Joensen [219] found that only 30·5 per cent. of the babies who were taken off the breast prematurely were below the average weight at the time of weaning.

Errors of Treatment

These include mismanagement of a depressed nipple during pregnancy or of a sore nipple later—in particular allowing the baby to suck when it is causing the mother great pain; delay in treating mastitis or abscess; failure to maintain lactation by expression when a mother acquires an infection such as influenza; putting the baby on to the bottle on account of irritability or inertia; mismanagement of overdistension of the breast, and taking him off the breast on account of hæmolytic disease of the new-born.

The commonest time at which babies are weaned is about the end of the second week, when the mother returns to her domestic work. This may be due to a combination of factors: partial involution of the breast as a result of inadequately treated overdistension, or fatigue and worry about her ability to manage her child. If the baby is tided over 2 or 3 days of insufficiency of milk by judicious complementary feeds and milk is expressed by hand, in the majority of cases the milk increases in quantity and the baby can be fully breast fed.

Lack of Provision in Hospitals for Nursing Mothers

This is a disgrace. Any hospital which is willing to admit young babies should have accommodation for mothers so that breast feeding can be maintained.

Justifiable Early Weaning of the Baby

Gross insufficiency of milk as a justifiable cause of weaning of the baby has already been mentioned. Other conditions include pulmonary tuberculosis, insanity, severe breast abscess and pregnancy of 3 months' duration. Other illness (such as nephritis and heart disease) have to be considered each on their merits, and no hard-and-fast rule can be made. It must always be remembered, however, that artificial feeding is a much more laborious method of feeding the baby than breast feeding.

Other Factors

Maternal toxæmia, early return to work, genetic and other factors may be related to the failure of lactation. Diet is probably not an important factor. Preoccupation with the baby's weight, on the part of the mother and her attendants, is a potent factor in leading to artificial feeding.

CHAPTER 6

DIFFICULTIES IN THE BREAST-FED BABY

Irritability in the New-born Period

IRRITABILITY when the breast is offered is a common condition in the new-born period and is a common reason for taking the baby off the breast and putting him on to the bottle. It causes a great deal of anxiety and distress to the mother and takes much of the nurse's time. It is surprising that so little is written about it. There is in fact little to add to the description given by Middlemore.[293]

The baby, a full-term one, who has had a normal delivery, behaves normally between feeds. He shows no sign of cerebral irritability and there is no suggestion of birth injury. When taken to the breast, as soon as he touches the nipple he screams violently and may refuse to suck, or else he may suck for a few seconds and withdraw to scream and fight. He may snarl at the breast and bite it hard, making the mother withdraw instantly in pain, so making the baby more annoyed. The more nervous and anxious the mother, the worse he becomes ; the calmer she is, the sooner he settles down. The whole feed is apt to become a fight and a thoroughly unpleasant and exhausting experience for the mother. The natural response of the nurse is to try to force the baby to take the breast, holding his head and binding his limbs down so that he cannot fight. Any attempt to discipline the child aggravates matters. A child knows where the breast is without being forced to it. When his cheek is touched the rooting reflex is initiated and he roots for milk. The holding of the child's head by the cheeks only annoys him further. Rough handling of any kind, even before the feed, makes him worse. A depressed nipple, which he finds difficulty in sucking from, increases his irritability. His irritability is also apt to be increased by excessive clothing, which makes him too hot, and a rigid feeding schedule, which keeps him crying for food.

The irritability is apt to arouse the suspicion that there is not enough milk for him. This seems to be confirmed by his defective weight gain. If a test feed is carried out the suspicions of the unwary are again apt to be confirmed, for it is likely to show that he has obtained only a small amount of milk from the mother. Many babies are taken off the breast for this reason or on the grounds that the breast milk is " not suiting " him, causing him to cry and to be irritable. This diagnosis, of course, is always wrong.

Gunther[174] thought that the irritability is usually due to the baby finding it difficult to breathe, either because his nose is embedded in the breast, or because the upturned upper lip is obstructing the nostrils.

Middlemore described the biting of the breast as due to "aggressive feeding." It is very likely, as Middlemore suggests, and as Edward Glover wrote in the Preface, that this early behaviour on the breast may give a good idea of the child's future character. Certainly none of the few which I have been able to follow up into later childhood could possibly be described as placid easy-going characters. They tended to be determined, active children who are apt to present feeding problems in the period of negativism between a year and 3 years.

The treatment is not entirely satisfactory. One should certainly see that the baby can breathe, by ensuring that the nose is not obstructed. A self-demand schedule is a rational approach to the problem, because it is likely that a child who is not kept waiting for a long time for his feed will be less irritable. It is certainly not the whole answer, however, for babies fed on this schedule may still show extreme irritability at feed times. It is also reasonable to suppose that it would help to have the baby constantly by the side of the mother rather than in a nursery, when his cries are apt to go unheeded. He should be picked up and cuddled by his mother as much as she wishes. It is particularly desirable that he should be cuddled for a fairly long time before a feed. He is more likely to approach the breast calmly in this case than if he is merely brought into the mother's room from the nursery and put to the breast immediately. He should be handled with the utmost gentleness and taken to the breast gently and without any forcing. The room should be quiet and interruptions should not be allowed. It is then purely a matter of patience. The less the nurse interferes the better. The nature of the problem should be fully explained and discussed with the mother. She must then fight her own battle. It is very difficult to stop the nurse interfering in an attempt to help the mother, but interference is undesirable. As Middlemore puts it, it is a matter of mutual adaptation between mother and child. The mother has to get used to the baby, and the baby to the mother. The nurse should be present at first to give moral support, but no more. As soon as possible she leaves the room. The child should not be stopped from licking the breast, and he should not be hurried. The whole feed may take almost an hour, though only a fraction of that time is spent by the baby in actual sucking. The essential thing is to reassure and encourage the mother. She must know that there is nothing wrong with her, her breast or the baby, and that it is purely a temporary phase which, though very troublesome as long as it lasts, will resolve itself in a very few days if only patience and tolerance are shown. If overdistension of the breast develops as a result of the poor sucking by the baby it should be treated by manual expression.

The role of drugs is uncertain. If all else fails the baby may be given chloral (1 grain) 20 minutes before each of about four feeds. Phenobarbitone is of doubtful value. By the age of 10 or 14 days, if not sooner, the child becomes reasonable and well behaved.

Inertia and Drowsiness

The problem of inertia in the new-born period was also discussed by Middlemore. In my experience it can be more worrying for the doctor than irritability, but it is less worrying for the mother. The baby does not seem to want feeding. He has no interest in it. If left on a self-demand schedule he does not demand feeds. Everyone is conversant with this behaviour in a small premature baby, but we are here concerned with the well full-term baby who, like the irritable baby, shows no evidence of birth injury. Gunther[174] ascribed it to inadequate protractility of the nipple. The presence of the normal nipple far back in the baby's mouth initiates sucking ; if it does not protract this stimulus to sucking is lost. Marked physiological jaundice may be a factor in some. In others underclothing or overclothing is responsible. A mentally defective child is particularly liable to be disinterested in feeds in the new-born period, but it would be a serious mistake to suppose that most babies with such inertia are mentally defective. Inertia may result from cerebral trauma, but most of the babies show no other sign of cerebral trauma and grow up to be normal children. They are frequently children of a particularly placid disposition.

A fairly rigid schedule is necessary until the child begins to be more alert and to demand feeds. Only patience and gentle coaxing without undue forcing will enable the child to suck adequately. As with the irritable child, the problem nearly always resolves itself by 10–14 days of age. Only very occasionally the baby continues to be disinterested in food and the maintenance of nutrition is not easy. It is of course always necessary to be sure that there is no infection.

Inertia in the baby is apt to lead to defective emptying of the breast. Unless manual expression is carried out during the period in which the baby is sucking badly, lactation may fail.

Sleepiness after the New-born Period

Many babies in the first 2 months or so fall asleep after they have sucked from one breast and before sucking from the second. Textbooks advise that they should be awakened by gentle slaps and other methods. Some apply pressure on the big toe in an attempt to awaken the baby. It is often, however, impossible to awaken him. The mother should avoid rocking while feeding the baby, but rocking is not usually the cause of the trouble. It may be that the baby obtains all that he requires from one breast and so falls asleep. It is largely a matter of immaturity, and it rights itself as the baby gets older (usually by 8 weeks or so). It is particularly annoying if the baby, having fallen asleep in this way, awakens in about 2 hours, feeling hungry and cries.

The problem may be caused by efforts to make the child suck longer than he wants on the first breast, because of a rigid rule that the baby should suck 10 minutes on each breast. If he is forced to go on sucking after he has obtained the milk, he is liable to fall asleep on the second breast because he is tired, and so he does not obtain enough milk.

An older baby may obtain the food so quickly that after about 5 minutes on each breast he falls asleep. This may worry the mother, but a study of the child's weight gain immediately enables one to reassure the mother and explain that he is obtaining a perfectly adequate amount of milk unusually quickly.

Overclothing as a cause of drowsiness must always be remembered. It is very common. At all times sleepiness of recent onset should arouse the suspicion of an infection.

Flatulence and Gastric Colic

Too many symptoms are ascribed to flatulence. It undoubtedly does occur in babies, but it is overdone. Crying for any reason—loneliness, desire to be cuddled, hunger—is ascribed to wind, and various medicines are given to bring it up. I have several times had older children (aged 1–2 years) referred to me on account of excessive wind. The excessive crying at night, which had been ascribed by the parents to wind, was simply a behaviour problem.

All wind which comes up from the stomach is wind which has been swallowed. The more immature the baby the greater the flatulence, because the greater is the amount of air which he swallows in sucking. The young baby in the first month or so is unable to approximate his lips closely to the areola of the breast, and milk consequently leaks out of the corner of his mouth as he sucks and air swallowing occurs. The older baby approximates his lips tightly to the areola, creating a vacuum in the process of sucking, and he swallows very little air. Provided, therefore, that none of the other causes mentioned below are found, the mother can be reassured and told that he will not be troubled with excessive wind in a few weeks, when he is older.

Flatulence may be caused by the baby gulping the milk down too quickly. It is usual to blame the baby for this, accusing him of being a greedy baby. He is then given chloral or boiled water before a feed in order to make him less hungry, or else the interval between feeds is increased. I feel that by far the commonest cause of this condition is an unduly rapid flow from the breast. It is easy to see that when a baby is suddenly disturbed while sucking at the breast and withdraws from it, the milk is squirting out of the breast. This is due to contractile myoepithelial cells between the secretory epithelium and the basement membrane.[350] Many mothers interpret the cause of the gulping correctly and note that it occurs particularly when the breast is distended, at the first feed in the morning. Some writers, recognizing the cause of the trouble, have recommended that the breast should be constricted by the mother's fingers during the feed so that the baby cannot obtain the milk so quickly. It is difficult, however, for the mother to regulate the flow properly. Either she does not constrict it enough and the flow is unaffected, or else she constricts it too much so that the baby swallows air, because he does not get the milk sufficiently easily. The best method is for the mother to express a small quantity of milk (e.g. an ounce) when the breast is distended, and after that to allow the baby to suck. By regulation of the quantity expressed excessive flow when the baby sucks is prevented.

Flatulence may be due to a wrong position in feeding the baby. If he is fed while almost horizontal, air tends to accumulate anteriorly and therefore does not come up until there is considerable distension of the stomach. Milk is then apt to be brought up with it. If the child is held well propped up during a feed the air rises to the cardiac end of the stomach and therefore comes up more rapidly. If when he is laid down, he is placed on his left side, air in the stomach tends to pass into the intestine, and so may cause discomfort. It is better to lay him on the right side.

Excessive wind is also due to the baby being allowed to suck on an overdistended breast. He is unable to obtain the milk and so he swallows air. Probably the commonest cause is sucking from the breast after all the milk available has been obtained. If there is an inadequate supply of milk the baby may obtain all the milk there is in much less than the 10 minutes commonly allowed for sucking and swallow air in the remaining time. The supply may be adequate, but the baby, who has obtained all the milk in about 3 minutes on each breast, may be kept on the breast because the mother has been instructed to feed the baby for 10 minutes on each side. Sometimes a mother feeds a baby for much longer than 10 minutes on each breast. This is nearly always wrong after the new-born period, for the baby merely swallows air and so suffers from flatulence and colic. The question of the duration of the feeds is discussed elsewhere (p. 20).

A baby of any age who is left to cry for a long time swallows air in the process, and may even vomit as a result. This is one of the reasons why a rigid feeding schedule may lead to feeding difficulties.

" Three Months' Colic "

The term " three months' colic " is an unsatisfactory title, but no one has thought of a better one, and at least it has the merit of being self-explanatory, in implying that it refers to colic which occurs in the first 3 months of a baby's life. As no one knows the cause of " three months' colic," it would be unwise to adopt any title which attempts to state its causation. One writer, for instance, coined the title " vagogenic gastroenterospasm." I am told that in parts of India it is called " sanjhana," and is ascribed to Evening Gods. Rosamond [359] wrote that " every layman and every doctor with experience knows about ' three months' colic ' " yet I have heard several pædiatricians deny its existence. I agree with Julius Hess [187] who wrote that " to appreciate colic fully one must be the father of a breast-fed infant with it." Brennemann [61] in his very full account of the condition, was himself the father of children with colic. I have reviewed the problem in detail elsewhere.[211]

The following is the typical story. A very few days after birth, though sometimes only on return from the Maternity Hospital, the baby, having been perfectly good during the day, has attacks of crying in the evening, mostly between 6 p.m. and 10 p.m.

In an attack his face suddenly becomes red, he frowns, draws his legs up, and emits piercing screams, quite unlike the cry of hunger or loneliness. These are likely to continue for 2 to 10 minutes, even though he is picked up. The attack usually ends suddenly, but sobbing is apt to continue for several minutes. He is just about to fall asleep, obviously tired out, when a further attack occurs. Attacks continue at regular intervals till about 10.0 p.m., when he lapses into sleep. During the attack one may hear loud borborygmi, and much flatus is passed per rectum, giving temporary relief. No unusual amount of wind is brought up by mouth. Gentle pressure or massage of the abdomen, or placing him in the prone position, gives some relief, and he obtains relief by sucking, though an additional feed does not give more than temporary relief. The attacks recur nightly, but almost always cease by the end of the third month.

Many have stated that the attacks do not begin in hospital. I think that the explanation of this idea lies in inaccurate observation in the maternity nursery. Thirty-six out of a series of forty-nine babies with colic observed by me had their first attack in hospital. Forty-four began in the first 15 days. True colic does not begin after 3 or at the most 4 weeks. According to Pierce [335] the onset in premature babies is delayed for a period approximating the degree of prematurity.

Forty-seven out of fifty babies in the series studied by me had their attacks after 5 p.m.

There are all degrees of severity of these attacks, and the description above applies to the severe one. In milder forms the baby is just mildly irritable in the evening, without definite screaming attacks. In mild forms the attacks cease by about the eighth week, while in the severest forms the baby may not be entirely happy in the evenings till the fourth month. The average duration in a series of fifty cases was $9\frac{1}{2}$ weeks ; 54 per cent. had lost the attacks by 2 months of age, 85 per cent. by 3 months and 100 per cent. by 4 months.

It is difficult to say exactly how frequent the condition is, but it is certainly very common. I am sure that Brennemann was exaggerating when he wrote that few children escape it. Jorup [222] claimed that 30 per cent. of 589 children attending a child welfare centre in Stockholm had it, but his description does not quite tally with that given above.

It appears to occur just as much in artificially-fed babies as in breast-fed ones.

The cause of the attacks is unknown. In my review of the literature I found an astonishing list of suggested causes. One writer [190] listed twenty causes. The suggestions include the following : overfeeding, underfeeding, too frequent feeds, too infrequent feeds, feeds too rich, feeds too weak, too hot or too cold ; excess of fat, carbohydrate or protein ; allergy, cod-liver oil, orange juice ; congenital malformations of the alimentary tract, inguinal hernia, urethral colic, appendicitis, foreign bodies in the alimentary tract, lead poisoning, anal fissures, imperforate anus, peptic ulcer, disease of the gall bladder, respiratory tract or osseous system, volvulus, syphilis, intussusception, renal colic, nasopharyngitis, otitis, pyelitis and hyperacidity, tension developed in utero from a hypothetical uterine handicap or transmitted from a highly strung mother's system, exposure to cold, chilling of the extremities, abdominal binders, fatigue toxins from the mother, acidosis, introversion, and accumulation of acid in the kidneys.

Several workers ascribe the colic to " hypertonicity " or " neuropathic constitution," whatever that means, claiming that these babies show a wide variety of signs such as vomiting, diarrhœa, constipation, abdominal distension, tetany and so on. There is no truth whatsoever in this. In my experience these babies are entirely normal apart from their colic. In my study of fifty babies with colic, whom I compared with fifty babies without colic, there was no difference with regard to their sex, birth weight, feeding history, their incidence of posseting, the number of stools, or their weight gain. Their mothers differed in no way with regard to their age, parity or pregnancy history.

White [452] studying forty-seven infants with colic, found that infants with colic in whom eczema develops later are three times more frequent than infants with either colic or eczema alone. He found that a family history of allergy was about equally frequent (30–40 per cent.) in infants with eczema, colic or both. White's picture of colic, however, including as it does diarrhœa and vomiting, is hardly the accepted picture of the condition. I have not seen three months' colic in association with diarrhœa. In my series there was no difference between the babies with colic and the controls with regard to the family history of allergy, or to the presence or development of other allergic manifestations in the babies.

Many blame the parents for the attacks. Parents are said to " pick the baby up too much, or to bounce him too much after feeds." They are said to convey their nervousness and anxiety to the baby. A psycho-analyst described colic as a combination of congenital hypertonicity in the baby with primary anxious overpermissiveness in the mother.[395] Wessel *et al.*[447] blamed family tension for twenty-two out of forty-eight cases. They wrote " Paroxysmal fussing is probably one of the earliest somatic responses to the presence of tension in the environment." The particular degree to which any infant reacts is probably determined by constitutional factors. In my opinion most of the so-called tension in parents of babies with colic is the result of the baby's colic, and not the cause of it. It is inevitable that severe colic in a baby will cause some degree of tension in a good mother. After careful observation of parents of these babies I do not believe that they are any different from parents of babies who have no colic. I do not see how family tension could produce these strictly rhythmical attacks of violent screaming with excessive borborygmi, attacks which should surely be due to pain from the nature of the scream and the fact that they continue unabated in the mother's arms.

Levine and Bell,[247] as a result of their observations on the use of a pacifier, suggested that colic is due to an unsatisfied need for adequate oral gratification. It seems unlikely, when it is so common in well breast-fed babies.

Jorup,[222] in his careful study of these babies, showed that there is no excess of wind in the bowel (a finding which I can confirm), but thought that the colon showed " excessive propulsive activity " ; when a barium enema was given it was expelled with unusual force. The attacks of pain coincided in time with violent colonic contractions. This would explain the excessive borborygmi which I have described.

Brennemann concluded : " It would seem to me that the more rational explanation of colic is found in the fact that the baby comes into the world more underdone than the young of other mammals ; that its intestinal tract is not yet equal in the earliest months to an unusual or even normal demand, either in the matter of digestion or of propulsion of its gaseous contents : that an excessive amount of gas accumulates in the intestines especially fostered by the highly fermentable contents of breast milk : that as a result the overdistended intestines become kinked and acutely obstructed at the bends : and that the effort to overcome this obstruction leads to colic on exactly the same basis as that of all the other types of colic enumerated above. This view and this view alone would seem to explain the relief that comes from an enema, or from a free spontaneous expulsion of flatus, from pressure, from the hot-water bottle, from adding powdered casein to the feeding to combat fermentation with putrefaction, and even from giving added food that naturally starts increased peristalsis that may help to push on the obstructed gas."

I believe that the attacks are due to temporary obstruction of gas in loops of the bowel.

As for the differential diagnosis, it must be remembered that there are many causes of crying other than "three months' colic." It is perfectly easy to eliminate hunger as a cause of crying. Rosamond [359] wrote that it is quite obviously due to hunger. The apparent relief given by sucking is a real cause of confusion here, and leads mothers to give very frequent feeds all through the evening. They are apt to conclude that the breast milk is not suiting the baby and to put the baby on the bottle ; but the colic continues unabated. In my experience these babies are in a good state of nutrition, quite up to or above the average weight for the age, and complementary feeds in the evening are either refused or taken badly, and do not give relief. Neither is there evidence of overfeeding. Efforts to reduce the feeds only lead to more crying.

Many babies cry merely because they want to be picked up, but such crying stops when the mother takes the baby into her arms. In the mild cases one can only guess that the slight restlessness in the evenings is a minor form of colic.

Treatment

A wide variety of treatments have been recommended for this condition. They include increasing or decreasing the frequency or quantity of the feeds, or their carbohydrate, fat or protein content : adding lactic acid or casein ; changing the mother's diet ; using protein milk, buttermilk, skimmed or evaporated milk, substituting banana powder for other sugars, giving warm cereal gruel before feeds, and thickening the feeds with cereal. Some have recommended a whole series of changes to be tried one after the other ; one feels that before one has reached the end of the series the child will have grown out of his colic. A wide variety of drugs have been suggested, including atropine, banthine bromide, prostigmine, opium, demerol, phenobarbitone, chloral, sodium bicarbonate, peppermint water, sodamint, tincture of cardamom, magnesium carbonate, "dill water," bismuth, sal volatile, sulphocarbolate of sodium, creosote, papain, nux vomica, salad oil, calcium chloride, calcium gluconate, and potassium citrate. Others suggest a culture of lactic acid bacilli, a glycerine suppository, dilatation of the anal sphincter, and the provision of a dummy. McGee [277] recommended that the baby be given whisky.

I have had no success with phenobarbitone. Jorup [222] found that methyl scopolamine nitrate (skopyl) gave relief. I did a controlled experiment with the drug, and found that it was quite useless.[212]

There is certainly nothing to be gained by taking the baby off the breast. An adequate dose of chloral would seem to be a reasonable approach to the problem. One would begin with a dose of 4 grains, increasing until sleep were obtained. As much as 10 grains or more might be needed. Until relief is given, the baby should be picked up in the attacks, even though it may create a habit which will have to be broken as soon as it becomes clear that the baby is crying for company, and not because of pain [398]. It would be cruel to leave a baby in pain without giving him that love and security which he needs.

Until we know more about the cause of the problem, we cannot expect to have a really satisfactory treatment.

Overfeeding

I agree with Wickes [453] that overfeeding is a problem only to those who take active steps to avoid it. Referring to artificial feeds, Wickes remarks that some prescribe milk mixtures as carefully as dangerous drugs. Vining [431] wrote that the fear of overfeeding is a potent cause of underfeeding.

I believe that overfeeding in a breast-fed baby in the first 4 months or so is excessively rare. Some textbooks give the impression that it is a major and important problem. Truby King,[235] for instance, wrote that "overfeeding is the commonest and most frequent cause of digestive and nutritional disturbance in early infancy." I have only seen one possible case in the last 23 years. The baby, who was 8 weeks old, was having up to 12 stools a day. The weight gain had been excessive at first (about 16 oz. per week) and then fell off and became less than the average. The child was treated by giving him 2 oz. of boiled water before each feed, and within a week all symptoms had disappeared. Thereafter he took breast feeds only and his weight progress was normal.

I believe that when vomiting, crying, colic, diarrhœa or other symptoms are ascribed to overfeeding, the diagnosis is almost always wrong, the cause lying elsewhere. Often, however, a child is thought to be overfed merely because his weight gain is greater than the average.

This idea is always wrong. Nothing should ever be done in the first 3 months or so about a greater than average weight gain. Wickes,[453] in a study of 503 infants, showed that 32 per cent. gained over 9 oz. per week. I commonly see a weight gain of 12 oz. a week or more in thriving babies. The largest weight gain I have seen is 25 oz. a week in a symptomless well 2-month-old baby who had been somewhat underfed before. I saw a 9 lb. baby who was admitted to the Children's Hospital, Sheffield, on account of excessive crying. He was given, as is our practice, as much milk as he wanted, and for several days he took 54 oz. per day (6 oz. per pound per day). All crying stopped and the baby was well and contented, with normal stools. He had been underfed, and after catching up to his expected weight he took a more usual quantity.

Some babies do become obese by about the fourth month. It is then time to wean them. Obesity in the older baby may justly be ascribed to overfeeding, but I believe that it would be more true to ascribe it to wrong feeding—to continuing full breast feeding far too long, or, in the case of a baby on a mixed diet, giving an excess of milk and starchy foods.

Posseting and Vomiting

True Posseting. An exact definition of posseting is difficult, and excessive posseting can be difficult to distinguish from vomiting. One may merge into the other. All would agree that the welling up of a little milk into the baby's mouth immediately after a feed should be called posseting and not vomiting. It occurs in all babies. It is harmless, though in some babies it happens so often that there may be a substantial loss of milk. Excessive posseting characteristically occurs in the highly active, wiry baby, the baby who exhibits unusually rapid movements of the arms and legs. It is not often seen in the slow, placid baby. It is much commoner in the first 2 or 3 months than later. It may, however, only become troublesome in the second six months of a baby's life.

It is very common for milk to be expelled, often with considerable force, when wind is brought up. Any causes, therefore, of excessive flatulence will lead to this loss of milk. It is a matter of opinion whether this should be called posseting or vomiting. The milk may clear the clothes, and some would therefore consider this vomiting. It does not matter what it is called, however, as long as its nature is understood. It is very commonly called "projectile vomiting," and it is in fact by far the most important condition which has to be distinguished from pyloric stenosis and which is most often confused with it. Mothers are very worried by such posseting and they tend to exaggerate the quantity brought up. The doctor assesses the truth of the mother's story by observation of the child's state of hydration and a study of the child's weight in relation to his age and weight at birth. Usually one finds that, in spite of the mother's complaint that there is severe frequent vomiting, the child is in no way below the expected weight.

The treatment of this sort of " vomiting " is the treatment of the cause. By far the commonest cause of excessive flatulence in the breast-fed baby is sucking after the milk has been obtained. This is due either to insufficiency of milk or to allowing the baby to suck longer than the time usually recommended. Apart from this the only treatment possible consists of proper care in bringing the wind up after feeds (see below).

Vomiting due to Improper Posture after Feeds. If the mother fails to bring the baby's wind up after a feed vomiting and colic are apt to occur. The baby should be placed on the knee, or (preferably) held up against the shoulder. Some mothers sit the baby on the right knee and lean him so far over the left knee that the stomach is pressed upon and the milk comes up. This defect of management will not be discovered unless it is specifically looked for.

Babies frequently pass urine or a stool after a feed, and the napkin has to be changed. It is easy in changing the napkin to tilt the child so far back that milk is brought up. This is due to the relative incompetence of the cardio-œsophageal sphincter in early infancy.

After a feed the baby should be placed on his right side, with the head slightly higher than the rest of the body.

Vomiting from Other Causes (with no Organic Disease). It is extremely rare for a breast-fed baby to take too much milk. It is said, however, that vomiting may result if too much milk is taken. I have never seen such a case. It is possible that if a breast feed is forced on a child a short interval after the previous feed, before the stomach has emptied, that some might be brought up. This is avoided by a self-demand schedule.

An excess of fat in the mother's milk is another extremely rare cause of vomiting, but I have never seen such a case. This question is discussed on p. 52.

Cod-liver oil may make a child sick. More commonly the " vomiting " described by the mother consists merely of a spitting out of the oil. It is a mistake to try to force the child to take it against his will, because of the danger of inhalation of the oil, and therefore of lipoid pneumonia. It should be given after a meal rather than before it, so that he is in a better temper. If the baby still rejects it one of the concentrated forms of vitamin D should be given, so that the quantity to be given is less. Some mothers prefer to give the oil to their baby when he is in the bath, so that his woollen clothes are not spoilt by oil which he spits out. Orange juice may also cause vomiting. A breast-fed baby does not need additional vitamin C as long as the mother is taking an adequate quantity of the appropriate foodstuffs herself.[238] If for some reason it is desired to give the baby vitamin C, it can be given cheaply and easily in the form of ascorbic acid (50 mg. per day).

A rare cause of vomiting in a breast-fed baby is allergy to human milk. This is very rare, and I have not seen a case.

The differential diagnosis of posseting and vomiting from the above causes is of extreme importance. The chief condition which has always to be borne in mind is congenital pyloric stenosis. This is commoner in males, but it cannot be excluded because the child is a female. The common age of onset is between the second and fifth weeks, but it can develop sooner and it may develop later, up to the end of the third month. The vomiting is usually projectile, but the fact that vomiting is projectile does not establish the diagnosis of pyloric stenosis. It has already been said that when milk is brought up with wind it may shoot out. In pyloric stenosis the story is that there is one big vomit during or at the end of a feed, the whole feed coming up. It is very rarely the case that the child with pyloric stenosis brings the milk up in several small vomits between the feeds. Examination often shows peristaltic waves passing across the upper abdomen from left to right, but this is not pathognomonic, for it occurs in other conditions too. In practically every case a pyloric tumour can be palpated on examination during a feed on breast or bottle. If the stomach is distended with wind, a gastric washout may be necessary before the feed is given. A properly taken X-ray will confirm the diagnosis if there is any doubt, but in the vast majority radiological confirmation is quite unnecessary. The diagnosis is made by feeling the pyloric tumour. This is a matter which must be left to the specialist, for no one else sees a sufficiently large number of cases to make his findings reliable.

A thorough examination of the child is always necessary to exclude other organic disease, such as urinary tract infection, otitis media or increased intracranial pressure. Vomiting may also be due to chalasia or achalasia of the œsophagus, or hiatus œsophageal hernia. These can readily be diagnosed by X-ray examination.

Rumination

Rumination, also called merycism, is a habit acquired by babies, usually after the age of 3 months. The child is brought to the doctor on account of " vomiting." The diagnosis can sometimes be made on the history alone, but it is usually made by observation of the child. The baby is usually a wide-awake, alert one. It is equally common in the two sexes. Examination shows that the baby hollows his tongue, champs the jaws, strains, arches the back, keeping the mouth open, and holds the head back. He contracts the abdominal muscles and may make sucking movements of the tongue, bringing milk up. Some of the milk dribbles out, while the rest is swallowed. The child shows satisfaction at his achievement, obviously enjoying it. The loss of milk may be considerable, so that the weight gain is unsatisfactory, and he may even lose weight.

As late as the end of the last century the skull was trephined for the complaint. The modern treatment is to thicken the feeds (e.g. with Farex, a tablespoonful in an average cupful of milk) so that they are not brought up so easily. The baby should be distracted when the characteristic movements are seen. The head of the cot may be raised so that the body is on a steep slope. In severe cases a bandage is taken from the head of the cot, passed under the mandible and tied again to the cot, so that in effect the child is suspended by his lower jaw. Others have tried a firm linen cap with a bandage at each side fitting firmly round the chin. Ylppo suggests that they should be kept in the prone position, for in this position it is much more difficult for them to bring the milk up. I saw one child successfully distracted from the habit by giving him a dummy.

The Baby's Stools

The great majority of babies pass the first stool during the first day of life ; 69 per cent. of 500 full-term babies passed the first stool in 12 hours, and 94 per cent. within 24 hours of birth.[378]

All who are responsible for the care of babies should be conversant with the normal changes in their stools. The first stool passed by the new-born baby may be the so-called meconium plug, which has a greyish-white or yellow appearance. Thereafter for the next 2 or 3 days he passes the typical meconium stool, which is dark green-black, tenacious, sticky and almost odourless. After 2 or 3 days this gradually changes to a less intense green-black and then to a green-brown greasy stool. There is then a gradual transition to the normal orange-yellow loose homogeneous stool of the fully breast-fed baby. This transition stage may take up to almost 3 weeks, and in this stage the stools contain mucus, are often explosive and may be quite frequent (up to twelve per day). They may, furthermore, be a bright green colour and they contain solid yellow soap plaques. A normal breast-fed baby may at times pass bright green stools for the first six weeks or so. An erroneous diagnosis of diarrhœa is readily made, but the child is well and thriving. According to Smith [389] and Bonar [53] examination of the new-born baby's stools frequently reveals the presence of blood. (This is quite apart from the presence of obvious naked-eye blood in melæna neonatorum.) Bonar examined 3,539 stools from 107 normal new-born infants and found a positive benzidine reaction in 55 per-cent. ; 67 per cent. of those examined on the fourth and fifth day gave a positive reaction. The reason for this was not known, but it was suggested that it was due to hyperæmia associated with bacterial invasion of the intestine.

The stools of the fully breast-fed baby remain very loose but change in character immediately after other foods are given. Even a small amount of cow's milk makes them much firmer. It should be borne in mind that when mixed feeds are given the stools readily show notable changes in colour. Certain fruits, such as bilberries, given to older babies, cause remarkable coloration of the stools.

Striking colours may appear in the napkin of a baby receiving phenolphthalein in teething powders.[18] The stool is surrounded by a salmon pink discoloration which turns a deep bright mauve when hot water is poured on to it. The alkalinity of the napkins causes the colour to change when the phenolphthalein is washed out of the stool.

Constipation

The vast majority of breast-fed babies who are said by their mothers to be constipated are merely having infrequent normal motions. There is a great deal of unnecessary anxiety about this. I was once asked to see a baby who had been given an enema by the doctor at the age of 24 hours on account of constipation. It is a strange fact that breast-fed babies often have periods in which they have very infrequent motions. At one time they have five or six motions a day. A few weeks later they are having a motion every 5 or 6 days. Such infrequency is extremely common. Hardly a day passes in a welfare clinic without a mother complaining about her child's "constipation." Gordon[162] described babies who had no stool for 7, 8 and 12 days without any sort of disturbance. I have frequently seen babies who only had a motion every 5 days. Such marked infrequency does not seem to occur in the first 2 or 3 weeks of life. It is exceptional to see a baby who has a motion as infrequently as every 10 or 12 days, but I have seen this, and it is certainly no cause for alarm. The baby rarely suffers any discomfort from infrequent bowel actions, though occasionally he seems to be a little restless for a day or two before the stool is passed. There is little abdominal distension. Flatus is passed as usual. The child is in every way perfectly well. The old explanation of the phenomenon was spasm of the anal sphincter. There is no evidence for this, and any attempt to dilate the sphincter is quite unwarranted. No treatment of any kind is needed. Mothers who are worried should be reassured. They commonly try various kinds of purgatives, usually in an unavailing attempt to make the child have a motion. They give enemas and pass soap sticks into the rectum. All those treatments are wrong. The mothers should be told that there is nothing wrong with the child, that this infrequency is extremely common in normal breast-fed babies, and that instead of being anxious they should be pleased that they have fewer soiled napkins to wash.

The reason for the infrequency of the motions is unknown. The condition does not occur in artificially-fed babies, and this should be emphasized. It seems as if the loose stools of the breast-fed baby fail to supply a sufficient stimulus to the bowel to lead to emptying. The phases are not usually long lasting, and the baby who for a few weeks had very infrequent motions gradually reverts to his former state of having two or three motions a day.

True constipation in a breast-fed baby is readily diagnosed. The child has the so-called " starvation stools "—small, often frequent, loose or semi-fluid stools containing mucus. They are often semi-transparent, dark green or green-brown, and have a faint old musty odour without any smell of fermentation or decomposition. In addition, the child shows defective weight gain and the appearance of an underfed baby.

The constipation of intestinal obstruction is diagnosed by the associated abdominal distension, illness of the child, absence of the passage of flatus and vomiting of material which is often green or fæcal. The diagnosis can be confirmed by a straight X-ray of the abdomen.

True constipation in a breast-fed baby is most often due to underfeeding. It may be due to vomiting, excessive posseting or to rumination. An occasional cause is gross overclothing, especially in hot weather, leading to dehydration and so to constipation. Organic disease must always be remembered, though it is a relatively rare cause of constipation. There is always a possibility, however, of megacolon or a semi-imperforate anus, and in any case of doubt a rectal examination should be performed, followed by a barium enema to eliminate megacolon. Rickets and cretinism may cause constipation, but they should be readily diagnosed.

Diarrhœa

When mothers complain that their breast-fed child has diarrhœa, by far the commonest finding is that the baby has perfectly normal stools. The motions of a fully breast-fed baby are very loose, and many mothers, not realizing this, think that he has diarrhœa. In the first 2 or 3 weeks of a baby's life there is very often obvious mucus in the stool and the expulsion of a stool may be quite explosive. The stool at this stage shows soap plaques and curds and is often bright green in colour, thus adding to the suggestion that food is going through the baby improperly digested. In the first 6 or 8 weeks of life some breast-fed babies have very frequent motions—up to 10 or 12 a day, or more. The unwary, therefore, diagnose gastro-enteritis, and I have known perfectly normal babies admitted to infectious disease hospitals on that account.

True diarrhœa can occur in a fully breast-fed baby, but it is very rare, for gastro-enteritis is practically confined to artificially-fed babies. There have been outbreaks of mild diarrhœa in nurses and mothers in maternity units which have led to infection of the babies, but these are uncommon. True diarrhœa in a fully breast-fed baby is difficult to diagnose with certainty. It would hardly be diagnosed without coincident loss of weight, malaise and evidence of dehydration. It is unusual for stools to be green when freshly passed after about 6 to 8 weeks, and there should not be obvious mucus after that age, unless some purgative has been given. An important point in the diagnosis would be the watery nature of the stools and their frequency, particularly if there had been a sudden increase in that frequency.

The looseness of the stools sometimes met with as a result of substances passing through the mother's milk has already been mentioned. Orange juice sometimes upsets a baby and causes diarrhœa. It is extremely important to distinguish the loose green mucus stools of starvation. Such stools often lead to the erroneous diagnosis of diarrhœa. This is a tragedy, for the baby is then likely to be starved still further, whereas all that he needed was more food. I have seen a baby develop diarrhœa as a result of licking ointment of zinc and castor oil placed on the lips, on account of soreness.

Defective Weight Gain

Though an average child after the first fortnight gains 6 or 7 oz. a week, some normal children gain more and some less. I would consider that a weight gain of 5 oz. a week was "normal" if the child were contented, had normal stools and looked well, and if the gain were maintained at that level.

The obvious cause of defective weight gain is insufficient food, and this diagnosis can readily be confirmed by test feeds. There are, however, other important causes which have to be considered. An important early cause is irritability or inertia in the baby, or poor sucking for any reason. It is easy to make a mistaken diagnosis of underfeeding in those babies, being misled by defective weight gain and a poor gain in test feeds. Expression of the breast after the baby has sucked shows that there is an adequate supply of milk, but the baby has not taken it.

Loneliness and separation of the baby from the mother may prevent a satisfactory weight gain. Prolonged crying due to a rigid schedule may prevent a satisfactory weight gain.

Defective weight gain may also be due to excessive posseting or to vomiting. It is extremely rarely due to overfeeding (p. 64). It is not uncommonly due to gross overclothing. In a baby whom I was asked to see because of failure to gain weight, a thorough search for infections had been made, with a negative result. Test feeds showed that the milk supply was adequate. The child was well but grossly overclothed, having fifteen layers of clothes in a room in which the temperature was 85°. When this was dealt with the child gained weight normally. Overclothing may prevent a satisfactory weight gain not only by causing excessive perspiration but by making the baby drowsy, so that he sucks badly. It must always be remembered that any infections, however slight, may prevent a young baby gaining weight adequately.

CHAPTER 7

THE ARTIFICIALLY-FED BABY

Historical

REFERENCE has already been made to the excellent series of articles by Wickes,[456] and to other papers. Sennert, in the seventeenth century, recommended broth made of beer mixed with boiled bread and butter when breast milk was not available. According to Meyer [292] the milk of the following animals is still used, or has been used, in countries abroad : the goat, ass, camel, llama, caribou, bitch, mare reindeer, sheep and water buffalo. In Paris babies were fed direct from asses, and in Malta direct from goats.

The Choice of Food

There is nothing to choose between the various dried foods, except in price. National Dried Milk is the cheapest, but if a mother buys this she will lose her right to obtain a pint of cow's milk per day at a reduced price, while if she uses other milk preparations she will preserve that right. *I have never yet had to change from one dried milk to another to find one which suits the baby.* It is a common practice to change from one dried food to another because the child is vomiting, crying excessively or presenting other feeding problems. In the case of pyloric stenosis, it is extremely common to hear that the baby was taken off the breast on the grounds that the vomiting was due to the breast milk not suiting the baby, and then tried on one dried milk after another in an attempt to find one which would not cause vomiting. This should never be done. The diagnosis is bound to be wrong.

There is little need for a half-cream milk, except in a premature baby, or one who, on account of an infection, has some looseness of the stools.

In countries in which cow's milk is not available, preparations of soya bean have been used. Other foods include preparations from peanuts and fish flour. Probably the best preparation is a sort of " meat milk " or soup, prepared by using strained meats as a protein base.[153]

The Quantity of Food

The first step in calculating the amount of food to offer a baby is to determine the expected weight, by adding 6 oz. per week (in the first 3 months) to the birth weight. For instance, the " expected weight" of an 8-week-old baby whose birth weight was 8 lb. would be 8 lb. + 6 × 8 oz. = 11 lb. The nearest convenient round figure above this is taken—in this case 12 lb.

Reference is then made to Table II, which shows the quantities of various foods which will give a caloric value of approximately 50 calories per pound.

TABLE II.

Quantity of Food for Baby, per Pound of Expected Weight per Day.

	Milk	Sugar	Water
Breast milk	$2\frac{1}{2}$ oz.	—	—
Cow's milk	$1\frac{3}{4}$ oz.	1 dr.	$\frac{3}{4}$ oz.
National Dried Milk. Half- or Full-cream; Full-cream Cow & Gate; Ostermilk No. 2	$1\frac{3}{4}$ measures	1 dr.	$2\frac{1}{2}$ oz.
Half-cream Cow & Gate; Ostermilk No. 1	3 measures	—	3 oz.

These figures are approximate, but near enough provided that the baby is given more if he wants it. Having worked out the calculated requirement for the 24 hours, the total quantity is divided by the number of feeds he receives in that period, keeping to a convenient round figure. For instance, if a baby's expected weight is 12 lb., and he is fed on cow's milk, the total quantity for the whole day would be

Milk . . $12 \times 1\frac{3}{4}$ oz. = 21 oz.
Sugar . . 12×1 dr. = 12 dr.
Water . . $12 \times \frac{3}{4}$ oz. = 9 oz.

If he has five feeds a day, one would offer at each feed

Milk . . . $4\frac{1}{2}$ oz.
Sugar . . . $2\frac{1}{2}$ dr.
Water . . . 2 oz.

There is no need to be more exact. The mother should be told that if the baby wants more he should be given more, but that he may want less than this, in which case a somewhat smaller quantity will be made up.

There is no point at all in using glucose in preparing the feeds, in place of ordinary sugar. It is more expensive, and there is nothing to be said for it.

If a baby requires feeds in the night, the milk should not be kept in a vacuum flask, for dangerous organisms may grow if that is done. Water should be kept in the flask and used for mixing the feed when required.

DIFFICULTIES IN THE ARTIFICIALLY-FED BABY

Flatulence and Colic

There are several causes of air swallowing in artificially-fed babies, most of them concerned with the teat of the bottle. Much the commonest is too small a hole in the teat. The hole should be tested for patency and adequacy before every feed. One often hears on questioning that the teat was tested when it was purchased, but not again. It is important to be conversant with the methods commonly used by mothers in testing the hole. A common and most undesirable practice is for the mother, having filled the bottle with milk and applied the teat, to suck it herself. She assumes that if she can suck milk the baby should be able to do likewise. Another method is to squeeze the teat when it is on the bottle, and still another is to fill the detached teat with water or milk and then to push a finger into it in order to determine whether milk can be expressed. These methods, of course, are wrong, because very considerable pressure is applied. Often the hole is tested when the bottle is filled with water. This is undesirable because water will flow more easily than milk. A common mistake is to test the hole when water or milk is in the bottle and then to fill the bottle with milk thickened with a cereal. I saw a 6-months-old child with extreme irritability, flatulence and loss of weight. Questioning showed that the mother had put the entire sago pudding into the bottle and expected the baby to be able to suck it out. There is no need to shake the bottle in order to test the hole. When the bottle is inverted the milk should drop out at the rate of several drops per second without any shaking. The patency of the hole should be tested before every feed, because it readily becomes blocked up, particularly if dried milks are used.

It is very common in the case of a baby suffering from excessive wind to find that the feed is taking 30 to 60 minutes. No feed should take more than 15 minutes if the hole in the teat is large enough.

Too large a hole in the teat is a rare cause of trouble. Some mothers enlarge the hole by cutting the teat with a pair of scissors, and the hole is then too large. If the hole is too large the baby is likely to gulp milk down and swallow air in the process.

If the bottle is not tilted so that the teat is kept full of milk the baby will swallow air. If the mother fails to withdraw the teat from the baby's mouth at frequent intervals, and certainly when it becomes flat as a result of the creation of a vacuum in the bottle, the baby will be unable to obtain the milk and will swallow air in his efforts. (This difficulty is easily avoided by using a boat-shaped bottle with a teat on the sucking end only.) It is largely for these two reasons that it is always wrong to leave a baby to feed himself from a bottle which is propped on a pillow. An old teat, or one which has been repeatedly boiled, readily becomes flat when the baby sucks.

It will be seen that in investigating the cause of excessive flatulence in a bottle-fed baby a careful detailed history is essential. It is always necessary to see the bottle to test the patency of the teat oneself.

The use of a dummy or pacifier might conceivably lead to air swallowing, but it is not an important cause of flatulence.

As in the breast-fed baby, prolonged crying as a result of a rigid feeding schedule may cause air swallowing.

" Three months' colic " has already been described (p. 60).

Posseting and Vomiting

Posseting occurs in a bottle-fed baby in the same way as it does in a breast-fed one. Excessive posseting or vomiting is often due to flatulence, which has been discussed above. If it still persists in spite of correction of the feeding technique, the feed can be thickened with cereal so that it does not come up so readily. Very rarely vomiting is due to the child taking too much food. In an artificially-fed baby there is always the possibility that it is due to the child being given unsuitable food, such as undiluted cow's milk, or even less suitable articles of diet. The possibility of infections and of other organic disease must always be borne in mind.

Constipation

When a mother puts her child on to cow's milk after a period of breast feeding she is apt to become worried about the much firmer consistency of the baby's stools and to think that he is constipated. The mother should be reassured.

True constipation in an artificially-fed baby is nearly always due to underfeeding. It may be due to making a feed up with too little water (i.e. giving less than 2½ oz. of fluid per pound per day). It may be due to failure to add sugar to a dried milk of low carbohydrate content (e.g. National Dried Milk). If undiluted cow's milk is given, the baby is apt to have dry, hard, greasy, foul soap stools or bulky grey ones. Constipation may be due to overclothing or excessive perspiration as a result of a high external temperature. It may be due to excessive posseting or vomiting. Organic causes of constipation (such as megacolon and early hypothyroidism) have to be remembered just as much as in the breast-fed baby. In some babies, however, true constipation does occur in spite of attending to all the above possible causes. The stools are hard and cause discomfort when they are being passed. It sometimes helps in these cases to change to a different carbohydrate, such as lactose or maltose. Brown sugar may be used instead of white. In the weaning period puréed prunes may be added to the diet. Purgatives are hardly ever required if attention to the above factors is given. If really necessary, milk of magnesia is safe and non-irritating. It is given in doses of 1 drachm two or three times a day, adjusting the dose to the child's needs.

Diarrhœa

It is a great deal more significant when a mother complains that her bottle-fed baby has diarrhœa than when a breast-fed baby is brought up with that complaint. Gastro-enteritis is very rare in fully breast-fed babies, the disease being almost confined to bottle-fed ones.

Diarrhœa may be due to excess of sugar in the feeds or to the practice of giving glucose between feeds. A common mistake is to add sugar to dried feeds which have a high carbohydrate content, such as half-cream Cow and Gate or Trufood. It may also be due to fat intolerance. There are considerable individual variations in the tolerance of both fat and carbohydrate. Looseness of the stools due to fat intolerance is usually remedied by changing from a full-cream preparation to a half-cream one. Diarrhœa may be due to orange juice. This can be remedied by giving the vitamin C in the form of ascorbic acid.

Very rarely diarrhœa may be due to overfeeding. The motions tend to be loose and frequent. There may be vomiting and the weight gain, which is sometimes excessive at first, falls off and weight may even be lost. It should be emphasized, however, that underfeeding is infinitely commoner than overfeeding.

In the United States allergy to cow's milk is regarded as a common cause of intestinal disturbances in babies, and in particular of colic, vomiting and diarrhœa. In my experience it is very rare.

Defective Weight Gain

The commonest cause of defective weight gain in an artificially-fed baby is underfeeding. This may arise in a variety of ways. It may arise simply from ignorance of the normal food requirements of a baby. It may arise from rigid ideas of the quantity of food which should be given. Many books about infant feeding give the impression that the quantities of food recommended at various ages must be strictly adhered to. This is wrong, for there are big eaters and little eaters. Some need more than the average amount of food to secure a satisfactory weight gain and to satisfy hunger. When advice is sought on account of excessive crying, the calculation that the food being given is adequate for an average child by no means implies that it is enough for the child in question. The child should have what he wants, whether it is more than the average or not. Rigid ideas of the quantity to be given are often based on totally unfounded fears of overfeeding the child.

Underfeeding may arise from feeding the baby by the actual weight rather than by the expected weight. Babies who have been underfed, perhaps as a result of defective lactation or for other reasons, have a compensatory increase of appetite which enables them to catch up to the expected weight. If extra food is not given to such children, excessive crying may result from hunger. It is for this reason, as well as on account of individual variations in appetite already discussed, that it is always wrong to feed babies by the instructions on the tin. Infant feeding should be much more individualized than that and the quantities given should be adjusted to the needs of the individual.

Another way in which underfeeding arises is reliance on a teaspoon as a measure of a drachm. Teaspoons vary considerably in size. I once saw a child in whom the weight gain was unsatisfactory in spite of attention to the quantity offered, and found that a teaspoon was being used to measure drachms. Four teaspoonfuls measured 160 gr., and not 240 gr. as intended. Another mistake is to use a tablespoon as a measure of $\frac{1}{2}$ oz. Tablespoons, too, vary in size and often measure $\frac{3}{4}$ oz. instead of $\frac{1}{2}$ oz. Feeds so made up would be too dilute and the quantity of actual food taken would then fall short of the requirement.

Defective weight gain may also be due to insufficient fluid in the feeds. In hot climates the quantity of fluid usually recommended in this country ($2\frac{1}{2}$ oz. per pound per day) is inadequate. I saw several babies in the Middle East who were failing to thrive for this reason. Excessive clothing will prevent the usual weight gain on account of excessive perspiration.

In bottle-fed babies separation from the mother has always to be remembered as a sufficient cause for a child not gaining weight. Bakwin [26] and others have described babies who refused to gain weight in spite of every attention to the feeding technique and without any infection being present. These babies tend to be kept longer and longer in hospital in an effort to make them gain weight, while if they are returned home they promptly put on weight and progress like a normal child. I have seen this on several occasions.

Defective weight gain may be due to excessive posseting, vomiting, diarrhœa or to any infection such as thrush.

One sees an occasional baby who, in spite of being given as much food as he wants, still gains weight unsatisfactorily. This can sometimes be remedied by adding a cereal to the feed or by adding an amino-acid preparation.

Refusal to take the Calculated Requirements

Some babies who are otherwise perfectly well refuse almost from birth to take the ordinary quantity of milk, and many are below the average weight as a result. It is impossible to find a reason for this behaviour. Such obvious causes as overclothing, coldness, too frequent feeds and infections are readily eliminated. They are not left crying excessively. They just do not take as much as they should. Still [404] called this condition "congenital anorexia." He had no particular explanation for the phenomenon. Gesell and Ilg [144] discussed it in their book on the "Feeding Behaviour of Infants." It seems to be an inherent characteristic of the child which is not due to any mismanagement, but food forcing is apt to result, and this aggravates the condition. It is rare and it is difficult to manage. The essential points in the management are patience, absence of forcing and absence of anxiety.

Excessive Weight Gain

This is hardly ever a problem of the first 3 months. An occasional baby of 4 months or so may become too fat. This is best dealt with by weaning the baby on to mixed feeds, taking care to avoid an excess of starch, as in cereal.

Excessive Crying

This is commonly due to underfeeding, and the causes of this have been discussed in the previous section.

Refusal of the Bottle and Refusal to Part with the Bottle

It is not at all uncommon for a bottle-fed baby suddenly to refuse to have food from a bottle any longer. The analogous refusal of the breast has already been discussed. The refusal is usually easy to deal with as soon as it is recognized, for such children are nearly always willing to take food from a spoon or cup. There need be no anxiety about the child's ability to use a cup. It is surprising how often mothers feed children with a spoon when a cup would be much quicker and easier to use. Most children can approximate their lips very adequately to a cup by about 5 months of age. They tend to manage thickened feeds from a cup sooner than ordinary liquids such as milk. Freeden [133] wrote an interesting account of 10 years' experience of feeding new-born babies from a cup. No serious difficulty was experienced.

A baby may refuse milk while he is very ready to take solids. I saw an 8-month child who had been on a mixed diet for 2 months, and who was put back on to the bottle by the doctor on account of a febrile illness. The baby refused to have anything to do with it and was brought up for a second opinion because of his quite marked loss of weight. He responded immediately to the return of a mixed diet.

A baby may refuse to part with the bottle. This is usually due to failure to offer the food by cup and spoon in place of the bottle. This should be done at the age of 5 or 6 months. Brennemann wrote that he had seen a girl of 18 years of age who could still only take milk from a bottle. No baby should have a bottle after the age of 12 months. It is better to discard it at about 6 months, before the baby has become too attached to it. It is quicker, furthermore, to feed the baby from a cup as soon as he can manage it.

The Age of Weaning (Artificially fed babies)

The age of weaning breast-fed babies was discussed on p. 21. There is a tendency to wean artificially-fed babies earlier. An interesting study by Butler and Wolman [79] in the United States indicated that there is a strong tendency to give babies mixed feeds early, including purēed meat, fruit and vegetables. In an analysis of 2,000 replies to a questionnaire sent to physicians dealing mostly with babies, it was found that 43 per cent. of the doctors were introducing supplementary foods by the fourth week, and 75 per cent. by the sixth week. Glaser [153] wrote that there was a potential danger in this practice, in that there might be an increased risk of allergic manifestations. The importance of the investigation lay in the fact that babies will tolerate early mixed foods in the first month or two, so that when there are indications for changing from milk to other foods, there is nothing to fear from introducing these early.

It seems reasonable to begin weaning from an all milk diet at about 4 months of age, unless there are other indications, such as incipient obesity.

As with breast-fed babies, cereals are usually added to the diet first, and then purēed meat, fish, fruit, and vegetables. One can give egg, grated cheese, mashed banana with milk, custard and jelly, or mashed potato with milk or gravy.

When the baby begins to chew, which is usually at about 6 months of age, solid foods can be given—a biscuit, raw banana, a piece of peeled apple, toast, or a piece of chocolate, and gradually more solid food is put on his plate, food which now has to be chewed. If a baby is given solid food before he can chew, he is likely to be sick.

Weaning Difficulties

Sudden Weaning. When it suddenly becomes necessary—on account, for instance, of some grave illness in the mother—to take the baby off the breast and put him on to the bottle, considerable difficulties may be met with in some babies. It probably depends largely on the personality of the baby as to whether there is trouble or not. With many babies there is no difficulty. With others there may be complete food refusal.

The basic principles of management have been discussed above. The management is very similar to that of the baby in the new-born period. It is particularly important to be patient and to avoid all forcing methods. He should be cuddled before he is fed unless he is crying vigorously for food, and the rest depends entirely on tact and patience. It may be wise to have a fairly large hole in the teat so that the food is obtained easily. It sometimes helps to give a dose of chloral (1 or $1\frac{1}{2}$ gr.) 20 minutes before the feed. A determined baby may refuse a feed, but it is very unlikely that he will refuse more than one. Capitulation usually occurs with increasing hunger.

Other Weaning Difficulties. The causes of food refusal when weaning is being attempted can be enumerated as follows :—

(1) Dislike of the food offered—because of taste or appearance.

(2) The child is being forced to take it or is being rushed unduly.

(3) The food is too hot or the child remembers a previous similar food which was too hot and which burnt him.

(4) He wants a drink first.

(5) He is not hungry, perhaps because he is tired.

(6) He is uncomfortable because of a wet napkin or because of teething.

(7) The food is being offered in a cup or dish other than his favourite one.

(8) He is not allowed to help to feed himself.

(9) He prefers a cup to a spoon.

Weaning difficulties are intimately bound up with the development of food refusal in later years (p. 249).

Looseness of the stools in the weaning period may be due to an excess of fruit in the diet, particularly rhubarb and pears.

Undue offensiveness of the stools may be due to excess of protein in the diet.

Section II

PHYSICAL PROBLEMS

CHAPTER 8

THE ASSESSMENT OF PHYSICAL DEVELOPMENT

A CHILD'S physical development is so intimately related to his health and nutrition that in any appraisal of these an assessment of his physical development is an essential part of the examination. Perhaps the most important single method of confirming the adequacy of a baby's food intake is his gain in weight. Frequent weighings are as a rule undesirable and unnecessary because they are liable to worry the mother. She becomes anxious when as a result of a cold, the eruption of a tooth or other simple complaint the weight progress is temporarily slowed. The more intelligent the mother the less necessary are frequent weighings. The less intelligent she is the more important it is to keep a careful watch on the child's progress by means of physical measurements. However intelligent she is, it is always wise to weigh a baby at intervals—say, once a week in the first 2 months, and thereafter at less frequent intervals—probably monthly—in order that in the case of an illness one has previous weights as a base-line from which one can observe the child's progress.

When a mother complains that her child is unwell, is posseting excessively or vomiting, has persistent diarrhœa or severe chronic food refusal, the child's physical development has to be assessed by the doctor in order that he can decide how much importance to attach to her story. When a mother or other person asks for an expert opinion about a child because of his appearance, or because he is unusually small for his age, the doctor must know how to assess his physical development. The child's measurements are then used to reinforce the doctor's clinical observations. When a child is unwell and under treatment or when he is convalescent from an illness, an essential part of his supervision consists of a careful regular examination of his progress in weight gain and other measurements. In the Welfare Clinic and School Medical Service a screening device is constantly needed to enable the nurse or doctor to pick out those children who are in need of expert medical examination. For a variety of research purposes accurate assessment of a child's physical development is essential. Below is a brief description of the main present-day methods used in the assessment of the physical development of children in the first 5 years. Basically they depend on single measurements or on the relationship of weight to height.

Single Measurements in Relation to the Average

Much the most important single measurement is that of the weight. The weight is a composite of other measurements and is an over-all measure of body size. It has the advantage of being very simple to record and it is at least partly understood by all parents. Other measurements commonly taken are the height, head and chest circumference, pelvic and calf girth and sitting height. The figures so obtained are compared with average figures obtained from the study of large numbers of children. Much more valuable than isolated readings are serial records showing the rate of increase in growth as judged by the various measurements.

The average weight gain in the first 3 months is 7 oz. per week (196 gm.), and 5·3 oz. (148 gm.) in the second 3 months. During the second year the average child gains weight at the speed of about $1\frac{1}{2}$ oz. (42 gm.) per week. It is wrong to suggest that a child's birth weight should be doubled at 6 months and trebled by a year. That is only true for a child of average birth weight.

Single Measurements related to the Percentage Distribution of those Measurements in other Children

Stuart and Meredith,[406] in Boston, U.S.A., worked out the percentage distribution (percentiles) of certain measurements in large numbers of children, so that the measurements of an individual child can be compared with them. They give figures for the weight, height, sitting height, pelvic and calf girth, and chest and head circumference, measurements which they think should be the minimum ones in any serious study. These figures are arranged in percentiles. The 25th percentile means that in 25 per cent. of the children studied the measurements fall below that figure. The range between the highest and lowest figures (the 90th and 10th percentiles) includes 80 per cent. of the measurements taken. When faced with the assessment of an individual child, the placing of each measurement in relation to the percentile is recorded on a chart as a figure (e.g. 25, meaning 25th percentile), so that not only can each measurement be compared with the corresponding measurement at the last visit, but it can be compared with those of other children. If, for instance, a child's chest circumference, pelvic girth, weight and height corresponded with the 25th percentile, while his head circumference corresponded with that of the 80th percentile, one would note immediately that the size of the head is out of all proportion to his body build. This would be all the more important if it were found by reference to the chart that the circumference of his head corresponded with a lower percentile, such as the 50th, when it was last measured. Such a child would need a careful clinical examination in order to determine the significance of the finding. To use their words: "To reach a reasonable judgment as to the significance of a given measurement at a given age, one should know not only what the average for that age is, but how

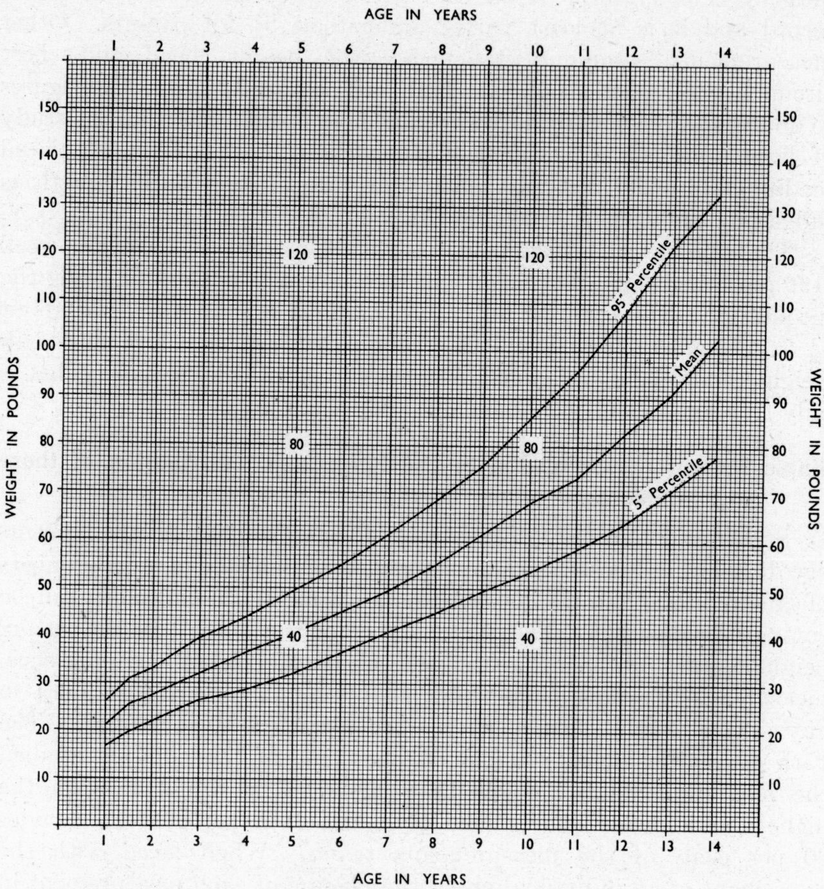

FIG. 5. Weight chart showing the mean with the 5th and 95th percentiles (based on figures by Gore and Palmer [163] of London school children).

widely normal healthy children deviate from the average. One must consider how normal the given measurement is, how it accords with other measurements of the same child and, if possible, how it compares with a similar measurement taken previously. The simple procedure of finding the place held by the child under study in the normal distribution in each of the measurements taken should call attention to the principal features of the child's size and build."

Tables III and IV show the percentiles for the weight and height of pre-school children in London, based on the paper by Gore and Palmer.[163] Fig. 5 shows the figures for weight in graphic form.

TABLE III

Percentiles of Weights of Boys and Girls in London *

(Pounds and Decimals)

Age	Boys Percentiles			Girls Percentiles		
	95th	50th	5th	95th	50th	5th
3 months . .	15·7	12·6	9·5	14·7	11·8	8·9
6 ,, . .	21·3	17·5	13·6	20·0	16·4	12·7
9 ,, . .	24·7	20·5	16·2	23·3	19·3	15·3
1 year . .	27·0	22·6	18·1	25·2	21·0	16·9
1 yr. 3 mths. .	28·8	24·1	19·3	27·0	22·6	18·1
1 yr. 6 mths. .	30·6	25·5	20·5	28·8	24·0	19·3
1 yr. 9 mths. .	32·2	27·0	21·6	30·5	25·5	20·5
2 years . .	33·9	28·3	22·7	32·2	26·9	21·6
2 yrs. 3 mths. .	35·4	29·6	23·8	33·8	28·2	22·7
2 yrs. 6 mths. .	36·8	30·8	24·7	35·3	29·5	23·7
2 yrs. 9 mths. .	38·2	31·9	25·6	36·6	30·6	24·6
3 years . .	39·3	32·8	26·4	37·8	31·6	25·3
4 ,, . .	44·0	37·4	28·6	44·0	35·2	28·6
5 ,, . .	48·4	41·8	33·0	50·6	39·6	30·8

* Calculated from the paper by Gore and Palmer,[163] which was based on figures for 5,684 London children.

TABLE IV

Percentiles of Heights of Boys and Girls in London (*cm.*)

Age in years	Boys Percentiles			Girls Percentiles		
	95th	50th	5th	95th	50th	5th
1½ . .	88	80	73	85	78	72
2 . .	92	85	77	90	82	75
3 . .	101	92	84	99	91	84
4 . .	108	100	91	108	98	91
5 . .	116	106	99	115	106	98

Weight-Height Ratio

Several methods of measuring physical development depend on the relationship of weight to height. Most of them concern children of school age. A popular method commonly used in the United States is the Wetzel grid.[450] Wetzel's "baby grid" [449] is shown in Fig. 6. At first sight the grid looks extremely complicated—and it is, in fact, based on advanced mathematical methods, but it is very easy to use, a single placement on the grid taking only a few seconds. The "physique" or "body build" of the child is determined by plotting the child's weight against his height on the left side of the grid. The figure so obtained is then plotted on the right of the grid against his age, so that his physique is shown against a background which depicts the percentage of children of his age possessing that physique. The second placing, in other words, shows his developmental level in relation to others. Serial readings are taken at intervals so that the pattern and direction of the growth curve is shown. Any illness or infection is likely to be shown by a deviation from the normal course of development and is clearly shown on the chart.

The grid is so constructed that certain other data are shown and recorded. The grid shows certain milestones of development—the age at which the child smiles, follows with his eyes, acquires head control, reaches objects, laughs, sits, stands, walks and speaks. It has subsidiary panels for the recording of his head and chest circumference, and a space for recording his immunizations and skin tests, such as the tuberculin reaction. It also shows the child's surface area and calorie needs and various other data.

It should be emphasized that the grid is intended to show the curve of the child's physical development so that alterations in his physique may be noted. He is compared, in other words, more with himself, with his previous growth, than with the growth of others.

The Interpretation of Measurements of Physical Growth

All the methods described above may indicate, some more clearly than others, that a child's measurements are unusual, but none of them tell *why* they are unusual. That depends on the history, clinical examination and clinical judgment, which involves a thorough knowledge of the normal and of the normal variations which may occur and of the various factors, other than disease, which affect growth. In all cases the following difficulties and fallacies have to be borne in mind :—

Errors in the Measurements. Scales are frequently out of order. It is never wise to compare the weight on one set of scales with the weight on another. In the case of a baby it is always important, in comparing his present weight with a previous one, to know that the conditions of weighing were identical in the two cases. He should be weighed naked in each case. If on one occasion he is weighed before a feed and on another he is weighed after one, a considerable error is introduced. An isolated reading is disturbed by the passage of urine or fæces immediately before the weighing.

It is easy to make mistakes in such simple measurements as the head circumference. In older children recumbent length is more accurate than standing height, because it eliminates postural factors.

Fallacies Inherent in Single Measurements. Single measurements cannot give an accurate idea of a child's physical condition. Isolated measurements may be taken at the beginning or end of a period of defective growth. They may reveal unusual features of his physique but they show nothing of his rate of growth. Much more important, therefore, than single measurements is the growth chart, which shows the child's growth in weight, height and other measurements.

The Average is not the Normal. Any doctor may be able to say what the average weight and height is for a child of given age and sex, but no one can say what the normal is, for it is impossible to define the normal. A child may be pounds below the average in weight and inches below the average in height and yet be perfectly normal. There are great individual variations in body build, but it is impossible to place a dividing line between the normal and the abnormal. Boyd [57] pointed out that weight charts which give average figures " represent the hypothetical . . . youngster who is a composite of all his mates, including the more fortunate as well as the less privileged." All children are individuals, and they have widely differing rhythms of growth. Some have unexplained slow and rapid periods of growth. Some are slow starters ; they grow slowly for a few years and then have a rapid spurt of growth and catch up to their fellows. This is particularly apt to happen at puberty. In general the large child matures early and the small child matures late, so that the small child, by having a longer period of growth, eventually attains the same build as his fellows who were much larger than he was in the earlier years of childhood.

It is logical to assume that the greater a child's deviation from his fellows in any of the measurements of body build the less likely he is to be normal. For this reason Stuart considers that his percentile charts afford the best method of assessing an individual child. His approach, however, which is probably the best and most rational one available, does not place the dividing line between the normal and the abnormal. The fact that a child's weight is below that of 80 per cent. of his fellows of the same age does not prove that he is abnormal. Table III, on p. 85, shows the range into which 90 per cent. of London children fall, but I would not like to say with certainty that, if a child's measurements fall outside that range, they are necessarily abnormal.

It cannot be assumed that maximum growth is necessarily the optimum. In the premature baby, for instance, it is dangerous to try to secure a rapid and large weight gain. This may be achieved for a time, but it is apt to be followed by a slowing of the weight gain, and later on by loss of weight. There have been several papers concerning the additional height achieved by giving vitamins in quantities greater than those normally recommended, but no one has proved that the children are healthier on that account. There is nothing to suggest that a child who is 5 or 10 per cent. above the average weight and height at any age is in any way better than a child who is 5 or 10 per cent. below the average, provided that the latter is free from infection or other known illness. Neither is there evidence that a child of 2 or 3 years who is increasing rapidly in weight and height is any healthier than the otherwise well child who is increasing in size at rather less than the average speed. In general, when a doctor is faced with an otherwise well child, who on account of constitutional reasons is smaller than the average, he should direct his efforts not at trying to alter his physique but at trying to persuade his parents and others to accept him as a normal child. One is reminded of the words of John Kendrick Bangs :

> " I met a little Elfman once,
> Down where the lilies blow.
> I asked him why he was so small,
> And why he did not grow.
> He slightly frowned and with his eyes
> He looked me through and through.
> ' I'm quite as big for me,' he said,
> ' As you are big for you.' "

Figures used for comparison must be valid ones. It is clearly wrong to use figures obtained in one country as a basis of comparison for children in another. American children, for instance, tend to be larger than British ones. In the same way it is unwise to use charts based on figures obtained many years ago. The physique of children varies from decade to decade.

Miscellaneous Factors. Various factors other than disease have an important bearing on the child's physical development, and these must always be borne in mind in the assessment of an individual child. These factors can be summarized as follows :

(*a*) GENETIC FACTORS. These clearly play an important part. It is commonly said that the child's growth potential is decided at the time of the fertilization of the ovum. Environmental factors subsequently may retard growth, but they have little effect in accelerating it. In some families the babies are small at birth, and in others they are large. In some families the children grow comparatively slowly for the first few years, and unusually rapidly later. It should be noted, however, that not infrequently smallness of build in child and parents is due to the effect of malnutrition acting on both.

(*b*) NUTRITION. Malnutrition has a considerable effect on growth, affecting the weight more than the height. Malnutrition may be due to poverty, ignorance, food fads, food refusal, excessive posseting or rumination as well as to actual disease. There is a voluminous literature on the effect of nutrition on growth, and this is not the place in which to discuss it.

(*c*) THE SIZE OF THE CHILD AT BIRTH. The weight at birth is related to the duration of gestation, to racial and genetic factors, to the parity of the mother and to her state of nutrition in the last 3 months of pregnancy, and to unknown factors. It is smaller in multiple pregnancies, the average birthweight of twins being 5¼ lb. and of triplets 4 lb. Later-born babies tend to exceed the first-born one in birth weight.

Mothers who have diabetes or who are going to develop it in years to come tend to produce large babies. Kritzer [239] carried out glucose tolerance tests on fifty-eight women of an average of 32 years, who had had babies weighing 10 lb. or more, and whose urine had been sugar-free 2½ years previously : eighteen (31 per cent.) had glycosuria and glucose tolerance curves characteristic of diabetes. Differences in the birth weight of twins may be due to differences in the vascularity of the implantation sites of their placentæ.[92] Cord blood examination showed differences in hæmoglobin concentration and in oxygen saturation. Social-economic factors are of considerable importance. It has been said that the mean birth weight of a country is a delicate measure of its health, and varies inversely with the infant mortality. Selber [374] found that the prematurity rate for European babies in Durban was 4·2 per cent. as compared with 18·3 per cent. in Indian babies.

The largest known birth weight of a living child is 17 lb., and of a still-born child 24 lb.

It was found [204, 205, 206] in Sheffield that there is a strong correlation between the child's size at birth and his subsequent body build. The smaller the size of the baby at birth, as shown by his birth weight, the smaller he is likely to be in later childhood, and the larger he is at birth the larger he is likely to be in later childhood.

The average weight of boys at one year who weighed 5½ lb. or less at birth was 20 lb. 12 oz., while that of boys who at birth weighed 9½ lb. or more was 24 lb. 7 oz. The average weight of boys at 2 and 3 years who weighed 5½ lb. or less at birth was 24 lb. 3 oz. and 28 lb. 9 oz. respectively, while that of boys who at birth weighed 9½ lb. or more was 29 lb. 1 oz. and 33 lb. 10 oz. respectively.

It was found in older children that all the various measurements taken—the sitting height, pelvic girth, chest and calf circumference, standing height and weight—were related in this way to the size of the child at birth. This work was confirmed by other workers.[101, 261, 278, 317]

TABLE V

The Relation of Birth Weight to Subsequent Weight
Mean Weight at Various Ages

(The figures in brackets indicate the number of children in each group)

Figures in pounds and ounces

	Group A (Birth weight 5 lb. 8 oz. or less)	Group B (Birth weight 7 lb. 2 oz. to 7 lb. 6 oz.)	Group C (Birth weight 8 lb. 8. oz. to 9 lb. 7 oz.)	Group D. (Birth weight 9 lb. 8 oz. or more)
Boys :				
Birth	4 lb. 14 oz.	7 lb. 4 oz.	8 lb. 13 oz.	9 lb. 15 oz.
1 year	20 „ 12 „ (51)	22 „ 5 „ (36)	24 „ 3 „ (104)	24 „ 7 „ (44)
1½ years	22 „ 6 „ (18)	26 „ 2 „ (23)	25 „ 15 „ (46)	27 „ 2 „ (22)
2 years	24 „ 3 „ (26)	26 „ 8 „ (26)	28 „ 15 „ (63)	29 „ 1 „ (22)
2½ years	28 „ 0 „ (10)	—	30 „ 14 „ (15)	30 „ 11 „ (10)
3 years	28 „ 9 „ (10)	—	—	33 „ 10 „ (18)*
5 years	40 „ 8 „ (57)	41 „ 1 „ (83)	43 „ 8 „ (125)	45 „ 12 „ (36)
Girls :				
Birth	5 lb. 0 oz.	7 lb. 4 oz.	8 lb. 13 oz.	9 lb. 14 oz.
1 year	19 „ 11 „ (59)	21 „ 13 „ (48)	22 „ 8 „ (73)	23 „ 3 „ (23)
1½ years	21 „ 15 „ (23)	24 „ 13 „ (15)	24 „ 10 „ (31)	25 „ 4 „ (9)
2 years	24 „ 12 „ (31)	27 „ 0 „ (28)	26 „ 15 „ (64)	29 „ 9 „ (19)
3 years	28 „ 1 „ (15)	—	—	32 „ 8 „ (20)*
5 years	37 „ 4 „ (69)	40 „ 0 „ (68)	42 „ 11 „ (68)	44 „ 4 „ (25)

Reproduced from the *Brit. Med. J.*, 1950, *i*, 96.

* Groups C and D combined owing to smallness of numbers.

In my experience by far the commonest finding in an otherwise well child who is unusually small in weight and height is the history that he was small at birth. Mothers connect the two more often than doctors, but many mothers are seriously concerned about the small size of their children and so try to force them to eat—with the opposite of the effect desired.

Owing to the tendency of large children to mature early and small ones to mature late, one would have thought that after maturation the adolescents' size would be unrelated to his birth weight. Blegen,[50] however, found that premature babies tended to lag behind in weight and height up to and including puberty, and that there was no tendency to compensation towards puberty. Alm,[13] who compared the physical development of 999 prematurely born boys with that of 1,002 controls, found that the former were statistically significantly smaller in weight and height than the controls at the age of 20. Douglas and Mogford,[117] though conceding that premature babies on the average do not reduce their initial weight handicap in the first 4 years, felt that the best guide to the expected height of a child was the height of his parents.

(*d*) UNKNOWN CONSTITUTIONAL FACTORS. In many children the

reason for the variation from the normal is not known. There are big children and little children, and there is no evident reason for the differences between them. In general the highly active child tends to be thinner than the placid, easy-going one. It is the great individual variations which make the assessment of an individual child so difficult.

Conclusion

It will be seen that there is at present no short cut to the assessment of the health of a child. An accurate assessment can only be made by taking a careful history, conducting a careful examination, studying the child's physique and then taking all the various factors which may have affected his growth into account. Investigations designed to compare the findings of clinicians with physical measurements have shown a disappointingly small correlation between the two. Weight alone is unreliable. On the one hand, an overweight child could be suffering from an avitaminosis ; on the other hand, an underweight child may be perfectly well. It is obvious that serial measurements of weight and height provide a great deal more information than single measurements, but even a steady weight gain does not exclude organic disease or psychological disturbances. There is much to be said for the use of charts showing the distribution of the measurements in large numbers of other children, but even those do not give certain information as to when a child is abnormal, and they certainly do not say why he is abnormal. Stuart and Meredith [406] remark that the Wetzel grid does not distinguish a well-nourished narrow-built child from a chronically malnourished average one. The physician must determine by other means whether skeletal build, muscular development or the amount of subcutaneous fat is the principal factor accounting for the unusual placing in the grid. One might add that, having found which of the three factors is responsible, one still has to determine *why* there is a deficiency in skeletal build, muscle or fat. The grid does not take into account the factors which affect growth. It was shown in Sheffield that children who were of small size at birth have in general a lower placing on the grid (a lower developmental level with regard to physique) than those of large size at birth. In addition the grid is costly to use.

In general, serial weight and height records provide the most useful information about a child's growth. It is desirable that in doubtful cases the figures obtained should be compared with those of others in terms of their percentage distribution. If due allowance is then made for all the various factors other than disease known to affect growth, then the measurements obtained give an invaluable pointer to the child's general state of health.

In the assessment of an individual child whose measurements are unusual, his size at birth and the build of his parents are the chief factors, other than disease, which have to be considered. *Of far greater importance than his weight and height are his well-being, abundant energy, happiness, freedom from infection and freedom from lassitude.* If he has these he is unlikely to have serious organic disease.

CHAPTER 9

THE SKULL

The Size of the Skull

THE measurement of the circumference of the skull is a routine part of the examination in a welfare clinic. Unusual growth in size may denote early hydrocephalus and so lead to the diagnosis and cure of a subdural hæmatoma. Examination of the skull may reveal premature synostosis of the cranial sutures—again a curable condition, for early operation may prevent the spasticity, mental deficiency and gross deformity of the skull which develop if early treatment is not given.

The effect of moulding in birth disappears in 2 or 3 days. Thereafter the measurements of the circumference of the skull should be a reliable figure. There is an increase of approximately 2 in. (5 cm.) in the first 4 months ($\frac{1}{2}$ in. per month), and of another 2 in. (5 cm.) in the next 8 months, so that in the first year there is an increase of about 4 in. (10 cm.) in the circumference. From the end of the first year to the age of 20 there is an increase of only 4 more inches (10 cm.).

The size of a baby's head, if unusual, may cause anxiety to parents, nurses and doctors. Some babies have small heads, suggesting the possibility of microcephaly, and some large heads, suggesting hydrocephalus, yet they may be perfectly normal, but unfortunately it is very difficult to define the limits of normality.

In assessing the head of an individual baby, one first of all inspects it. It may give an immediate impression of hydrocephalus, but one should remember that a bulging forehead may be simply a familial trait, and of no importance. When a baby has an unusually large or small head it is always as well to see both parents, for one of them may have a similar head, so that further anxiety about the baby need not be felt.

The next step is to palpate the fontanelle and sutures.

In hydrocephalus the fontanelle may be found to be bulging or unduly wide for the age, and the sutures may be found to be abnormally separated. Parmelee [327] thinks that the squamous suture is the most reliable place to examine for undue separation of the sutures. A good deal of experience, however, is necessary in the interpretation of one's findings, because the normal variations which occur in the fontanelle and sutures are considerable. It should be remembered that ossification of the sutures is delayed by rickets. Microcephaly is usually

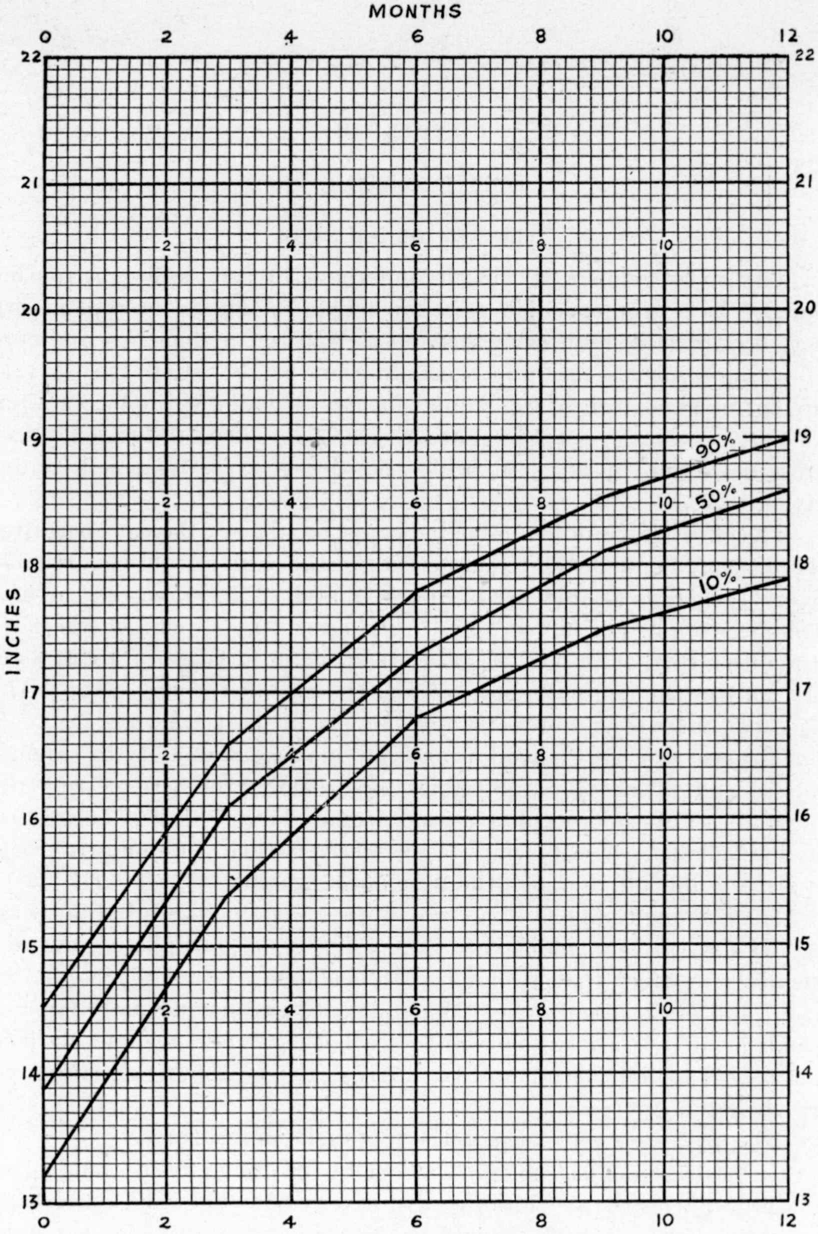

FIG. 7. Head circumference chart as used at The Children's Hospital, Sheffield.

due to defective growth of the brain, but it may be due to premature synostosis of the cranial sutures—a condition curable by operation—and this can be found by the experienced finger ; in place of the usual

TABLE VI

Circumference of Head

(Westropp and Barber [448])

Age	Boys Mean			Girls Mean		
	Inches	Cm.	σ	Inches	Cm.	σ
1 month . .	14·7	37·3	1·54	14·3	36·5	1·41
3 months . .	16·1	40·7	1·43	15·6	39·8	1·39
6 ,, . .	17·2	43·6	1·45	16·7	42·5	1·42
9 ,, . .	18·0	45·7	1·40	17·6	44·6	1·41
1 year . .	18·4	46·8	1·40	17·9	45·6	1·30
1½ years . .	18·9	47·9	1·40	18·5	47·0	1·32
2 ,, . .	19·4	49·1	1·47	18·8	48·0	1·35
3 ,, . .	19·8	50·4	1·35	19·6	49·5	1·45
4 ,, . .	20·1	51·2	1·41	19·9	50·7	1·50
5 ,, . .	20·4	51·8	1·47	20·2	51·2	1·37

slight separation of the sutures one feels a rim of bone where they have prematurely fused.

The circumference of the head is then measured, taking the mean of two or three readings, and compared with Table VI.

The figure is then recorded on a graph (Fig. 7) so that at subsequent examinations the rate of increase in the head circumference can be plotted. Only by so doing can one make a reliable assessment. The average skull circumference of a full-term baby is 13·8 in. at birth, and it increases by 2 in. in circumference in the first 3–4 months, and 2 in. in the subsequent 8 or 9 months. Even if the baby is born with a mild degree of hydrocephalus, the condition may no longer be progressive, so that the future prognosis will be good. On the other hand if a head is found to be enlarging at more than the usual speed, the prognosis is much less hopeful. A progressive shift upwards from one percentile to another may well indicate progressive hydrocephalus.

One must remember that the head of a prematurely born child is larger relative to the rest of the body than that of a full-term child. I have seen the diagnosis of hydrocephalus wrongly made in premature babies because of ignorance of this fact. The circumference of the head of the prematurely born baby is as follows [188] :

28–32 weeks' fœtus		10·2–11·8 in.
32–36 ,,	,,	11·3–13·0 in.
36–40 ,,	,,	13·0–14·6 in.

There have been many attempts to relate the head circumference to the circumference of the chest and to body length, but I have not found them of much value in assessing an individual baby. The head measurements, like other measurements, are related to the size of the baby at birth, so that in general the body proportions of the child who was a large baby are larger than those of a child who was a small baby at birth.

A developmental examination should be included in cases in which one feels doubtful. A microcephalic baby will show retardation in development. A baby developing hydrocephalus sooner or later begins to slow in his development, and defective head control becomes manifest as the head enlarges. Radiological examination for the so-called " digital impressions " in the skull as a result of increased intracranial pressure is not likely to help before clinical signs are obvious.

In conclusion, in the assessment of an individual child whose head measurements are unusual, one will consider familial traits, feel the fontanelle and sutures, assess his development, and make serial measurements of the circumference of the head in order to determine whether the rate of increase in circumference is normal or not.

The Shape of the Head

A common source of worry to the mother and doctors is a flattening of the skull of the baby on one side and a corresponding bulge on the other. This is perfectly normal and is simply due to the baby always lying on one side. Babies often prefer one side, and it is pointless to attempt to make them lie on the other side. The peculiarity disappears shortly after the first birthday.

When other peculiarities of shape are noted, the first step is to see both parents. Very often the peculiarity in the shape of the skull is familial. It is not due to moulding at birth, because the effect of moulding disappears a few days after birth.

Sometimes the peculiarity of shape is such that the question of craniostenosis, or premature closure of the cranial sutures, arises. This condition is rare, but early diagnosis is important for successful operative treatment. The expert can feel the ridge of the abnormal suture line. Expert radiology confirms the clinical diagnosis.

Asymmetry of the face may be due to the condition known as hemiatrophy or hemihypertrophy.

The Fontanelle

The anterior fontanelle is small at birth, and enlarges considerably during the first 2 or more months. After this period it decreases until it is closed on palpation. Aisenson [5] studied the age of closure in 1,677 infants, and found that this varied from 4 to 26 months : in 90 per cent. it closed between 7 and 19 months ; in 41·6 per cent. it closed in the first year. In another study [3] the age of closure was studied in 550 children: at the age of 1 year it was closed (clinically) in 30·5 per cent. of boys and 18·8 per cent. of girls; at 18 months in 90·6 per cent. of boys and 70·3 per cent. of girls; at 2 years in 98·1 per cent. of boys and 96·9 per cent. of girls. It was closed in all the boys by the age of 3, but not in all the girls till the age of 4½.

It is very important to be aware of these normal variations. It is true, of course, that variations in the age of closure are associated with certain diseases. Premature closure occurs in microcephaly and craniostenosis. Delayed closure occurs in hydrocephalus, rickets, hypothyroidism and cleidocranial dysotosis; but in the vast majority of cases of delayed closure there is no underlying organic disease and the mentality is normal. The posterior fontanelle is usually closed to palpation after the second month.

The sutures tend to be somewhat separated in the neonatal period, and there is often a continuous gap from the forehead to the posterior part of the posterior fontanelle which may cause anxiety in those not accustomed to palpating the skull of normal new born babies.

The sutures close rapidly and become ossified at or about the age of 6 months.

The Caput Succedaneum

This is an exudation of serous fluid in the soft tissues of the presenting part during delivery. It disappears by the second or third day. There may be some residual blood pigment for a few days but no permanent mark is left even if the caput is over the face.

Cephalhæmatoma

Cephalhæmatomata occur in up to 1 per cent. of deliveries. They are rare in premature babies. They consist of an extravasation of blood between the bone and periosteum. The swellings are therefore limited by the sutures. They may be unilateral or bilateral. They are usually found in the region of the parietal bones, but may be elsewhere. During the first few days the cephalhæmatoma is often obscured by an overlying caput. This disappears after a day or two, revealing the underlying cephalhæmatoma. It may increase in size in the first few days as a result of further hæmorrhages.[427] By the second or third week a rim of bone may be felt round the periphery of the cephalhæmatoma due to new bone formation at the site of the detachment of the periosteum. The hæmatoma is cystic and an erroneous diagnosis of a depressed fracture is readily made. An X-ray does sometimes show, however, a non-depressed fracture underlying the cephalhæmatoma.[230]

Small swellings subside by the third or fourth week, but large ones may be visible for 3 months or more. When extensive ossification occurs the swelling may be visible for many months or even years.[151]

Von Reuss suggested that they are due to the tearing of veins as a result of the to-and-fro movement of the scalp with the uterine contractions. They are more likely to occur if the pelvis is roomy than if it is a constricted one. Though they may occur in forceps deliveries, they are sometimes found after Cæsarean section and they bear little relationship to difficult labour. Hartley and Burnett[183] suggest that there is often an underlying defect of bone, due to incomplete ossification, and that this may be a factor in the tearing of vessels.

They are very occasionally associated with hæmorrhagic disease of the new-born, or with other blood diseases.

The treatment is entirely conservative, except in the rare case in which bleeding persists after birth, necessitating transfusion. Even if there is an underlying fracture, nothing is done about it. They should on no account be aspirated. They disappear if left alone and do no harm to the baby. Suppuration is a very rare occurrence if they are not tampered with. If they are in the mid-line in the occipital region they have to be distinguished from occipital encephalocœles. The rim of calcium which can be seen in the X-ray in most cephalhæmatomata after 2 or 3 weeks helps to establish the diagnosis.[215]

Craniotabes

This condition was reviewed by Bille.[44] He found that one in three infants, who had no rickets at all, had craniotabes at some time in the first year. He ascribed it to pressure of the skull against the pelvic bones of the mother, on the grounds that it is very rare after breech or Cæsarian deliveries, and the craniotabes is found on the right in right vertex presentations and on the left in left presentations. It is three times commoner in first-born children than in subsequent ones, presumably because of the lower position of the head *in utero* in the last few weeks of pregnancy. Though admitting that craniotabes is common in rickets, Bille regards it as a normal condition in the great majority of infants.

CHAPTER 10

THE TEETH

Normal Dentition

THERE are considerable variations in the age at which teeth erupt. On the one hand, the child may be born with a tooth or teeth (see below); on the other hand, the first tooth may not appear until the child is 13 or 14 months old. In neither case is there any need to suppose that there is any disease. As a milestone of development teething is quite useless. It is true that occasionally dentition is late in mentally retarded children, but more often the time of dentition is normal in such children. It is useful, however, to know the average age at which teeth appear, as long as one remembers that individual variations are considerable. Table VII shows the average age of eruption of the first teeth.

TABLE VII

Average Age of Eruption of First or Deciduous Teeth

(After Harold Stuart)

Order of Eruption	Average Age in Months	Usual Range
Lower central incisor . .	7½	5½–10
Upper ,, ,, . .	9½	7½–11½
Upper lateral ,, . .	11½	8 –14½
Lower ,, ,, . .	13	10 –17
Upper first molar . . .	15½	13 –18
Lower ,, ,, . . .	16	13½–18
Upper canines	19	16 –23
Lower ,, ...	19	16 –23½
Lower second molars . .	26	22 –31
Upper ,, ,, . .	27	23 –32

Note (1) In girls teeth tend to erupt earlier than in boys.
,, (2) The range given covers two-thirds of normal children. Dentition falling outside this range is not necessarily abnormal.

Dentition in the Neonatal Period

Every maternity unit occasionally sees babies which are born with teeth (Fig. 8). It is said that Julius Cæsar, King Louis XIV, Mazarin and King Richard III were among famous people who had a tooth or teeth when born. In Poland children born with teeth were considered to be monsters.[272]

It is not possible to give the exact incidence of neonatal teeth,

There were 2 cases in two Chicago hospitals in 2,000 births.[272] In the Jessop Hospital at Sheffield four children were born with teeth in 3,000 births. A premature baby was born with 3 teeth. The teeth found at birth are usually lower central incisors ; rarely they are canines. They are very rarely supernumerary teeth. They are usually merely prematurely erupted normal teeth. The reason for such premature dentition is unknown. There is often a strong familial or hereditary factor.

Certain difficulties and dangers arise from premature dention. The teeth are usually loose owing to poor root formation, and there is therefore a danger that the tooth will be inhaled or swallowed. They sometimes cause sublingual ulceration and damage the mother's nipple.

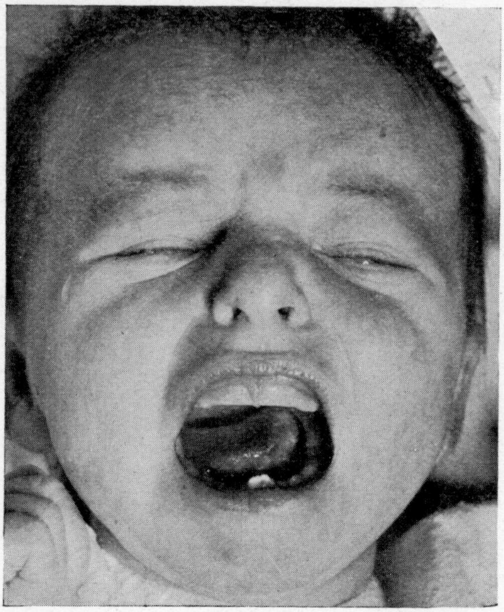

FIG. 8. Lower central incisor tooth in new-born baby.

If possible, the teeth should be left alone. If left they become more firmly fixed. Excessive bleeding may occur if they are removed, though this may perhaps be prevented by administration of vitamin K before the extraction. Their removal, furthermore, is apt to interfere with subsequent dentition. Nevertheless, if there is serious danger that they may be inhaled, extraction must be performed.

The Symptoms of Dentition

The symptoms of teething have occupied the attention of writers for generations. Guthrie [176] wrote a very interesting review of the subject. Hippocrates * in the twenty-fifth aphorism of his third book said that : " Teething children suffer from itching of the gums, fever, convulsions, diarrhœa, especially when they cut their eye teeth, and when they are very corpulent and costive." Jean Scultet (1675) * treated the pain of teething by application of the actual cautery to the occiput. Popular remedies of the Middle Ages included necklaces made of the roots of henbane, peony, the wild gourd and other vegetables ; blistering and leeches behind the lower jaw ; rubbing of the gums with hare's brain and the hanging of the tooth of a dog

* Quoted by Guthrie.[176]

or wolf round the neck. Ambroise Paré introduced gum lancing in the sixteenth century as an improvement on the practice of nurses "who with their nails and scratchings tear and rend the children's gums in order to liberate their teeth." Hurlock * nearly 200 years later alluded to the mischief caused by "meaner people who with their thimbles and monstrous wedding rings hack and bruise the gums in attempting to bring the teeth out." Clendon * in 1862 wrote: "Trace the nerve to its source in the Pons Varolii and floor of the fourth ventricle, where it is in close proximity to the glossopharyngeal, pneumogastric and spinal accessory and spinal nerves, and at once the whole train of evils—difficult breathing, immoderate diarrhœa, convulsions, squinting, effusion on the brain are easily accounted for." Arbuthnot * in 1732 wrote that "above one-tenth part of all children die in teething by symptoms proceeding from the irritation of the tender nervous parts of the jaws, occasioning inflammation, fevers, convulsion, looseness with green stools, not the worst symptoms, and in some gangrenes." Charles West in 1842 quoted the Registrar-General's reports that teething was the registered cause of death in 4·8 per cent. of all children who died in London under 1 year old, and in 7·3 per cent. of those who died between the age of 1 and 3 years. Guthrie says that the Registrar-General's report of 1839 showed 5,016 deaths in England and Wales attributed to teething. Guthrie concluded that there was no proof that any of the constitutional symptoms were due to dentition.

Several authors of papers have attempted to prove that dentition causes fever,[119,299] but none of those seen by me gave any satisfactory evidence of this. They all give theories as to its causation. Some suggest that "teething fever" is due to liberation of organisms into the blood from infected tooth sockets. Others think that it is due to the inflammation of the gums. During the eruption of a tooth the gums certainly do look red and inflamed, but Heinemeyer[185a] by means of 137 histological studies of teeth in 30 patients showed that in fact there was no histological evidence of inflammation. Guthrie and others suggested that if true inflammation did occur it was due to the introduction of infected materials into the mouth, but that it was not the direct result of teething.

It is obvious to any clinician that there is no justification at all for ascribing the great majority of these conditions to teething. It is evident from the Registrar-General's returns in the last century that teething was a convenient diagnosis to make when the cause of death was unknown. Cautley[87] thought that many of the symptoms ascribed to teething were due to rickets. I attempted to find the evidence in the literature that general conditions, such as fever, bronchitis,

* Quoted by Guthrie.[176]

convulsions and diarrhœa, are caused by teething. The search included British, American, Italian, German, New Zealand and South African journals, but the search was fruitless. No such evidence was found. Most of the workers apparently relied on the mother's diagnosis of teething. This, of course, is hopelessly fallacious. It would, in fact, be extremely difficult to conduct a scientifically acceptable piece of research on the subject because of the difficulty of making a satisfactory definition of teething. Some teeth come through a great deal more quickly than others, and in some children the eruption of the teeth takes a great deal longer than it does in others. The investigation could hardly be based, therefore, on a study of the child an arbitrary number of days before the eruption of the tooth. Careful observation of babies in an institution, where daily temperature recordings and accurate health records are kept, and where the mouth can be examined daily for changes in the gum, might supply the answer. One can certainly say that at present there is no evidence that teething causes fever, convulsions, bronchitis, diarrhœa or any general disease. It is natural that mothers should ascribe those conditions to teething. It is obvious that colds, coughs and other complaints will occur during the many months in which dentition is occurring. It is not possible to see how these conditions could be related on a pathological basis. *In the present state of our knowledge no general conditions should ever be ascribed to teething. Many serious mistakes are made as a result of ascribing convulsions and other general symptoms to teething, and some of those mistakes cost lives.*

It is obvious that dentition does cause considerable discomfort in some babies. Some are upset more than others. It is natural to suppose that when the gum becomes red and congested, as it does when a tooth is about to erupt, and when the gum finally begins to split, pain and discomfort is likely to occur, and that earache will be associated with the eruption of some of the back teeth. Pain in the mouth causes salivation, and it is easy to see that a baby with a painful gum rubs the gum with his fingers in an attempt to obtain relief from it. It is obvious that such pain will make the baby irritable. Even slight discomfort at night may be enough to awaken the baby or to keep him awake. Sometimes the pain is so severe that the baby screams even when he is picked up. It is clear that the baby, though tired and wanting to go to sleep, is unable to do so. More often the discomfort is only slight, for the crying stops when he is picked up. The pain is enough to disturb his sleep and to make him demand the company of his parents. Once he is given that he is happy and good tempered. When the gums are painful, hard items of food may be refused by the baby, and if the discomfort is severe the child may refuse almost everything. Some have suggested that gastro-intestinal disturbances are caused by the baby bolting the food, because he does not wish to chew solids with his tender gums.

A strange result of teething sometimes seen is refusal to sit on the chamber. This may recur in the 3 or 4 days preceding the eruption of each tooth. I have seen this, and it is described by Arnold Gesell. The reason for it is obscure.

Teething should be regarded as a natural though sometimes painful process, and no specific treatment can be given for it. In my opinion lancing of the gums is always wrong. It is dangerous and may cause infection of the mouth. The diet should be suitably modified if the baby shows reluctance to eat hard foods. If the baby cries because of pain he should be picked up even though there is some risk of habit formation. If he has severe pain at night, chloral should not be withheld. The dose needed to produce an effect varies from child to child. A child 1 year old could begin with 3 gr. and increase by 2 gr. each night until sleep is produced. It would be cruel to withhold it if the child has severe pain and is unable to go to sleep even though obviously tired. No local applications help. Teething powders are useless.

The Prevention of Dental Caries

For at least 3,000 years man believed [91] that caries was due to the gnawing of worms. This was believed in ancient Egypt and Mesopotamia, right through Roman times and the Middle Ages. Jaques Houllier (1498–1562) [244] first cast doubt on the existence of dental worms, but Gottfried Schulz, who lived at the same period, declared that the gastric juice of a pig would expel worms, some even as large as an earthworm, from a decayed tooth.

It is known that caries is caused by bacteria, but it is likely that there are many related factors, hereditory, developmental and dietary, amongst others. Rats can be bred with a high or low susceptibility to caries [361] ; this may be related to the bacterial flora in the mouth. It seems clear that refined carbohydrates such as sugar are more harmful than complex carbohydrates such as starch, because acid is formed more rapidly by bacteria from the former.[65] On the other hand a greatly increased sugar intake in diets of children in institutions in three cities in England had no significant effect on the institution or spread of dental caries.[290] Yet rats fed by stomach tube and animals fed on a carbohydrate free diet do not develop caries[361]; and there was a great increase of caries in Eskimos when refined carbohydrate was added to the diet.[244] There was a sharp drop in the incidence of caries in 1939–1945, when sugar was rationed, followed by a rise subsequently.

Massler [270] wrote that "Sugar control is to-day the only rational and therapeutically successful method in the dietary control of caries."

The role of fluorine in the prevention of caries seems to have been firmly established. Fluoridation of water supplies reduces the incidence of caries by 50 to 65 per cent.,[186] and is absolutely safe. Efforts to inhibit the harmful organisms by ammonium urea dentifrices and by inclusion of alkalies in dentifrices has not proved effective.[65]

Although human teeth formed in a period of suboptimal vitamin intake are particularly susceptible to caries, there is no evidence that the giving of vitamins in quantities larger than the normal ones is of any value in caries prevention. The subject of dental caries was well reviewed by a panel of experts in a symposium in the *Quarterly Review of Pediatrics*.[341]

The most effective methods of preventing caries at present [65] seem to be:

(1) Avoidance of sweets between meals, because of the fermentation of the sugar and acid formation, and the avoidance of excessive amounts of refined carbohydrates at any time. Pacifiers sweetened with honey or glycerine are thought to be particularly harmful to the teeth.

(2) Removal of fermentable carbohydrates from the mouth before conversion into acid.

The care of the teeth should begin when the first tooth comes through. It is brushed morning and night. By the age of three the child learns to brush his teeth without help, but under supervision.

(3) Elimination of areas where food stagnation occurs, and of developmental defects on the surface of the enamel. A child should first be taken to the dentist when he is 2 years old, and thereafter he should attend regularly in order to have his teeth inspected and treated.

(4) Increase of resistance of teeth to caries by fluorine, in the water supply (preferably), or possibly by topical application.

Orthodontics

A child should be taken to a dentist shortly after his second birthday.[164] This enables dental caries to be treated promptly so that the deciduous teeth can be preserved, for the premature loss of deciduous teeth is a major cause of malocclusion; and if malocclusion is found, or teeth are becoming overcrowded, steps can be taken to remedy the defect. One frequently sees older children and adults with unsightly malocclusion and with seriously overcrowded teeth, defects which could readily have been prevented.

Alveolar Frenum

The midline membranous labial frenum, which normally extends from the upper lip to the labial surface of the upper gum, may continue on between the upper central incisors to the lingual side of the upper

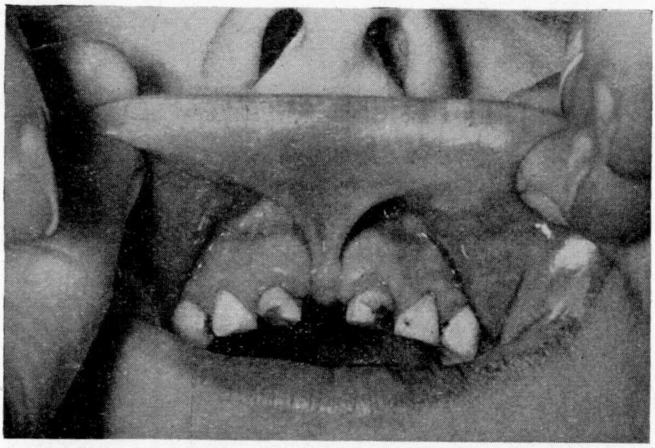

(*By courtesy of Mr. Michael Oldfield, F.R.C.S.*)

FIG. 9. Alveolar frenum.

gum, and may lead to spacing between the central incisors [165] (Fig. 9). As the alveolar ridge grows downward in later childhood, the attachment of the frenum normally migrates from the alveolar margin so that the spacing of the incisors is corrected.[88] Occasionally plastic surgical treatment is required,[319] but this must be very rare.

CHAPTER 11

THE SKIN AND UMBILICUS

Perianal Soreness

SOONER or later the majority of babies develop some perianal soreness or ammonia dermatitis, however careful the management is. Perianal soreness is particularly common in the new-born period, especially in artificially-fed babies. When the baby is older, and therefore more tolerant of a wet or soiled napkin than he is in the earlier weeks, he may lie or sit with a soiled napkin for a long period, especially in the night, before it is removed. In the new-born period

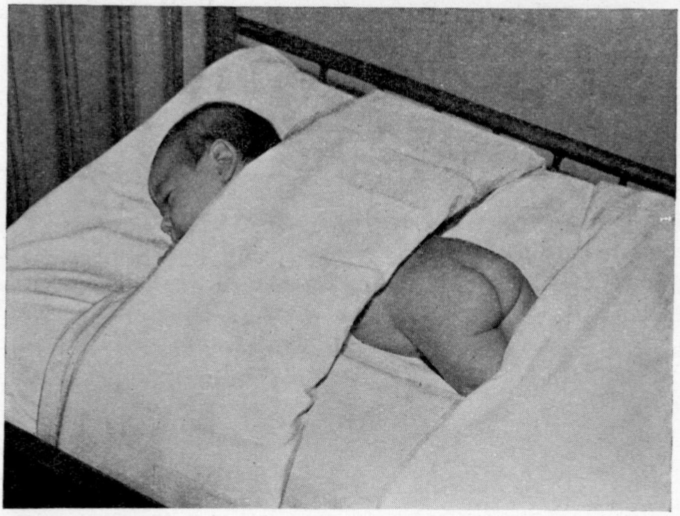

FIG. 10. Method of treating perianal soreness by exposure to the air.

the best treatment is exposure of the buttocks to the air, the baby being kept in the prone position (Fig. 10). This, however, can only be done in a warmed room. An alternative treatment is the liberal use of a baby cream or zinc and castor oil ointment. With this treatment the skin usually rapidly clears.

Ammonia Dermatitis

This is a dermatitis affecting the napkin area, and therefore largely avoiding the creases in the groin and the perianal region. The prepuce is often severely involved. In severe cases the hands may be affected. At first there is a simple erythema, but subsequently the skin becomes thickened and rough, resembling the skin of the scrotum, and it often desquamates and cracks. Vesicles may form, and they may become secondarily infected and even form ulcers. There may be a great deal of swelling and local heat. Sometimes with secondary infection oozing of serum occurs and scabs form. In the circumcised baby there may be ulceration at the urinary meatus, which causes severe pain on micturition especially if the urethral orifice is unusually high on the end of the glans. Meatal ulceration only rarely occurs in uncircumcised babies, because the prepuce usually fully protects the glans. The ulceration is followed by scabbing and scarring, and sometimes by narrowing of the urethral orifice.

Ammonia dermatitis is due to urea-splitting organisms, including the *Bacillus ammoniagenes*, which is a normal inhabitant of the fæces.[429] The organisms cause the liberation of ammonia from the urine, and the napkins smell strongly of ammonia. The condition should be distinguished from simple erythema due to contact with alkalies or soap residue left in the napkins.

The treatment of the condition should begin with a discussion with the mother about the washing of the napkins and the frequency with which they are changed. It is wise to ask her in the first place how many napkins she possesses. Some mothers from particularly poor social conditions only own a dozen napkins in all because of their high cost. Even two dozen would not be nearly enough for a baby, because of the frequency with which babies pass urine or stools and the time taken to dry the napkins after they have been washed. Some mothers do not usually wash them out at all when they have been wet. They merely hang them up to dry and reapply them to the baby. It is important also to advise the mother about the thorough rinsing of the napkins after they have been washed, for no alkali soap material must be left in them. The babies' buttocks should be sponged after they have been very wet with urine and thoroughly dried and powdered. It is particularly important to remove all traces of a stool from the buttocks. Simple exposure to the air, leaving the baby lying on a napkin, is often effective without other measures. Baby cream, or zinc and castor oil ointment applied to the affected part will, with these steps, rapidly cure the mild cases. In the severe forms a lotion containing 4 per cent. tannic acid with 0·1 per cent. proflavine, applied several times a day, is very useful. Waterproof pants are undesirable because they retain moisture and aggravate the condition. A plastic napkin holder avoids this difficulty. In the severest forms, with acute inflammation and oozing, simple saline dressings are desirable until the inflammation has subsided. The tannic acid lotion may then be applied. In all cases the mother must be instructed to change the napkin as soon as she reasonably can after it has been wet.

In resistant cases the napkins may be impregnated with certain substances which prevent the growth of the *Bacillus ammoniagenes*, such as quaternary ammonium compounds (e.g. Domiphen bromide*). The napkin is thoroughly washed and rinsed, and then passed through a solution of 3 dr. of domiphen bromide in 1 pint of water, and not re-rinsed. Mercuric chloride solution should not be used, because it may lead to pink disease Erythroedema.[280]

Boracic crystals should never be used for the purpose, either in solution or, worse still, sprinkled into the napkin, because of the serious risk of boric acid poisoning.[158] This is a highly dangerous condition, manifested by diarrhœa and vomiting, generalized erythema with desquamation, especially of the palms and soles, meningism, hæmorrhages, convulsions, circulatory collapse and death. The mortality in one series of 113 cases was 55 per cent.

Boracic ointment should never be used, especially when the skin is macerated or excoriated. On the other hand the small amount of boric acid (5 per cent.) in dusting powders does not do any harm,[221a] though it might be unwise to use it if there were severe excoriation.

A meatal ulcer should in addition be treated by the application of Tulle Gras. If there is severe pain on micturition a local anæsthetic ointment (e.g. Nupercaine 1 per cent.) may be applied to the ulcerated area. An older child may be persuaded to pass urine in his bath if pain is severe. As meatal ulcers are merely a part of the ammonia dermatitis, this must be treated as already described.

When ammonia dermatitis proves resistant to treatment, a monilia infection should be suspected. Holzel[198] and Bound[54] have given good descriptions of this condition, which is common. Flat superficial vesicles may be found on the buttocks, thighs or genitalia. These are often followed by desquamation. Flexural intertrigo or seborrhoeica dermatitis predisposes to the infection. Scrapings of the skin lesions should be cleared of débris by partly heating with 10 per cent. potassium hydroxide, and examining under the microscope without staining, when the yeastlike cells and branching mycelia may easily be seen. Scrapings may also be cultured on Sabouraud's medium. Treatment consists of the application of nystatin ointment.

Intertrigo

For intertrigo 1 per cent. brilliant green, applied three or four times a day, is an effective treatment, though it is a nuisance for the mother on account of the colour.

Scurfy Scalp

Some scurfiness of the scalp occurs in most babies in the first few weeks of life. In the mildest forms no treatment is necessary. In the

* Trade name "Bradosol."

rather more severe forms the scalp should no longer be washed in soap and water ; the scalp should be washed daily in a lotion of 1 per cent. cetavlon. It may also be cleaned by applying olive oil instead of soap, or by the application of equal parts of emplastrum plumbi and Vaseline.

Other Skin Lesions in the New-born Period

Most new-born babies show white or yellow punctate pinhead lesions on the nose ("Miliaria"). They are due to the retention of secretion in the sebaceous glands and should not be confused with pustules. They may occur elsewhere on the face, and the distinction from pustules is not always easy. A red areola round them should suggest the presence of an infection.

Peeling of the skin, especially of the hands and feet, is normal in the new-born period. It sometimes occasions some anxiety in mothers.

The falling out of the hair after 2 or 3 weeks is normal. Baldness over the occipital region should not cause alarm. It will be temporary only. Some normal babies are born with an unusually large amount of hair.

Small capillary dilatations or nævi on the inner corner of the upper lid, above the nose and on the occiput are so common that they should be considered to be normal. Those on the eyelid are sometimes called "stork bites." No treatment is required, for they disappear spontaneously in a few months.

Petechiæ may be seen on the face in a new-born baby as a result of delivery. They should not cause alarm.

In dark-skinned races one frequently sees irregular bluish pigmented areas over the buttocks, sacrum, upper part of the back and extremities. These are termed "Mongolian blue spots." They disappear during infancy.

Koilonychia is sometimes seen in young babies, and is of no importance.

Cyanosis

Cyanosis may be due to conditions other than serious organic diseases. There have been several papers on cyanosis in babies due to methæmoglobinæmia resulting from nitrites from well water, and from the marking ink used in laundries to mark napkins and other clothes.[224] It only occurs if the laundry mark is applied after washing, instead of before. It is rapidly cured by an intravenous injection of 1·5 mg. methylene blue per kilogram as a 0·1 per cent. solution. There is sometimes local cyanosis of the face for a few days after birth. The cyanosis of the head and neck may be quite marked. Parmelee [327] thinks that the common cause of this is delay in delivery of the shoulders after the birth of the head. The cyanosis disappears spontaneously after a few days.

A new-born baby may have quite marked cyanosis of the arms below the elbow, and the legs below the knees, the hands and feet being particularly blue. It is of no importance, and disappears in a few days.

Harlequin Colour Change

Neligan and Strang [307] described episodes, lasting up to 20 minutes in which an exact half of new-born babies became paler than the other half. The distribution of colour appeared to be related to gravity, for the picture became reversed by turning the baby on to the opposite side during an attack. The attack was brought to an end by turning the baby on to his back. There was no evidence that it was associated with any particular disease, and it appeared to have no particular clinical or pathological significance. Herlitz,[186a] in describing further cases, pointed out that unilateral vasoconstriction may be induced experimentally through irritation of the vasomotor centre in the medulla oblongata on either side, and suggested that the colour changes in babies might be due to local vasospasm in the medulla, possibly associated with small petechial hæmorrhages.

The Umbilicus

The umbilical cord usually separates by the fifth to the ninth day. It tends to separate early if it is kept dry and there is no daily bathing. It sometimes separates later than the ninth day in spite of being kept dry and free from infection. Moistness after separation should be dealt with by cleansing with spirit, and in some cases by the application of aureomycin in kaolin powder. Small granulations or polypi, which are said to consist of intestinal mucosa, should be touched with a silver nitrate pencil.

There is a difference of opinion as to the best method of caring for the umbilicus in the new-born.

In many hospitals, including the Jessop Hospital at Sheffield, no dressing of any kind was applied, and no binder is used. Evidence,[52] however, that the umbilicus of the new-born may harbour hæmolytic streptococci, without itself showing disease, with consequent danger of infecting the mother, has led to a reconsideration of the problem. Colebrook [96] suggested that penicillin cream (1,000 units per gm. in a lanette wax and castor oil base) should be applied to the umbilicus, which is then covered up and left undisturbed for 10 days or more. It may well be shown that the old method of applying a sterile dressing is the best.

Umbilical hernias are so common that they can hardly be considered to be abnormal, especially in premature babies. On the Gold Coast a large hernia is thought to be beautiful and decorative, and such hernias are produced by traction on the umbilical cord.[100] The vast majority cure themselves if left alone. Crump [100] found an umbilical hernia in 26·6 per cent. of 1,237 negro infants, but less than 1 per cent. of them had a hernia by the time they were 4 years old. Woods [462] studied the natural history of 283 umbilical hernias. She thought that breech presentations, prematurity, a high birth weight, an unusually long umbilical cord, or mild sepsis, were predisposing factors. 93 per cent. cured themselves spontaneously by the end of the first year. Spontaneous cures occurred in others by the age of 5 or 6 years. She thought that the local application by strapping may delay the disappearance of a hernia. On the other hand Denis Browne [69] distinguishes the true umbilical hernia through the centre of the umbilical scar, from the semi-umbilical hernia, whose sac emerges through the upper border of the umbilical scar, so that half the bulge is covered by the umbilicus and half by the skin above it. The former cures itself, and operation is never necessary ; the latter requires operation. Haworth [185] conducted a controlled study on 100 babies with umbilical hernia, applying strapping to half of them. None had a hernia of the supra-umbilical type. The strapping was applied as follows : two pieces of 2 in. non-elastic plaster were applied, threading a tongue cut in one through a hole cut in the other. An assistant reduced the hernia by binding the skin into a vertical fold over the hernia and the plasters were then pulled tight. A strip of 3 in. plaster was then applied on top of the 2 in. plaster. The strip of 2 in. plaster extended to the baby's back. The strapping was changed after two weeks. He found that a protrusion of $\frac{1}{4}$ in. or less disappeared just as quickly without treatment, while larger protrusions disappeared more quickly when strapping was applied.

My own feeling is that in any but the largest hernias no strapping (or binder) should be applied. Strapping may irritate the skin, and sepsis may occur under it. There is no danger at all from strangulation. In the case of large hernias, there is no doubt that many of these cure themselves if left alone, but it is impossible to say whether the very few who eventually require surgery would have been cured by early strapping. Although Haworth showed that the large hernias clear up more quickly if strapped, this is of no particular value to the child provided that if left they eventually cure themselves. I have certainly seen some supra-umbilical hernias undergo spontaneous cure. It is possible that strapping would lead to closure in more of them. There is no doubt that the more usual methods of applying strapping, with or without the use of a penny or button, are useless. " Binders " serve no useful purpose.

Divarication of the recti cures itself when the baby gets older.

Inguinal hernias should be operated on as soon as diagnosed, because of the ever-present risk of strangulation.

CHAPTER 12

THE BREASTS AND GENITALS

Changes in the New-born

It is very common for the breasts of babies of both sexes to enlarge 2 or 3 days after birth. This does not occur in premature babies. The exact frequency cannot be stated, because minor degrees are often overlooked. It is certainly not an inflammatory condition, as the term "neonatal mastitis" would imply. It is probably related to the secretion of œstrogenic substances from the ovary, and prolactin from the anterior pituitary gland. The breasts secrete a fluid closely resembling colostrum, which is commonly called "witches' milk." Forssell,[130] in a study of 1,000 babies, found that 99 per cent. of full-term babies and 50 per cent. of prematures secrete "milk," beginning usually about the second, third or fourth day. He observed that both swelling and secretion may continue up to the third or even the fourth month of life. According to Parmelee [327] the swelling persists longer in girls than in boys. He mentions a case in which the swelling was visible for fourteen months. Prolonged swelling of this nature could not be due merely to substances derived from the mother via the placenta. No treatment is ever required, because it is a normal condition, and no attempt should be made to massage or foment the breast.

Enlargement of the external genitalia is equally common in the new-born period. In the female the labia and clitoris are often so prominent that it may even be suggested that the baby is a pseudo-hermaphrodite. The enlargement subsides by a month or so of age. Smith [387] described the occurrence of small tags or excrescences about the inner surfaces of the labia, which are sometimes so prominent that the question of their surgical removal arises. They always disappear if left alone. The vulva becomes moist and congested and there is a thin glairy discharge from the vagina, becoming thicker and milky white after 2 or 3 days, disappearing by the fourth to the fourteenth day. At about the seventh day there may be some blood in the vaginal discharge of a full-term baby. This arises from the endometrium. The vaginal discharge is due to the hypertrophy of the vaginal epithelium in the new-born period and the subsequent desquamation of the squamous cells. It is also associated with the invasion of the vagina by organisms. The genital changes are due to œstrogenic substances received from the mother via the placenta. No treatment is indicated, because the changes are normal.

Labial Adhesions

Labial adhesions, completely closing the vaginal orifice, are not uncommon, and may lead to a diagnosis of absence of the vagina. The adhesions can be easily broken down by a probe.

Circumcision

An excellent review of the subject of circumcision was written by Gairdner.[140] An interesting section on the historical aspects of the operation was written by Gordon.[160] According to Gairdner the operation is practised over a wide area of the world by about one-sixth of its population. It is probably the oldest surgical operation known to man, dating some 6,000 years back to antiquity.[297] The operation was practised by the ancient Egyptians, as is shown by wall carvings in the Temple of Karnak, near Luxor. According to Voltaire, circumcision among Jews arose from an earlier Egyptian religious custom, and later it became a blood covenant. It was a form of tribal marking, enabling the nomadic Jews to produce a secret sign of the fact of belonging to one tribe.[233] The Arabs practised it before the time of Mohammed. There is no reference to the operation in the Koran. It is said that Pythagoras had to submit to circumcision before he was allowed the privilege of studying in the Egyptian temples. Bergmann holds that circumcision was originally a method of marking slaves, which was a development from an earlier practice of amputating the organ. Saul instructed David to bring 100 foreskins as evidence of killing that number of Philistines, in order that he should prove that he was worthy to be his son-in-law.* He brought 200. In various African tribes and in New Guinea circumcision is part of an initiation ceremony at puberty. After puberty, "It is part of the ritual of mutilation, by which the young male, and less often the young female, is called upon to give proof of courage, by which they are admitted to the privileges of the tribe or estate of manhood or womanhood." [451]

It is not clear when the operation largely changed from being a religious rite to a widespread surgical procedure.

Gairdner, after a study of the embryological development of the prepuce, showed that the prepuce is still in the course of development at birth, and so is usually incompletely separated from the glans penis. Prior to birth there is no separation of the prepuce from the glans. The term "preputial adhesions" is therefore a misnomer. Gairdner studied 100 new-born babies and 200 boys of varying ages up to 5 years, and found that only 4 per cent. of the new-borns had a fully retractable prepuce. In 54 per cent. the glans could be uncovered enough to reveal the external meatus, and in the remaining 42 per cent. even the tip of the glans could not be uncovered. The prepuce is non-retractable

* 1 Samuel xviii, 25.

in 4 out of 5 normal males of 6 months, and in half of normal males of 1 year. By 2 years about 20 per cent., and by about 3 years about 10 per cent., of boys still have a non-retractable prepuce.

In a National Sample of 2,428 children, 24 per cent. had had the operation by the age of 4 years.[276] It is likely that 100,000 operations for circumcision are carried out in the United Kingdom every year.[67] It is interesting that the operation has the same sort of social incidence as that of tonsillectomy,[276] affecting as it does the upper classes more than the lower ones ; 84 per cent. of 73 students at Cambridge, coming from the best-known public schools, had been circumcised, compared with only 50 per cent. of 174 coming from grammar or secondary schools.

Most practising pædiatricians have seen unfortunate consequences from the operation of circumcision, and seen or personally heard of a death directly resulting from it. The Registrar-General's returns show that every year there are about 16 deaths from the operation. Browne [68] described some of the operations which he has had to do in order to correct mistakes made by others. The mistakes included ; (i) Removal of too much skin. Browne said that he had known a case in which skin grafting was necessary to relieve pain on erection due to this cause. (ii) Removal of too little mucosa, causing obstruction to the flow of urine. (iii) Untidy tags of skin. (iv) Eight cases of fistula of the urethra. (v) Amputation of part of the glans. (vi) Amputation through the body of the organ. (vii) Sewing the skin edge to the glans, with consequent burying of the corona. (viii) Circumcision in a case of hypospadias. This removes the reservoir of skin on which the surgeon depends for making a new urethra.

I have twice seen partial amputation of the glans during the operation, several cases of severe hæmorrhage and prolonged sepsis, and various strange cosmetic results. Freud [136] and others have shown that meatal ulcer is almost confined to circumcised male infants and is only occasionally seen in the uncircumcised child when the prepuce is unusually lax and the glans is consequently exposed.

Gangrene of the penis has occurred as a result of over-enthusiastic bandaging of the organ by the parents. In the Thousand Family Survey [393] at Newcastle, 22 per cent. of the children circumcised developed complications from the operation, including infections, and hæmorrhage severe enough to necessitate transfusion.

It is a common practice to perform circumcision on young babies without an anæsthetic. This is a cruel practice.

Enthusiastic efforts to stretch the foreskin by forcibly opening sinus forceps inserted into the preputial orifice are painful and completely unjustified. Efforts forcibly to withdraw the foreskin cause bleeding, and are equally unjustified and unnecessary, considering the fact that it is not usual for separation of the prepuce from the glans to have been completed by the time the baby is born. Every casualty department is well used to seeing babies with paraphimosis, which results from the mother's efforts to retract the foreskin on someone's wrong advice.

The operation should certainly not be done because of enuresis. There is not the slightest reason to believe that the operation will help. It should not be done because the foreskin is a long one. There is no justification for this. It should never be done on account of masturbation. It will make no difference. It should not be done because the foreskin is involved in ammonia dermatitis (unless it has resulted in scar formation. Even then circumcision should not be performed until the dermatitis has been cured.) This dermatitis has nothing to do with the uncircumcised state of the child. The operation should never be done because the mother or the father or the general practitioner has asked that it should be done. The child is the only one who matters in this regard. It is he who should be considered and no one else. If it is in his interests that the operation should be performed, it should be done. If there is no particular reason from his point of view for doing the operation, it is quite unjustifiable to do it. The child has to suffer the pain and discomfort of the operation and the unpleasantness of the anæsthetic. If the technique is faulty and there are any of the unfortunate results described by Denis Browne, which have been seen by most other pædiatricians, then it is the child who is the sufferer and no one else.

The only serious argument in favour of routine circumcision is the theory that the presence of a prepuce predisposes to penile cancer. This was discussed by Gairdner and others. It is agreed that circumcision in the first 5 years of life protects from penile cancer. Gairdner, however, suggests that penile cancer may well be due to the poor hygienic standards of patients with this condition, which has been noted by various workers. Gairdner concludes : " It may reasonably be contended that if the uncircumcised male has a prepuce which he can retract and which he keeps clean, he is likely to enjoy the same immunity from penile cancer as his circumcised brother."

Other reasons which I have seen adduced for circumcision include the prevention of venereal disease and the reduction of sexual desire. It used to be performed to make men better warriors, to make men more chaste husbands, to increase their libido, to reduce masturbation, to give them longevity and increased physical vigour.

Some consider that the operation has to be done because the prepuce causes obstruction to the flow of urine. In the last 15,000 babies born in the Jessop Hospital at Sheffield, we have not seen one such case.

More than a third of circumcisions are performed in the first month of life at a time when faults or diseases of the prepuce itself are practically non-existent.[276]

After the first 5 or 6 months it may be found that a neglected chronic ammonia dermatitis has, as a result of secondary infection, caused such severe scarring in the prepuce that retraction when he is older will be impossible. Circumcision is then clearly indicated. Rarely a baby develops a balanitis (apart from that due to ammonia dermatitis) and pus formation may occur behind the prepuce. Circumcision is then necessary to drain the infected parts. Recurrent paraphimosis may be another indication, but this is usually due to unwise and determined efforts on the part of the mother to retract the foreskin before separation of the prepuce from the glans is complete. Very occasionally the orifice in the prepuce is so small that it is obvious that retraction will never be possible. Circumcision should be performed in such a case.

There is no need for the mother to retract the foreskin in the first year or two, and certainly there is no need to make determined efforts to retract it in this period. Gentle efforts may be made by the time the boy is 2 or 3, and if by the age of 3 or 4 it is still not retractable, then a blunt instrument may be passed through the orifice in the prepuce and round the glans to separate the strands of tissue remaining between the two structures. It is only in a very small number of children that this manœuvre fails, and circumcision may then have to be considered in order that smegma can be removed and the glans can be kept clean.

Manipulation of The Penis—Erection

When a baby learns to grasp objects it is natural that he should grasp the penis and pull at it. No attempt should be made to stop it.

The subject of erections of the penis was discussed by Conn and Kanner.[98a] It may be seen in very young babies, and it is certainly common by a year or two. Conn and Kanner suggest that it may be associated with local irritation such as balanitis. Usually there is no discoverable cause. It certainly should not cause any alarm.

Undescended Testes

In a study of 1,700 new-born boys, incomplete descent of the testis was found in 3·4 per cent. of full-term babies and in 30·3 per cent. of prematurely born ones.

No treatment is required until the age of 9 to 11 years, when operation will be carried out in select cases.[169]

CHAPTER 13

SOME MISCELLANEOUS PROBLEMS

Tongue Tie (Ankyloglossia)

THE frenum linguæ arises from a thickening of the geniohyoglossus muscles meeting in the midline of the tongue to form a vertical fold. The tongue is always short at birth, but as the infant grows the tongue becomes longer and thinner towards the tip until eventually the frenum is placed well behind the tip.

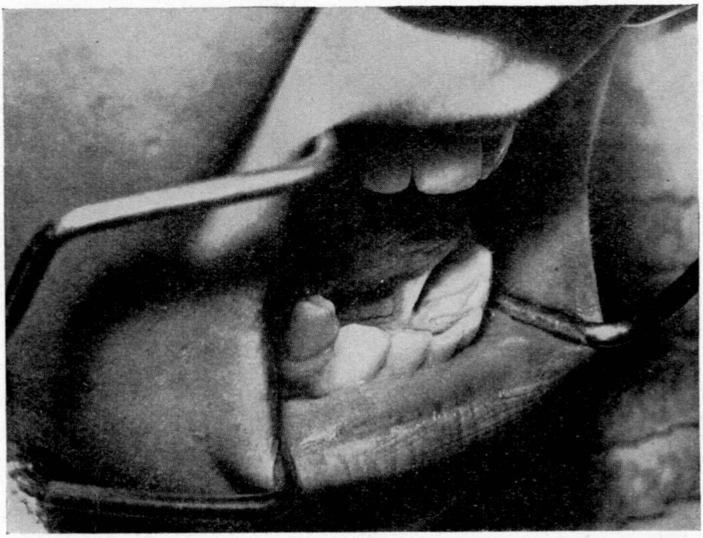

(By courtesy of Mr. Michael Oldfield, F.R.C.S.)

FIG. 11. Tongue tie.

Many mothers ascribe their child's feeding difficulties, lateness in speaking or indistinctness of speech to tongue tie. This diagnosis is almost invariably wrong. In my experience true tongue tie (Fig. 11), sufficient to produce symptoms, is very rare, but I certainly do not deny its existence.

Some think that if the child is unable to protrude the tongue or to touch the palate with the tongue, he may have difficulty in pronouncing the letters N, L, T, D and Th, especially if the palatal arch is high. It has been said that intelligent emotionally stable healthy people can overcome such a slight physical handicap without operation or speech therapy.[426] Dyslalia is common, and it is easy to ascribe indistinctness of speech to tongue tie when it is due to no such thing. I have certainly never seen any feeding difficulty in the first year as a result of tongue tie, and I doubt whether it is ever necessary to carry out an operation on it till the age of 2 or 3. The operation should certainly not be performed if the tongue can touch the palate. A guide to the severity of the tongue tie is a marked midline depression at the tip and the child's inability to lick his upper lip.

There are still doctors who cut the frenum in the new-born period. This is always wrong. There is apt to be hæmorrhage from the profunda linguæ vein, and infection may complicate the operation. The operation in the new-born period is always due to ignorance of the normal appearance of the tongue of the new-born. If it has to be done at all the operation should be done by a pædiatric or plastic surgeon when the child is 2 or 3 years old.

White Tongue

One often sees a uniformly white furred tongue in a baby in the first few weeks of his life. There is no sign of stomatitis. It is quite unlike the appearance of a monilia infection, in which the white areas are discrete. It is of no significance and disappears as the baby grows older.

The Lips

In the first few weeks of life one often sees so-called " sucking pads " or "sucking blisters " on the lips. They are well demarcated areas of cornified epithelium separating off from the underlying mucosa. As they are shed, new ones are formed. They are normal.

The Gums

Inclusion cysts (" epithelial pearls ") and sometimes larger mucous cysts may be found on or near the margin of the gum in young babies. They shed themselves spontaneously in a few weeks, and require no treatment.

One sometimes sees a fringe of membranous material with a serrated edge extending along the gum margin in a new-born baby. It disappears if left alone.

The Palate

Inclusion cysts (Epstein's pearls), mostly pinhead size, commonly form close to the median raphé of the palate in new-born babies. They last a few weeks, and are of no importance.

Snuffles

A nasal discharge, other than that associated with coryza, or following a spell of crying, is very common in young babies. The problem has been well reviewed by Apley, Laurance and MacMath.[21] They studied ninety-nine babies with snuffles in the new-born period, and observed them until the discharge cleared up. In most of them it began between the age of 2 and 12 weeks. The discharge was usually serous, but in some it was purulent or serosanguineous. None were due to syphilis. In most of them there was no evidence of infection. In only a few was there any evidence of allergy, and there was no seasonal variation. Cultures of nasal swabs failed to grow pathogenic organisms. They suggest that some babies have a larger than usual amount of mucous in the nose, without any apparent reason, and that this is responsible for the " snuffles." The condition was not responsible for any other symptoms of note. It may be concluded that in the young baby snuffles, in the absence of coryza, is of little significance.

Tonsils and Adenoids

The tonsils are often quite large by the age of 3 or 4, but there is practically never any need to remove them in a child as young as this. They tend to become smaller after the age of 6 or 7.

Adenoids may cause trouble even in an infant. They may lead to post-nasal obstruction, excessive snoring, a persistent nasal discharge, a " nasal " speech, with substitution of B for M, a troublesome cough from post-nasal discharge, and recurrent otitis media. If found they should be removed.

Impatency of the Nasolachrymal Duct

Incomplete patency of the nasolachrymal duct in young babies is so common that it can hardly be regarded as an abnormality. Cassidy [83] describes the development of the duct as follows : " In the 12 mm. embryo the nasolachrymal duct starts from a thickening of epidermal cells which grows down into the mesenchymal tissue and detaches itself from the surface ectoderm. This epithelial cord begins to develop by the third month. The ocular end establishes the lumen long before the nasal end, and the latter is delayed approximately till birth or a little later. The last portion to become patent is the site of coalescence between the nasal sprout of the mother cord and the nasal mucous membrane." Schwartz * examined 207 ducts in 8–10-month fœtuses and found atresia in 35 per cent. Kendig and Guerry [232] found an incidence of 5·7 per cent. in 1,000 consecutive full-term infants.

Most babies do not produce tears till about the age of 3 weeks,

* Quoted by Cassidy.[83]

though there is considerable variation in this. When tears are produced and the duct is not patent, epiphora occurs and the eye may become infected (dacrocystitis or conjunctivitis). For some months after birth epiphora is apt to occur when the child has a cold, presumably as a result of swelling of the nasal mucosa and consequent obstruction of the ostium of the duct.

There is a difference of opinion about the treatment of this condition. Many ophthalmologists advise that the duct should be probed as soon as the condition is diagnosed before secondary changes in the mucosa occur from chronic or repeated infections.[245] It should be noted that ophthalmologists are apt to see the severe cases only, the mild cases of epiphora never reaching them. Others (e.g. Kendig and Guerry) and many pædiatricians strongly advise conservative treatment. Kendig and Guerry [231, 232] advised that no probing should be carried out for 6 months, any infection which occurs being controlled by massage upwards over the duct and the use of penicillin ointment three times a day (1,000 units per gram of ointment). Many ophthalmologists advise that the child should be observed for a full year before operative treatment is carried out. The vast majority treated in this way clear spontaneously.

I prefer to leave these cases for at least 6 months in the hope that they will cure themselves, as the great majority do. I have not yet had to refer a baby to the ophthalmologist for probing of the duct. Probing necessitates the use of a general anæsthetic. I have seen one death from post-anæsthetic pneumonia after an operation for this condition. In my opinion it would have cured itself if only the child had been left alone.

Absence of Tears

In some normal babies tears are not produced for some months after birth. It must be borne in mind that in the rare condition termed familial dysautonomia (Riley's syndrome) [301] there is an absence of tears, in association with excessive salivation and drooling, severe pulmonary infection and various other manifestations.

Puffiness of the Eyelids

Puffiness of the eyelids may be merely the result of crying. It is sometimes noted when a baby wakens up after a sleep. It may occur as a result of any septic place near the eyes. Lastly, the possibility of nephritis will not be forgotten.

The Sclerotics in babies for the first few months are often notably blue. This should not lead one to diagnose Albers-Schönberg disease, or osteogenesis imperfecta.

Retinal Hæmorrhages in New-born Babies have been studied by several writers. Millan and San Martin [294] found them in 19·35 per cent. of normal new-born babies. They are not related to other hæmorrhages in the new-born period and they leave no sequelæ.

Squint

Infants in the first few weeks of life very commonly show slight degrees of strabismus, but it disappears by the age of 5 or 6 months. If strabismus is noted after the age of 6 months, the baby should be examined and treated by an ophthalmologist. It is a common mistake to postpone treatment till later, thereby delaying the resolution of the squint.

Transitory Fever of the New-born (" Dehydration Fever ")

By transitory fever of the new-born is meant a sudden rise of temperature, especially on the third or fourth day, with an equally rapid subsidence of the temperature within 12–13 hours, and often less, in a baby who is otherwise well and free from infection. The fever hardly ever lasts beyond the fifth day. The maximum temperature is usually 100°–102°. The child may be apparently unaffected or be a little sleepy and lethargic. The fever corresponds with the lowest point of the weight curve, after the loss of weight characteristic of the new-born period.

The cause of transitory fever is unknown. Von Reuss [427] summed up the question as follows. It may be due to " replacement of meconium flora by milk flora in the intestine, to the irritant effect of bacterial products of decomposition or toxins and of nutritive ingredients on the intestinal cells, unaccustomed to these irritants, and of the products of absorption on parenteral cells ; to the presence of products of the breaking down of tissue, such as occurs during the first days of life ; to deficiency of water due partly to an inadequate external supply of fluid and partly to internal causes, and the resulting concentration of tissue fluid and restriction of diuresis ; and finally to the backwardness of the mechanism of heat regulation." Tyson [419] showed that transitory fever was commoner in children who had an unusually large weight loss. The loss of weight in 200 babies who did not have fever averaged 7·7 per cent. In 224 babies who had fever the loss averaged 10·3 per cent. of the body weight. He thought that the fever was unrelated to the heat of the room, and that it was probably due to bacterial invasion of the bowel. Bakwin [25] showed that the serum protein concentration was higher in babies with dehydration fever than in those who did not have it. Administration of fluid caused a fall in the level of the serum proteins and a fall in the temperature.

Whatever the cause of the fever, it is harmless to the baby. It will probably never be known about unless routine temperatures are taken.

Its importance lies in the differential diagnosis, for a diligent search for infection must be made immediately a rise of temperature occurs. If, for instance, there is a persistently raised respiration rate, one would be particularly careful to exclude the presence of pneumonia or of multiple areas of atelectasis. If in doubt the baby should be treated as if infected. Otherwise no treatment is necessary other than the giving of boiled water.

Temperature Variations after the New-born Period

Pædiatricians are sometimes faced with the problem of the child who appears to be perfectly well but has been found to have a slightly raised axillary or sublingual temperature (99°–99·8°). When a very careful history has been taken and a thorough examination has been performed, the finding has to be checked by personal observation. One then has to do various special investigations, including the tuberculin reaction, X-ray of the chest, blood sedimentation rate, red and white cell count, microscopy of the urine, culture of the stools for pathogenic organisms, and agglutinations for brucellosis and other infections. All investigations are usually completely negative, and one is safe in telling the mother to stop taking his temperature. The boy is then seen at intervals to check progress and to weigh him.

The cause of this abnormality is not known. It seems that for some children the "normal" temperature is a little above the usual figure of 98·4° F. Van der Bogert and Moravec [51] discussed the temperature variations in normal children. They conducted a series of experiments to show the effect of excitement and exertion in causing a rise of temperature. They concluded that oral readings slightly above 99° F. and rectal readings over 100° F. need not in the absence of other findings be considered to be evidence of disease.

Bakwin [27] described a condition in infants which he termed "psychogenic fever," with five case records. These infants had a persistent low-grade fever while in hospital separated from their mothers, and this defied all efforts at diagnosis and treatment. In each case the temperature settled immediately on the baby's return home.

The various fallacies in temperature recording were fully set out in Talbot's monograph.[409] He showed the differences in temperature in different parts of the body (e.g. trunk, face, extremities), the relation of the skin temperature to the environment, the rise of temperature after exertion and other factors. Talbot [410] stated that the rectal temperature varies with the depth to which the thermometer is inserted. It should be inserted 5 cm. in infants. He mentions the well-known effect of hot and cold drinks on the oral temperature.

Rappaport [343] described a series of 25 exceptional patients who showed a persistent high temperature when the readings were taken by mouth, while the rectal temperatures were normal. It is certainly much commoner to find the reverse—a rectal temperature higher than the oral temperature.

Heart Murmurs in the New-born Period

Routine examination of new-born babies sometimes reveals a precordial murmur, which naturally suggests the possibility of congenital heart disease. In the majority the murmur is heard all over the precordium, but it is usually loudest at the apex or in the third left space close to the sternum. Lyon, Rauh and Stirling [264] found heart murmurs in 147 of 7,673 babies (1·9 per cent.) in the first week of their life. There was no relationship between their incidence and the sex or birth weight of the child. They followed up 92 of those babies. Four died, and autopsies in two of these showed that the heart was normal. In 14 babies (16 per cent.) the murmurs persisted. Of the remaining 74, 71 were found to be free from any cardiac abnormality. In 3 there were functional murmurs or extra systoles. In 41 of the babies (49 per cent.) the murmurs had disappeared by the third to the sixth day. In 23 (27 per cent.) the murmurs were not heard on the first day and were only heard between the fifth and the eleventh days.

Richards *et al.*[347] found a murmur in the immediate postnatal period in 1·7 per cent. of babies. With repeated examinations at 6 and 12 months, murmurs were heard at some time in 7·0 per cent. of 5,017 full-term single birth infants and 9·9 per cent. of 364 premature single birth infants. Of 353 murmurs in full-term infants, 166 were ultimately thought to be functional, and 25 organic. The remaining 162 were inconstant, and probably all functional. They felt that murmurs heard at birth carry a 1 in 12 chance of being due to congenital heart disease. The chance was increased to 1 in 3 if it was heard again at 6 months. When a murmur is first heard at 6 months, and it persists till 12 months, the chance of its being organic is 1 in 7. When a murmur is first heard at 12 months, the chance of it being organic is 1 in 50.

It follows that one must not diagnose congenital heart disease merely on the basis of a systolic murmur in the new-born period. When one hears such a murmur, and there is no cyanosis, it is wise to wait for a period before radiological studies are carried out, because so many murmurs disappear spontaneously.

Venous Hum

A common source of confusion in ausculating a heart is a continuous basal hum, passing right through systole into diastole, and therefore simulating the murmur of a patent ductus arteriosus. It is heard best in the erect position, and it decreases or disappears when the child lies down. It can be heard on both sides, and the point of maximum intensity is usually the supraclavicular region. It is accentuated on inspiration, and on turning the head to the opposite side, especially if the chin is raised.[168] It is obliterated by compression of the jugular vein. It is distinguished from the murmur of a patent ductus arteriosus by the change in intensity on rotating the head, and by its diastolic accentuation. It is heard to some extent in 50 per cent. of children under the age of 9, and is of no significance.

Pulse Rate

The pulse of new-born babies is notably irregular. The average rate is about 120 per minute, but when the child is crying a rate of up to 180 per minute or more may be found.

Intracranial Bruits

Hughes and Todd [200] heard an intracranial bruit in 15 per cent. of children under 5 years of age suffering from common clinical conditions. The murmur was best heard in the temporal region, and in some it could only be heard when the child stopped breathing.

The importance of this observation lies in the fact that when an intracranial vascular anomaly is suspected, the finding of a bruit does not prove the presence of such an anomaly.

Respirations in the New-born Period

The average respiration rate in the first 2 weeks is about 45 per minute, but there are great individual variations. The rate under ordinary resting conditions may be as low as 20 per minute. I noted a respiration rate of over 150 per minute in a normal 3-month baby who was feeling very pleased at the time.

Irregularity and periodicity of the respirations is common. If there is marked irregularity in the new-born period the baby should be given oxygen.[199] This usually increases the breathing volume and restores regular respiratory rhythm.

A young baby in the first 2 or 3 months frequently grunts a great deal in breathing when asleep. Mothers are often worried by this and think that the baby has "catarrh" or some obstruction at the back of the throat. The noise is not that of a snore. It is possibly due to vibrations produced in respiration by the soft palate.

Hiccough is almost universal in young babies after a feed.

Sneezing is very frequent in young babies and should not suggest that the child has acquired an upper respiratory tract infection.

Postmaturity

The importance of postmaturity lies in the heavy fœtal risk with which it is associated. Clifford [93] in his full review of the subject, found that after 300 days of gestation in a primipara, the fœtal death rate is 1 in 10. In this section the problem is discussed only in so far as it affects the living baby. Clifford describes three stages in the development of the features characteristic of the postmature child. In the first stage there is a loss of vernix, and the skin is dry and parchment like. The child looks old and worried, long and thin, with skin too big for the body, as if he has recently lost weight. The skin later peels. In the second stage there is a large quantity of meconium in the amniotic fluid, so that the skin is covered by meconium. In the third stage the nails are bright yellow, as a result of changes in the colour of the meconium.

The birth weight is not necessarily a large one. In one series [192] 25·2 per cent. were under 7 lb. at birth, and 40 per cent. weighed between 7 and 8 lb.

Motion Sickness

Motion sickness is very common in children. It occurs particularly on car and train journeys, and it causes considerable inconvenience to the parents. Sea-sickness is also very common in small children. According to Bakwin [31] it has been estimated that under severe conditions only 20 per cent. of unacclimatized children will remain entirely free from sea-sickness. Sea-sickness is said to occur in dogs, cats, horses, monkeys and birds. Brooks * said that fish transported from the Galapagos Islands to the New York aquarium were sea-sick !

The cause of motion sickness is unknown. It is unrelated to mealtimes. There is a strong familial factor in many cases. It has been suggested that it is due to a disturbance of the autonomic nervous system, that it is a disturbance of vestibular function, that it results from circulatory changes in the large vessels of the neck stimulating the carotid sinus, and that it results from gross movements of the abdominal viscera.

The usual age at which motion sickness begins is the second or third year, but it may begin in the earliest infancy. The child becomes pale, quiet, looks unwell and then vomits. The excitement which is so common before a journey predisposes to it and may even cause vomiting before the journey begins.

A variety of drugs prevent motion sickness.

Glaser and Hervey [152] compared three drugs—hyoscine, promethazine hydrochloride (" phenergan ") and diphenhydramine hydrochloride (" Benadryl "), in a controlled experiment involving 68 men. The

* Quoted by Bakwin.[31]

protection afforded was respectively 96 per cent., 61 per cent. and 44 per cent.

An American Team [23] compared twenty-six compounds, and found that meclizine (" Ancolan ") was the most effective, especially for continued use. Cyclizine and promethazine were placed second and third. Hyoscine when used repeatedly gave troublesome toxic reactions (dryness of the mouth and blurring of vision).

In my experience hyoscine, given in the form of Kwells, is very effective when given half an hour before a journey. A child of 7 takes half a tablet, and a child of 3 to 7 a quarter of a tablet. Each tablet contains 0·0046 gr. of hyoscine hydrobromide. I have also found mepyramine maleate (" anthisan ") useful, but the elixir (1 drachm dose containing 25 mg.) has the disadvantage of being very unpleasant to the taste. Dimenhydrinate (dramamine) is also effective

It is probable that a stuffy atmosphere and reading in the car predispose to sickness, and so they should be avoided. It has been said that the child should be encouraged to look forward rather than through the side window.

When vomiting is threatening, the child's attention should be immediately distracted and, if possible, the car should be stopped so that he can have a walk before continuing the journey. Every effort should be made to avoid suggesting sickness by anything one says. When sickness occurs there should be a minimum of fuss about it, for vomiting readily becomes an attention-seeking device. The less that is said about it either before a journey or after an attack of vomiting the less likely he is to have trouble again.

The Periodic Syndrome

It seems likely that so-called cyclical vomiting, migraine and certain cases of unexplained recurrent abdominal pain are basically the same condition, or at least very closely related, and a convenient term is " the periodic syndrome." Some children have attacks of pallor, followed by fever and vomiting, lasting usually a day or two. There is loss of appetite, and often acetone in the breath. The urine may contain ketone bodies and the stools may be pale and even loose. Others have recurrent fever and abdominal pain with or without vomiting. Others have vomiting and headaches, or even headache without associated symptoms. Migraine may begin in infancy with attacks of nausea and vomiting, and it is only later that it becomes clear that the attacks are associated with headache.[305] The attacks tend to occur in active intelligent children, and to be precipitated by punishment, worry about a strict teacher or about bullying, friction at home, excitement, an accident, a fit of temper, an infection, or even undue fatigue. The onset is usually between 6 months and 10 years.

The attacks recur at irregular intervals ; in some children the attacks occur monthly or even more often. In the majority of cases there is a family history of migraine. There is often an unduly high incidence of motion sickness in siblings.[126, 388]

There has been much discussion as to the cause of the syndrome.[134, 229, 242] It bears no relationship to the diet, though there are still doctors who prescribe a low fat diet, because of the erroneous idea that acidosis is the cause of the attacks. It is, of course, the result of the attacks, and not the cause. Some have suggested that allergy is a factor and Glaser [154] claimed good results with histamine desensitization and elimination diets, but Friedman and van Storch,[134] in a study of 1,400 cases of migraine, could find no evidence of allergy. Wallis [437] ascribes it to epilepsy, but I feel that this is only a rare cause of the syndrome. Errors of refraction and antrum infection are only rare factors in the ætiology.

The treatment of the attacks is largely symptomatic. The child is given as much food as he can keep down, particularly in the form of sweetened drinks. As soon as an attack begins he should be given a tablet of Caffergot (Ergotamine tartrate 1 mg., caffeine 100 mg., at the age of 6 years). This is said to give relief in up to 86 per cent. of children if taken early in the attack.[134] The dose is repeated in an hour if no relief is obtained. After a few trials the initial effective dose is determined. Some have found phenindamine tartrate (" thephorin ") effective if given at the beginning of an attack, and it may be tried as a prophylactic if given continuously in a dose of 25 mg. twice a day at the age of 5 in an effort to prevent attacks. Promethazine hydrochloride (phenergan) in a dose of 10–20 mg. three times a day in a five-year-old, or 20 to 25 mg. three times a day in an older child, is said to be effective in preventing attacks.

Some have said that excitement should be avoided. This is impossible in a child and any attempt to bring it about are likely to lead to further emotional disturbance. Any cause of insecurity should be treated, and it is essential that as little fuss as possible should be made when an attack occurs. The parents should not talk about their own attacks in the child's presence.

Œdema of an Arm

Œdema of an arm often occurs in young babies in the first month of their life. The mother is dismayed when she picks her baby from his cot in the morning and finds that one arm is swollen, cold and perhaps blue. It is not due to the baby lying on the arm, for it may be found when he is lying on his back and when one knows that he has been on his back all night. It is more likely to occur in cold weather than the hot. In a series of twenty-five cases [128] the attacks occurred in the winter in twenty-four. It occurs in the arm which has been uncovered by bedclothes and not in the arm which has been under the blankets. It seems to be due partly to posture and partly to cold, but the part played by each is not clear. The œdema usually subsides in a few hours but occasionally it may last for a day or two. It may recur night after night. I do not know how to prevent it. No treatment seems to be necessary.

Physiological Jaundice

It is not possible to give the exact frequency of physiological jaundice. Neither would it help to make a precise statement on the matter. At least 50 per cent. of all babies show it. It is detectable in doubtful cases if the skin is pressed with a glass slide. Jaundice usually appears on the second to the third day and reaches a maximum by the third or fourth day. Physiological jaundice usually disappears by the end of the first week, but it may last longer. If it lasts beyond the second week, serious doubts about the accuracy of the diagnosis should be entertained. The colour of the urine and stools is unchanged, though there is sometimes a trace of bilirubin in the urine. The liver and spleen are not enlarged. The jaundice is due to a combination of slight hæmolysis with immaturity of the liver. There is an excess of bilirubin in the blood of every infant at birth, and this reaches a peak on the second to the fourth day.

The Urine of the New-born Baby

It is commonly stated that the urine of new-born babies frequently contains albumin. Doxiadis [118] showed that this is not the case. When urates are removed before the urine is heated it is found that there is either no albumin at all or that there is a mere trace (less than 20 mg. per millilitre).

Haworth and McCredie [184] tested the urines of fifty normal male babies for reducing substances by paper chromatography, and found that twenty-four excreted either lactose, galactose, or xylose, or a combination of these, at some time during the first seven days.

About one in ten babies do not pass any urine for the first 24 hours.

A Large Abdomen

After a child has begun to walk and until the age of about 3 the abdomen often seems to be unduly large, and this often worries the mother. As long as a simple physical examination reveals no abnormality the large size of the abdomen should be ignored. It is normal.

Bow-legs and Knock-knee

Many mothers note with anxiety the bowing of the legs of their 1–2-year-old child, and the appearance of knock-knee in their 2–4-year-old. In the majority of children these conditions are self-righting. The great difficulty, however, as with so many other problems in children, is to place the dividing line between the normal and the abnormal and so to decide when treatment is necessary. Bowing of the legs must be distinguished from the broad base of the toddler which is due in part to the napkin. Price [340] remarked that " a very casual observation of the posture of normal children will refute the suggestion that the legs should be straight." He wrote that there is first a varoid phase, occupying the first two years of life. The child's leg shows an outward curve and an inward twist in the lower end. This is due to the shape of the bones, and it disappears before the age of 2 years. The foot is affected secondarily ; it tends to turn in and the weight is borne on the outside edge. Bowing of the legs is merely an exaggeration of the normal varoid phase. It is likely to be first noticed when the child walks, particularly if he is rather heavy and walks early. It may increase in the first 6 months after walking begins. There are corresponding X-ray changes in the tibia and femur. Later there is usually a spontaneous improvement and disappearance of the bowing. Price thinks that if there is still bowing by the time of the second birthday the condition is unlikely to cure itself and treatment should be instituted. He thought that mild cases, in which there is less than $\frac{1}{2}$ in. of separation of the knees when the malleoli are together, usually cure themselves, while those with a greater separation should be treated. On the other hand it has been shown[197] that bowed legs may not completely straighten till the age of 4 or 5. According to Denis Browne* if treatment becomes necessary, it should consist of manipulation, and in severe cases the Denis Browne walking splint. No operation should be performed and plaster of Paris should never be applied.

Price wrote that the varoid phase is followed by a valgoid phase, beginning shortly after the age of 2 years. It is due partly to the straightening of the tibia, but chiefly to increasing ligamentous laxity and consequent hypermobility of the knee and ankle joints. Pes valgus develops secondarily. The degree of valgus is usually maximal at the age of $4\frac{1}{2}$, but by 6 years it has usually righted itself spontaneously. He says that knock-knees are rarely noted before the age of 2. They are merely an exaggeration of the normal valgoid phase. If the knock-knee is marked there is pronation of the foot and the weight is borne on the inner side of the foot, and in-toeing occurs. He thinks that if there are more than 2 in. between the malleoli in the recumbent position when the knees are together, treatment should be given.

* Personal communication.

Some [265, 266, 414, 466] think that faulty foot alignment may be due to postural errors in the early months of life. They blame the common habit of sleeping in the prone position on the knees. Thelander and Fitzhugh,[414] studying the foot and leg alignment of 246 children mostly aged 18 months to 3 years, found the largest group of deviations in these " knee-chest " sleepers. One-third of those children slept with their toes turned in, and two-thirds with the toes turned out. The deformities usually, but not always, righted themselves. They suggest that the knee-chest position should be prevented by padding the legs so that extension is maintained. Macnamara [265] suggests a moulded cardboard splint or a malleable metal splint on the extensor surfaces of the knees to maintain extension and so prevent prone sleeping. It was also suggested that " toeing-out " may result from allowing the baby to stand for long periods on soft surfaces (such as the mattress in his cot). This causes hyperextension of the knees and eversion of the foot. When the child sleeps on his back, tightly tucked in bedclothes may cause excessive abduction of the foot. Macnamara [265] thinks that the habit of sitting on the feet or of squatting has a harmful effect on the feet. She also thinks that knock-knee is largely prevented by footwear which does not force the foot into the everted position. If the inner side of the shoe shows wear, support should be given.

I have no personal knowledge of the importance of the factors mentioned by Thelander and Macnamara. It would certainly seem that further investigation of those factors would be well justified. Orthopædic surgeons with whom I have discussed this question do not think that the sleeping position bears any relationship to postural deformities of the feet.

When treatment is given for knock-knee, it should consist of wedging of the inner side of the heel by a $\frac{1}{4}$-in. wedge. According to Denis Browne, wedges, exercises and manipulation cure almost all cases Osteotomy should never be performed and plaster of Paris should never be applied. Price wrote that splints are used too frequently and too soon ; they are hardly ever required in the first 3 years.

Flat Foot

A flat foot is normal in infancy, because of the foot pad in the region of the longitudinal arch. The arch does not become apparent till about the third year.

Toeing In

When a young child turns his toes in when walking, the question of corrective measures arises. Nothing is done if it is found that there is a full range of ankle movements without stiffness. The condition corrects itself.

The Prevention of other Foot Deformities

An important step towards the prevention of foot deformities in later life is the provision of properly fitting shoes. Shoes should only be obtained from a good firm which measures the foot. It is essential to ensure that the feet are measured at frequent intervals, so that the shoes being worn are not allowed to become too tight.

Owing to radiation hazards X-ray apparatus should not be used in shops.[289]

The Effect of Cold

Mann and Elliott* have drawn attention to the effect of chilling of young babies, especially new-born ones, due to inadequate clothing in cold weather. The syndrome is manifested by the onset of lethargy, swelling of the extremities, a deceptive facial erythema, and often by hæmatemesis. It is diagnosed by the finding of a subnormal temperature with a low reading thermometer. At autopsy massive pulmonary hæmorrhages may be found.

* Mann T. P., and Elliott, R. I. K., (1957). *Lancet,* **1,** 229.

CHAPTER 14

THE PREVENTION OF INFECTION

The Care of Babies in Hospital

When honest and accurate records are kept it is found that a very large number of babies acquire infection in maternity units and in hospitals. In a British hospital known to me 158 babies under 1 year of age were admitted to medical wards for treatment in the first 6 months of 1947. Of these 44 (27·8 per cent.) acquired infections in hospital, and 8 died as a result of those infections. More than 5 per cent. of the babies, therefore, who were admitted for treatment died of infections acquired in the hospital. A similar record was kept of cross-infections in older children in the medical wards, and an attempt was made to assess the number of extra days which they had to spend in hospital as a direct result of those cross-infections. The number of bed days lost as a result of these infections was 1,243. Apart from the suffering caused to the children and the anxiety to the parents, this represents a considerable expenditure of money.

It is very difficult to compare accurately the incidence of infections in different maternity units, because the standard of accuracy in recording them varies so greatly. It seems clear, however, from published work, annual reports and other sources that it is common for 10–20 per cent. of all new-born babies to acquire infections—most of them admittedly very trivial ones—while in hospital. This is a very high figure and much can be done to lower it. In the pages to follow I have summarized the most important measures necessary to prevent infection.

The Mode of Spread of Infection

The main sources of infection are patients, attendants or visitors. Some of these persons are carriers, having no signs or symptoms of disease themselves. The infections are spread by secretions, excretions or discharges. The main modes of spread are by contact, droplet, ingestion and air-borne infection. Contact infection is direct (e.g. from a nurse with a septic hand) or indirect (e.g. by dust or thermometers). Air-borne infection usually reaches the child by contact. The principal methods of preventing infection will be discussed under the three headings—contact, droplet and ingestion—though there is some overlapping between them.

Contact

The first essential is to wash the hands thoroughly before and after handling a baby. After washing the hands nothing whatsoever, other than the baby's clothes and adjoining bedclothes, must be touched before handling him. There is dust everywhere, and dust is infected, so that it follows that every object may harbour pathogenic organisms. The attendant must not touch the tap handle, temperature chart, mask or mask strings, gown strings, cot side, window, door, toy on the floor, or laboratory specimen bottle, before touching the baby. He must not rub a tickling nose. He must not pull the bedclothes down in order to see a baby's face without first washing the hands.

Hand lotions are better avoided. Rubenstein and Foley [364] cultured a hand lotion of 95 per cent. ethyl alcohol used in this way and found 150,000 organisms per ml. These organisms were chiefly *E. coli*, *B. subtilis* and *Staphylococcus aureus*. Antiseptic lotions for the scrubbing brush may also be dangerous. There is some evidence that an antiseptic cream (" Hibitane ") may be useful. After the hands have been washed, they must be dried on a clean roller towel from a machine, pulled out section by section, or by sterile paper towels (which are liable to be expensive).

Every effort must be taken to avoid unnecessary infection by dust. Napkins and bedlinen should never be placed on the floor after bed making or for counting purposes. Dry dusting or sweeping should never be allowed. Wood or linoleum floors should be oiled, and other floors should be washed and never swept when dry. A nurse may convey infection from one cubicle to another by a duster. The role of the oiling of blankets and clothes in the reduction of dust is uncertain.[241, 444,] Air disinfection by ultra-violet light may be of value,[17 285] though there is no unanimity about this. The walls of a nursery should be washable and have rounded corners, so that dust does not accumulate. Oxygen should be piped, so that dirt is not carried into the nursery on oxygen cylinders. The ventilation arrangements must be such that dust and infected particles are carried away from the babies and not towards them. Fly-proofing is essential.

Napkins and clothes for the baby should be autoclaved and delivered to the ward wrapped in sterile packages, and then distributed to each baby's locker in the morning. The baby is changed in his mother's room if separate rooms are provided. If there are several mothers with babies in a ward, no napkins should be changed when other babies are being fed. The buttocks are cleaned with wet cotton wool and not with the napkin. The soiled napkin is then placed into the baby's bin, where the lid is opened by the foot pedal. The bin has an internal container, which is removed from the room or nursery for emptying into a hamper. Napkins should not be counted by any nurse who looks after babies. They should go uncounted to the laundry. Checking should not be carried out in a corridor or room where babies clothes are stored.

Gowns should be worn. On no account should a nurse don a gown and go from one baby to another in it. Each baby's locker contains a gown for those who will attend to it. No one should touch the baby without washing the hands and donning the gown. Gowns should not be left on coat hangers, one gown infecting another.

The communal trolley should be abolished. A communal ointment pot, gentian violet bottle, olive oil or thermometer is a menace to the lives of babies. A communal bath should never be used. Each baby should have his own locker and equipment and his own sterilizable plastic bath. The whole is thoroughly scrubbed out with 1 per cent. carbolic on discharge of the baby. Communal scales alone are necessary, but the " pan " must be *completely* covered by a sterile towel so that the child does not come into contact with any part of the scales. The nurse requires an assistant for the purpose of weighing, so that she does not touch the weights, for this would spread infection from baby to baby. On no account should the baby be taken to the scales in a nursery. The scales are taken to the baby.

The baby's thermometer and container must be thoroughly cleaned after his discharge. So-called antiseptics into which thermometers are placed may be the source of serious infection. Green and Penfold [164a] recovered 40 million organisms per ml. from a jar of glycol thymol co. used for thermometers in a ward round.

The greatest care must be taken in handling the umbilical region. Absolute sterility must be insisted upon. The dusting powder must be sterile—and in some hospitals this is not the case. Tetanus has been caused by dusting powder, and other less serious infections could readily be spread by it.

It is better not to bath the new-born baby every day. The committee of the American Academy of Pediatrics [14] made the following recommendation : " It is recommended that no water or oil bath be given during the first week or ten days after birth. The vernix may be gently wiped away from the folds of the infant's skin with warm sterile mineral oil or wet sterile cotton wool." Sanford [367] showed that the incidence of skin infections is very much lower if the baby is not bathed till the ninth or tenth day. Bruce* found no difference in the incidence of skin infections in two groups of babies, one of which was bathed daily with soap and water, the other being left unbathed, 1 in 500 cetrimide being used to wash off blood, excess vernix, meconium, and stools from the buttocks. She suggested, there-

* Bruce, L. (1956). *J. Obstet. Gynæc., Brit. Emp.*, **63**, 735.

fore, that as there is nothing to be gained from daily bathing, it saves valuable time if the cetrimide no-bath technique is used.

The baby wears a minimum of clothing, and blankets are never allowed to touch him. Excessive clothing causes sweat rashes, and these readily become secondarily infected. It is wrong to wrap a blanket round and round the baby. He should be allowed free movement of the arms and legs, and blankets so wrapped round the baby prevent it.

New-born babies readily scratch the skin, and the scratches quickly become infected. For this reason the nails should constantly be kept short. Nails often have to be cut within a day or two of birth, and thereafter every few days. The skin may also be damaged by the removal of the vernix with dry cotton wool instead of with wet wool. Spots around the neck may be due to chafing by blankets, which should never touch the skin. Spots around the mouth and below the ear are often the result of saliva and posseted gastric contents irritating the skin, which then becomes secondarily infected.

The danger of infection of babies by contact is ever present and very real. A very great deal can be done to prevent it by proper techniques.

Droplet Infection

Droplet infection affects the baby in various ways—through the inhalation of dust, or by direct infection of the respiratory tract. Although many advocate routine nose and throat swabs in all personnel attending babies, their value is uncertain. A real difficulty is the grave shortage of nursing staff, which would make it difficult or impossible to exclude from duty large numbers of persons found to harbour dangerous organisms. Wegman [443] suggested that routine swabs may cause false confidence. They cannot detect viruses. At the best they can only reveal organisms present at the time of culture. They do not show what organisms will be present on the following day. Wegman considered that of greater importance was the indoctrination of personnel that no one with any sort of illness should attend a baby.

There is some difference of opinion about the value of masks. A mask consisting of three or four layers of gauze of not fewer than 44 threads per inch, covering nose and mouth, or a mask containing a piece of cellophane, is fairly effective in the prevention of infection. Such masks are, however, uncomfortable to wear for long periods. They must never be put into the pocket. If touched by the hand, the hand will be infected. They are apt to give a false sense of security and reliance cannot be placed on them to prevent infection if the wearer has an infection in the nose and throat. They cannot replace the absolute rule that no one with a cold or sore throat should attend to a baby in hospital. The mask should not be worn for more than 2 hours at a stretch.

In several maternity units with a high standard of care masks are no longer worn. It is probably wise, however, for anyone actually attending to a baby to wear a suitable mask.

Ingestion

There can be little doubt that an extremely common cause of infection of babies, and almost certainly the chief cause of gastro-enteritis, is the ingestion of infected foodstuffs. There is a great deal of carelessness in the handling of infant foods. Wright [463a] cultured breast milk after expression in various hospitals. In a pooled sample from one hospital eight million organisms per ml. were cultured. She showed that the common methods of expressing breast milk were dangerous and that pasteurizing or boiling of the milk was essential before it is given to babies. In a subsequent investigation [463b] she cultured artificial feeds from 300 infants' feeding bottles in various hospitals when the feeds were ready for the babies. Fifty of these were sterile. In 38 bottles there were over one million organisms per ml.

Breast milk is by no means necessarily sterile, however carefully it is collected. Knott and Blaikley [237a] found the *Staphylococcus aureus* in the milk of 36 out of 50 mothers examined. There was some doubt about their pathogenicity. Nevertheless, dangerous organisms are very frequently found on the mother's nipples, and if there is a fissure in the nipple it is the usual thing to find *Staphylococcus aureus* in the milk. I found that some mothers prepare the breast for the baby by spitting on their hands and then rubbing the spittle into their nipples. I also noted that in one hospital the design of the nightgowns was unsatisfactory in that they did not enable the mother to bare the breast without being pulled up over the body. Contamination of the breast by fæcal organisms was therefore liable to result. It is essential that breast milk should be pasteurized before it is given to the baby.

The Milk Kitchen. In a maternity or children's unit in which babies are housed there should always be a milk kitchen devoted entirely to the preparation of infants' feeds. There is no need for a large or elaborate room. It must be fly-proofed. If there is only a single room available, the bottles and teats must be thoroughly washed out in a detergent after use and then placed in a steam sterilizer (Fig. 13) or autoclaved. The crates of bottles are then taken to the milk kitchen, ready for the preparation of the feeds. The bottles and teats must be thoroughly washed (the teats being inverted for the purpose), for it has been shown that bottles which are used day after day without proper cleaning can produce contaminated feeds in spite of autoclaving.

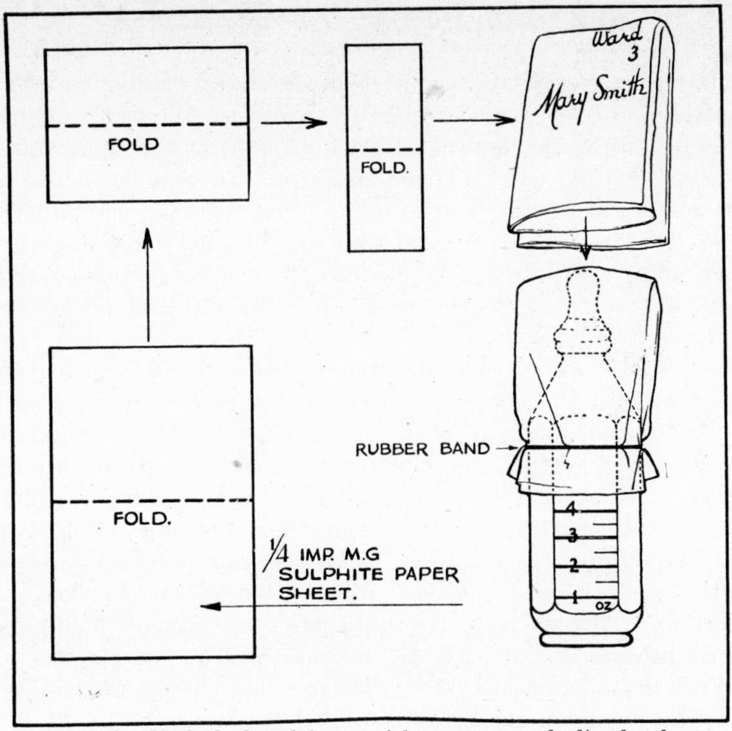

FIG. 12. Method of applying special paper cap to feeding bottles.

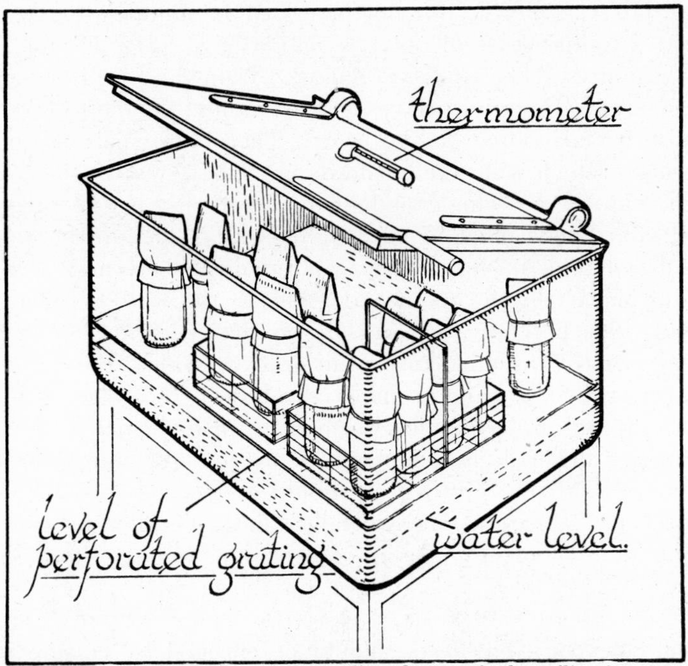

FIG. 13. Bottles in steam sterilizer for terminal sterilization.

(*By courtesy of Dr. J. L. Emery*)

If there are two rooms, or one room which can be divided into two, the bottles and teats can be brought to one of the rooms for washing—preferably with a mechanical bottle washer—and the teats and caps are washed and placed in a steam sterilizer. There must be one nurse in one room and another nurse in the other, with no communication between the two rooms except that the cleaned bottles are taken through from the "dirty" room into the "clean" room or passed through a hatch. There the feeds are made up and placed in the bottles.

The feeds in either case are then mixed with an electrical mixer and poured into the bottles. The sterile teats are applied and over them are placed caps of glass or metal or water-resistant paper (Fig. 12). The bottles are then placed in racks into a sterilizer or autoclave. Rourke,[362] in an investigation of various methods of sterilizing infant feeds, found that boiling in an ordinary water sterilizer for 10–15 minutes was efficient. Such a sterilizer has the advantage that the milk is easily cooled rapidly before being placed in a refrigerator. Alternatively the feeds are sterilized by high-pressure terminal heating at 230°–232° (7 lb. pressure) for 10 minutes. The New York State Sanitary Code [315] declares that there must be terminal heating by steam under pressure of not less than 15 lb. at 121° C. (250° F.) for not less than 5 minutes, or at a pressure of not less than 6 lb. at 110° C. (230° F.) for not less than 10 minutes, or by flowing steam at a temperature of not less than 100° C. (212° F.) for not less than 30 minutes. The feeds are removed from the sterilizer, and after rapid cooling (if an autoclave is used) they are transferred to a refrigerator and stored at 40°–45°. There are specially designed refrigerators which will take hot feeds immediately after their removal from the autoclave. The attendant in this room must be gowned and masked, and hands must be thoroughly washed before the crates are removed from the sterilizer. Crates are collected by nurses or others through a hatch in the room and taken to the ward refrigerators as required. The hatches are necessary so that personnel do not enter the clean part of the milk kitchen in order to collect the crates. The feeds are warmed in pans or similar heaters in the ward as required. They should on no account be warmed in wash-basins. The caps are kept in place until the last moment before the baby takes the feed.

It is essential that one person should be in constant charge of the milk kitchen. Nurses have to be trained in its working, but continuity is essential. A constant change of personnel would otherwise invite disaster. A sister may be employed for the purpose. The services of a bacteriologist are constantly required for bacteriological checking by frequent cultures. The feeds should be checked by culture not less frequently than once a week. No nurse helping in the milk kitchen should have any contact with patients. At least, if there is not enough work for her in the milk kitchen, she must never attend to any sick child.

Cereals and lactic acid milk cannot be given terminal heating in this way. The milk and containers into which the feeds are put must, however, be sterile. Colostrum or breast-milk mixed with colostrum may coagulate when sterilized by heat.

Ward Arrangements

If the maternity unit is part of a general hospital it should be entirely separate from all other parts of the hospital, so as to minimize the spread of infection. I am very strongly against the use of large nurseries for babies in maternity units. Not only is it unnatural and undesirable psychologically for the baby to be separated from the mother, but the risk of infection is greater in a large nursery than in a room containing only mother and child. Ideally, every baby should be with his mother day and night, unless it is a premature one and unless there is some special reason, such as birth injury, which makes it desirable to nurse him separately from his mother. For this reason separate rooms, in which mother and child are alone together, are desirable in maternity units. The baby is then not moved from his mother's side for any purpose, such as bathing or napkin changing, unless there is some special reason, such as undue noisiness at night which does not respond to a feed and which is exhausting the mother. This system minimizes the risk of infection passing from baby to baby. Unfortunately such accommodation is not always available. Even if there are no separate rooms, the babies should still be with their mothers day and night as long as there is a room for an occasional noisy baby at night. The babies should not normally be moved to a nursery at night, for this increases the risk of infection. A common treatment or examination room is equally undesirable, for this can easily cause infection to spread from one baby to another.

A small sick nursery is required. The accommodation for premature babies will not be discussed here.

If there is a nursery, overcrowding must be prevented. The New York State Sanitary Code [315] requires that no nursery shall contain more than 12 babies. Each infant must have a minimum of 24 sq. ft. of floor space. The provision of floor space, however, is not enough. It is common to see a row of cribs side by side, touching each other, in a nursery in which the floor space is adequate. At least 2 ft. should separate the cribs.

The Out-patient Department

It very often happens that one standard of asepsis is found in the wards of a hospital and a very different one in the out-patient department. It is almost impossible to prevent some cross-infections occurring in an out-patient department, but much can be done to reduce the risk. The pan of the scales can be properly covered by a clean sheet of paper for each child. A small sheet can be provided for each baby to lie on while being examined. Instruments can be properly sterilized. Thermometers can be cleaned after use, and the rectal route must be avoided. Care can be taken in the collection of urine and stool specimens. Supervision of the canteen should ensure a high standard of cleanliness. By means of an appointments system something can be done to separate babies from older children. Well babies can be separated from the ordinary out-patient clinic and concentrated in a well-baby clinic.

Personnel

A pædiatrician should be responsible for the care of the new-born babies in every maternity department. He should not merely be called in to see a sick baby when asked. That arrangement is totally inadequate. He should be responsible for the maintenance of health and not merely for the treatment of disease, much of which is due to infections resulting from the carelessness of others. Under him, unless the number of babies is very small, there should be a resident assistant, who is responsible for the day-to-day care of the babies and who is responsible to his chief for the prevention of infection. He must know the exact details of the technique used by the nurses in the handling of babies. He has to know, for instance, exactly what happens to soiled napkins, what happens to napkins after they have left the laundry and before they are put on to a baby, and what happens to feeds after they have been made up in the milk kitchen. When he is doing his rounds he has to watch the work of others and to take action when he sees rules being broken. He must always set a good example himself.

Every effort should be made to ensure that the nursing staff is as adequate as possible, day and night. There is a particular danger that lapses will occur at night when the staff is a small one.

The nurses must be under continuous supervision, and the pædiatrician should be constantly interested in their training and its application. He should personally take a part in the training. A children's training for the nurses is most desirable. Nurses in a children's hospital should spend a time in the maternity unit. When a children's ward is part of a larger hospital there are likely to be less nurses trained in children's work and the standard of pædiatric care is likely to be correspondingly lower.

Nurses should have instruction in the prevention of infection before they enter the wards. All too often this instruction is given after, sometimes months after, they have started ward work. The instruction should include emphasis on the importance of cross-infection by concrete examples of its results. The modes and the routes of infection must be thoroughly taught and cinematographic and other visual aids should be fully utilized.

Many teachers are in favour of written instructions and rules. The difficulty is that they are apt to go unread. They are no substitute for constant supervision. I do not think that they serve a useful purpose. An infection chart, kept by the nurses themselves, is valuable, as long as every case of infection is accurately recorded, for it serves as a constant reminder of the ever-present danger of cross-infection. Frequent discussions over infected cases are of value. Ward rounds for nurses, are of value when taken by the doctors, as at the Children's Hospital at Sheffield.

A monthly or quarterly report, in which infected cases are cited, is an invaluable method of maintaining interest in the prevention of infection, and it enables one to compare one's incidence of infection with that of other hospitals.

Nurses should be taught the vital importance of reporting infections of the skin, upper respiratory tract infections, including colds and diarrhœa, immediately. The danger of going on duty with these complaints should be emphasized. The nurses should be under a proper health service, and X-rays of their chests for tuberculosis are done at regular intervals—not less than yearly.

Nurses should not have any cleaning duties. They should not count soiled linen or napkins. A proper use of the nurses' time is important. In one hospital known to me, where there was a severe shortage of nurses, routine test feeds were carried out at every feed of every baby every day. This inevitably took them away from more important duties. The arrangement whereby one nurse does one task, such as the feeding or napkin changing or bathing of all babies, is a wrong one, for it might well lead to infection of a very large number of babies. It is a rule at the Children's Hospital, Sheffield, that if a baby has a loose stool, the nurse looking after that baby is not allowed to look after any other baby, but she may look after other children.

The remaining personnel must also be supervised and given elementary instruction in the prevention of infection. These include laboratory assistants, assistant nurses, orderlies, cleaners, maids and porters. Laboratory workers in particular are apt to handle babies without the usual asepsis. Maids and others must be forbidden to play with babies or touch them. The kitchen staff in any hospital must be instructed to report any bowel disturbance immediately. Detailed instruction about the prevention of infection is an important part of the medical students' teaching.

The constant co-operation of a bacteriologist is essential. He is required to check techniques, especially in the milk kitchen.

The training in the prevention of infection must extend to health visitors, for they have an important part to play in the home.

Mothercraft lessons play a part in a maternity unit. Mothers are given talks and encouraged to take part in discussions during their pregnancy.

Other Steps to Prevent Infection

Admission of Babies from Outside the Hospital. The practice of admitting sick babies, especially premature babies, to a maternity unit is to be condemned on account of the risk of introducing an infection. They should be sent to a children's hospital or unit.

Visitors. No one but the father should be allowed to visit the new-born baby. He should be warned not to visit if he has a cold or other infection.

The Eyes. Many hospitals, including the Jessop Hospital for Women at Sheffield, no longer use any prophylactic treatment for the eyes, relying on proper antenatal and postnatal supervision.

Action when Epidemic occurs. When an epidemic occurs it is notified immediately to the Public Health Laboratory Service. A full bacteriological investigation is then carried out. This includes nose and throat swabs and, in the case of gastro-enteritis, rectal swabs or stool cultures from the staff. The maternity unit is then closed and the walls, floors and all equipment should be thoroughly scrubbed and, where possible, sterilized. Blankets and mattresses are stoved.

Action to be taken when a suspected or actual Infection occurs. In a maternity unit the best place for a baby suspected or known to be infected is with its mother in her own room. The nurse who attends to the baby should not attend to any other baby. If single rooms are not available it must certainly not be allowed to remain in the ordinary ward. A suspected case must be transferred to a special room kept for the purpose. A proved case of infection in those circumstances is better away from the maternity unit altogether and may be transferred with the mother to the isolation unit of a children's hospital. If this is impossible, it will have to be nursed in the maternity unit, but no nurse looking after it should have anything to do with other babies or with the preparation of feeds. The sick nursery should not be used for proved infections. A very important measure is prompt immediate reporting and treatment of any infection, however trivial. The new-born contacts should be quarantined if possible and the ward should be thoroughly scrubbed out. If the baby has gastro-enteritis, special precautions must be taken to prevent the infection spreading. It would be extremely dangerous to retain the baby in the maternity unit.

Summary and Conclusions

In my opinion the commonest causes of cross-infections are failure to wash the hands before handling the baby, attending to babies in spite of suffering from colds, throat, skin or bowel infections, communal bathing and napkin changing, dry dusting, and absence of a properly supervised milk kitchen. A very important cause of these infections is a lack of interest in the subject on the part of the medical staff.

Elaborate equipment is not necessary for a good standard of hygiene. Hand washing takes time. Nurses should be brought to realize that the care of infected children takes much more time and that infections cause a great deal of morbidity and worry.

It is essential at all times for the pædiatrician to be reasonable in his demands and not to ask for that which is neither feasible nor economically possible. In a maternity unit every possible precaution must be taken to prevent infection. In a children's hospital the same precautions should be taken for babies. It is obvious, however, that absolute asepsis is neither possible nor feasible for older children. For all children, however, of whatever the age, such elementary precautions as the use of individual thermometers should be insisted upon.

It would be undesirable psychologically to insist that every child, of whatever age, should be isolated in a separate cubicle and that no child should be picked up by a nurse unless absolutely necessary. Theoretically visiting should not be allowed at all in a children's hospital. In fact, exclusion of parents from their children is inhuman both to parents and child. What one gains in the partial prevention of infection is lost by the adverse psychological effect on the child. Some writers have lost sight of these matters in discussing the prevention of infection. Conrad,[98] in discussing infections in new-born babies, says : " The mother is cautioned about inspecting the baby unnecessarily." I once set a question in the Final Medical Examination concerning the prevention of infection in young babies. A medical student, referring to droplet infection, wrote : " On no account must the mother be allowed to kiss her baby in his first six months " !

Some measures are desirable theoretically but economically impossible. The provision of nothing but paper towels and destructible napkins, though desirable in theory, is economically difficult or impossible on account of the cost involved. Excessive demands for nursing personnel may be impossible to meet. One must at all times, therefore, balance the importance of the prevention of infection with practical, economic and psychological factors.

It should be borne in mind that the incidence of cross-infection is very much less in fully breast-fed babies than in artificially-fed ones. There would not be nearly as much need for milk kitchens if proper attention were paid to the essentials of breast feeding.

Many make the serious mistake of thinking that such measures as those described above are excessive and quite unnecessary. They have got along quite well without such precautions and are daily making the mistakes outlined above. It is likely to be found that such people have no idea of the actual incidence of infection in babies under their care, and that they have never taken the trouble to compare the mortality of the premature and mature babies in their unit with that of other hospitals. They have a false sense of security. Even if their figures are good, the fact that for a long time they have not experienced serious infections does not mean that one day they will not have an extremely serious epidemic of gastro-enteritis or other infection which will kill a large number of babies in a very short time. They are sitting on dynamite.

Finally, the importance of not admitting babies to a hospital unless it is absolutely necessary cannot be over-emphasized. The risk of cross-infection is a great one, and far too many babies are exposed to that risk by totally unnecessary admission to hospital for observation and investigations which could perfectly well be made in the out-patient department. In the case of the new-born and of babies who have to be admitted to hospital, the more the mothers are able to care for their babies themselves the less will be the risk of cross-infection.

Prevention of the Common Infectious Diseases

The Role of Quarantine

The term quarantine implies the restriction of movements of contacts of a case of infectious disease for a period equal to the longest incubation period of that disease. This must be distinguished from surveillance, which implies the practice of observing contacts during the incubation period without imposing restrictions on their movements.[391] It is now widely recognized that quarantine has proved an ineffective weapon in the prevention of infectious disease.[19, 390, 391]

It is a matter of opinion whether quarantining of contacts is advisable in the case of poliomyelitis.[156, 157] The difficulty is the fact that the relative importance of the different modes of spread of infection are not known. Contacts of a case of poliomyelitis in the home are likely to harbour the organism in the nasopharynx and to excrete it in the stools, and excretion in the stools may continue for some weeks —long after the quarantine period has expired, so that isolation hardly seems rational. Strict isolation was applied in a small outbreak in a country district,[156, 157] but community infection occurred nevertheless. The virus was found in sewage from homes in which there was no contact, and it was clear that the infection was widely disseminated in the community, and must have been spread by other means than by the patients and contacts. On the other hand, knowing the frequency with which contacts harbour the organism in the nasopharynx, there is something to be said for the quarantining of child contacts of a case in the home, and adult contacts of such a case if they come into contact with other children. This would accord with the recommendations of the Ministry of Health that a child contact should be isolated for 21 days. In other diseases, with the possible exception of smallpox, there is no case for the use of quarantine for the whole of the incubation period. It is certain that in no other disease should contacts who have themselves suffered from the disease be quarantined.

There is sometimes something to be said for partial quarantine—the isolation (e.g. from a nursery school) of a child during that part of the incubation period in which infectivity may develop. For instance, when a child is exposed to mumps, whose incubation period is 12 to 26 days (usually 16 days) one remembers that a child is infectious for 2 days before the swelling appears, and if isolation is to be carried out at all, it would be for the period of 10 to 26 days after exposure, because he could not be infectious before then (unless he were exposed to the original source of infection) and he cannot carry it. He would certainly not be isolated at all if he had already had it. This alone would be a rational method of quarantining, but in fact it is hardly ever necessary. It is now widely recognized that quarantine achieves very little, and that in the past it led to a great deal of unnecessary absence from school. It seems much more sensible to tell parents when their child has been in contact with a case of infectious disease, to keep him under special surveillance at the time when the disease is liable to develop (e.g. in the case of mumps, any time after the twelfth day until about the twentieth day after exposure). It is not necessary to take the temperature if the child is well. Unless he is unwell, he should be allowed normal activity, though friends should be warned that the child may be about to develop an infectious disease.

An important point against quarantine is the fact that however careful the precautions most children will acquire whooping cough, measles and chickenpox. By the age of 14 about 90 per cent. of school children have had measles, 70 per cent. have had chickenpox and whooping cough, and 50 per cent. have had rubella and mumps. In any case there is much to be said for acquiring the infectious diseases during childhood. Mumps, for instance, rarely causes orchitis before puberty, but it frequently does later. Rubella is well known to cause serious anomalies in the fœtus if a woman acquires the infection in the first 4 months of pregnancy. Chickenpox, measles, rubella and other infectious diseases are often more severe in adults than they are in children.

Another fallacy in the practice of isolating children from a nursery or other school lies in the fact that such children are very liable to mix with the others at and around the home at play. In poor social circumstances with overcrowding strict isolation is almost impossible to achieve.

When a child acquires one of the acute infectious diseases one has to decide what policy to adopt with regard to isolating him from his siblings. Each case has to be decided on its merits. It should be borne in mind that the most infectious period is probably the day or two before the rash develops in the case of the exanthemata, or before the parotid swelling develops in the case of mumps, or before the signs of poliomyelitis develop in the case of that disease ; in other words, it is very likely to be too late to achieve anything by isolation. Isolation, furthermore, is apt to lead to quite a lot of unpleasantness except in the case of older children, because it is difficult to prevent younger ones going to the bedroom of a sibling. Lastly, as far as the common infectious diseases go, there is a lot to be said for getting them over, except when a sibling is a baby. In general, therefore, one does not usually try to prevent contact with siblings.

The Duration of Infectivity

Table VIII shows the incubation period of the common infectious diseases, with the duration of infectivity. The table is based largely on the booklet published by the American Public Health Association [16] on the control of infectious diseases. In the case of chickenpox, it used to be held that a child was infectious until all scabs have separated. A joint memorandum of the Ministry of Health and the Ministry of Education considers that a child should be considered infectious for 14 days after the appearance of the rash, but one feels that there is no need for such excessive caution, and that the American attitude seems more reasonable.

In the case of rubella, it is so desirable that a girl should acquire the infection so that she cannot subsequently acquire it during pregnancy that it is quite wrong to do anything to prevent girls acquiring it. It should be encouraged. The same applies to mumps in boys.

In poliomyelitis the duration of infectivity may be longer than that mentioned in Table VIII, because the virus may be excreted in the stools for some weeks. It is felt that the chief period of infectivity lies in the day or two before the onset of symptoms and the 7 to 10 days after.

Infectivity within the Home

The infectivity of the common exanthema varies considerably. The Newcastle Survey [393] found that 87 per cent. of those exposed to whooping cough in the home acquired the infection. The corresponding

TABLE VIII

Incubation Period and Duration of Infectivity of Common Infectious Diseases

Disease	Incubation Period (Days)	Period of Infectivity
Chickenpox	15–18	1 day before rash to 6 days after start of rash.
Diphtheria Scarlet fever	2–5	Till swabs negative.
Enteric group	7–21 (especially 14)	2 days before symptoms, till stools and urine negative.
Measles	10–15	5–6 days before rash till 5 days after temperature becomes normal.
Mumps	12–26 (especially 18)	2 days before swelling, till swelling has subsided.
Poliomyelitis	4–30 (especially 7–14)	3 days before symptoms start to 2 weeks after onset if temperature is normal (see p. 146).
Rubella	10–21 (especially 18)	1 day before rash till 2 days after start of rash.
Whooping cough	7–10	2 days before start, 5 weeks after start.

figure for measles (in the first year of life) was 71 per cent., and for chickenpox 64 per cent. Measles is rare in the first 6 months. About 75 per cent. of contacts of chickenpox in the home will acquire the infection as compared with a figure of 20 per cent. of those exposed to mumps.

Secondary cases of poliomyelitis in the home are common. When the first case is paralytic, three quarters of contact cases are paralytic; when the first is nonparalytic, most contact cases are nonparalytic.*

The Role of Immunization

It is my practice at the Jessop Hospital for Women at Sheffield to immunize babies against diphtheria, tetanus and whooping cough at the age of 1 to 2 months. No one will dispute the need to immunize children against diphtheria. Some are reluctant to immunize against tetanus. The following are the relevant arguments in favour of such immunization.

(i) There are more deaths from tetanus each year in England and Wales than there are from diphtheria.

(ii) The administration of tetanus antitoxin may be fatal in an allergic subject. About 1 in 40,000 will show anaphylaxis to it. If a child has been immunized by tetanus toxoid, and subsequently receives an injury potentially dangerous from the point of view of tetanus, he should not be given tetanus antitoxin, but he should be given a booster dose of tetanus toxoid (1 ml.). This is safe, while tetanus antitoxin is dangerous. The duration of immunity conferred by tetanus toxoid is unknown, but there is good evidence that a booster dose as much as 10 years after immunization will give a satisfactory antitoxin level.[258, 418]

* A recent study (Spicer, C. C., McDonald, J. C., 1957. *Lancet*, **1**, 470) did not confirm this.

(iii) The addition of tetanus toxoid, to form the triple vaccine adds nothing to the risk of untoward reactions from the vaccine, neither does it reduce its efficacy. There is, therefore, nothing to be lost from using it and everything to be gained.

There are still some who do not immunize children against whooping cough. It has now been adequately proved that whooping cough vaccine is of great value. In the Medical Research Council trial [287] in which 7,558 children were inoculated, 18·2 per cent. of vaccinated children who had been exposed to the infection in the home acquired whooping cough, as compared with 87·3 per cent. of the controls who were exposed ; and the infection was considerably milder in the vaccinated.

The immunization should be carried out early, because of the fact that the chief risk of whooping cough is in the first months of life. In the Newcastle survey 100 children acquired whooping cough in the first year ; 15 per cent. of those acquired it before 3 months and 44 per cent. before 6 months. Almost all deaths from whooping cough occur in the first year, and there is a serious risk of sequelæ, in the form of bronchiectasis, in others. It seems obvious, therefore, that steps should be taken to prevent it as soon as possible. It has been shown by numerous workers that immunization at the age of 1 to 4 months is effective. The American Academy of Pediatricians [15] recommends that all infants should be given the triple vaccine at the age of 1 to 2 months. A booster should be given at the age of 12 to 18 months and again at 3 to 4 years.

If a child has not been given tetanus toxoid, a triple vaccine should not be given as a booster, for interference may lead to an unsatisfactory response to the tetanus component, unless the mixture has been preceded 4 weeks before by tetanus toxoid.[325] The maximum period between the three immunization doses should be 3 months ; ideally it should be 1 month.

B.C.G. may interfere with responses to other prophylactics.[325]

Vaccination for smallpox should be carried out when immunization for the above has been completed, i.e. at 4 or 5 months. Vaccination before this is rather less likely to give a satisfactory "take." It is obvious that in England the risk of whooping cough is far greater than that of smallpox, and it is therefore reasonable to suggest that the triple vaccine should be given first.

There is much to be said for giving all new-born babies B.C.G.

At the time of writing this, the supply of poliomyelitis vaccine is insufficient for all babies, but it seems likely that in the very near future all babies will receive protection against poliomyelitis.

The multiplicity of vaccines suggests that all parents should have an immunization card, which records all the immunization procedures.

This is particularly important in the case of tetanus immunization, so that tetanus antitoxin will not be inadvertently given in place of toxoid.

Complications of Immunization Procedures

Any immunization procedure carries with it a minute risk of an encephalopathy—a sensitivity reaction involving damage to the nervous system.[296] The risk has been thought to be greater with whooping cough vaccine than with diphtheria immunization. Some have felt that the very rare encephalopathy after whooping cough vaccine was more frequent in children who had had convulsions in the past, or who had a strong family history of such disorders. This matter was discussed by Melin [291] and in a subsequent Editorial. Melin felt that the risk of a convulsive child developing serious neurological complications after whooping cough was greater than the risk of such a child developing complications after the vaccine ; he recommends that whooping cough vaccine should not be withheld from such children. This was the opinion of several experts, whose opinions were sought by the Editor of the Journal.

The American Academy of Pediatrics [15] recommended that if a child has a history of febrile fits, the first dose of vaccine should be a small one—0·05–0·1 ml., phenobarbitone and acetyl salicylic acid being given by mouth. If there is no reaction a full dose is given a week later. It recommended that if a convulsion occurs with the first injection, no further injections should be given for several months, and then single antigens should be used, beginning with a dose of 0·05–0·1 ml. to test tolerance. I would feel that if a convulsion occurred with the first injection, it would be unwise to risk a second. The Academy recommended that in a child with brain damage, immunization should be postponed till the baby is past his first birthday. Single antigens rather than the usual multiple antigens would be used.

It is usually said that an immunization procedure should not be carried out when a child has an infection, or when vaccination for smallpox is being carried out. I am not aware of the evidence for this recommendation.

It may be felt that an immunization procedure should be withheld in an allergic child. The reverse is the case, especially with regard to tetanus and diphtheria. An allergic subject might react badly to antitoxin, and it is therefore all the more important to protect such a child by immunization.[325]

In the case of an older allergic child who has not been previously immunized, it should be remembered that T.A.F. (toxoid antitoxin floccules) contains a small amount of horse serum. Diphtheria F.T. (purified formol toxoid) may be used as an alternative.

When a child has a marked febrile reaction after the first dose of vaccine, one is anxious about the possible effect of the second. I have never seen any ill results in such a case, though as a precaution I give an antihistamine drug (e.g. mepyramine maleate) half an hour before the injection and half an hour after, and I instruct the mother to give aspirin if there is a rise of temperature. It is sometimes wise after a severe reaction to give a smaller dose for the second injection.

We *never* give a vaccine to any child without having adrenaline at hand in case of an immediate allergic response.

A risk carried by any injection in the poliomyelitis season is the introduction of the poliomyelitis virus. A Medical Research Council Report* showed that the risk is greater if alum precipitated vaccines are used. (British vaccines do not contain alum.) The risk is not reduced by giving it subcutaneously instead of intramuscularly. The risk was greatest in the second quarter of the year.

In the early summer months one has to strike a balance between the risk of whooping cough and the risk of poliomyelitis. The advent of the poliomyelitis vaccine may solve this difficulty.

It sometimes happens that a nodule remains at the site of the injection for some months. Some have termed this an "antigen cyst." It is of no importance.

Sometimes an area of fat necrosis develops at the site of injection Such necrosis is less likely to occur if the injecting needle is not coated with antigen—i.e. if one needle is used for withdrawing the material from the syringe and another for injecting it.

Vaccination for smallpox should never be carried out on a baby suffering from infantile eczema, neither should it be done on the sibling of a baby with that condition. The danger lies in the development of generalized vaccinia, which may be fatal.

It is not always fully appreciated that the absence of a "take" on smallpox vaccination, even after repeated attempts, certainly does not imply immunity. It sometimes happens that a child will not "take" when the scarification method is used, but he does "take" with multipuncture.

Other steps in the Prevention of Infectious Disease

Colds

There are no known means of preventing frequent colds in young children. It has been adequately shown that the removal of tonsils has no effect in preventing colds. Ultra-violet light has been shown to be useless as a preventive measure.[288]

Children are especially liable to frequent colds in the first 2 or 3

* *Lancet,* 1956, **2,** 1223.

years after starting school, but after that they almost all acquire considerable immunity. It follows that when a child begins school he is likely to bring colds back home and infect siblings.

Parents can do much to prevent the spread of colds by ensuring that if their child has a cold they do not allow his friends to visit the house during the infectious stage. When a child has a cold it is impossible to prevent siblings from coming into contact with him.

Sore Throats

Only about half of all cases of acute tonsillitis in children are streptococcal. Burke [77] showed that when 0·5 gm. sulphadimidine was given daily, the incidence of acute throat infection was reduced. I prefer to use continuous prophylactic penicillin tablets (100,000 units twice a day) in children who are suffering from frequent attacks of tonsillitis, and find that many tonsillectomies can be avoided by this treatment. The child is tided over a year or two until he develops immunity himself. Tonsillectomy should only be carried out when prophylactic penicillin has failed.

In any child who has had acute nephritis, continuous penicillin prophylaxis should be given until the kidney has completely healed, and usually for not less than one year after the acute attack. When a child has had acute rheumatic fever, continuous penicillin prophylaxis should be given for an indefinite number of years, possibly till adolescence.

Measles

Passive immunization is achieved best by gamma globulin. The dose depends on whether complete prevention is desired or merely an attenuated attack. If complete prevention is achieved, no active immunity is developed by the child. If the child has an attenuated attack he develops full immunity to the disease. Normally, therefore, it is desirable to give a child a modified attack. The dose recommended [284] is as follows :

	Dose in Milligrams		
	Modification desired	Prevention desired	Prevention essential
Age 6 to 23 months .	150–225	450	675
,, 24 ,, 59 ,, .	225–300	675	900

These doses must be given within 72 hours of the appearance of the rash in the primary infecting case.

The danger of hepatitis as a result of gamma globulin is almost *nil.*

Chickenpox, Mumps, Rubella

No special methods of prevention are necessary or desirable. In a hospital outbreak, a ward should not normally be closed on account of these infections.

Poliomyelitis

The Salk vaccine appears to provide definite but not complete protection against paralytic poliomyelitis. By the end of 1955 ten million American children had received the vaccine,[425] and 80 per cent. protection against a paralytic form of the disease was provided.

Possible measures which should be taken in the face of an epidemic of poliomyelitis were discussed by Sabin.[366] He thought that the bulk of evidence points to human fæces from patients and healthy carriers as the chief source of infection, and that the infection therefore reaches the body by means of food and drink, possibly with flies as vectors. He wrote : " Available evidence indicates that the virus which is occasionally present in the throats of patients and healthy carriers does not ordinarily reach the outer environment in significant amounts of droplets from the mouth or nose."

Exclusion from school and avoidance of crowds is unnecessary, but avoidance of wading and swimming pools may be desirable. Flies should be excluded from food. Hands should always be washed before eating. Intimate association—kissing, hand shaking, the use of communal eating utensils—with members of a family in which a case has occurred in the last 3 weeks should be avoided even though the case was moved to hospital.

Other measures to prevent poliomyelitis during an epidemic are the avoidance of immunization procedures, the avoidance of tonsillectomy and the avoidance of violent exercise and over-fatigue. If a contact has a raised temperature, however slight, he should be kept strictly in bed until it is normal.

Tuberculosis

This is not the place for a discussion on the prevention of tuberculosis. The use of B.C.G. has already been mentioned. The family doctor can do much to see that an infected adult does not visit a house containing children, and that parents do not take their child to the house of an infected person or allow him to visit such a house for play or other purposes. The early diagnosis of tuberculosis in adults lies largely in his hands, and his early diagnosis is essential for the prevention of childhood tuberculosis.

Section III

DEVELOPMENTAL PROBLEMS

INTRODUCTION

In pædiatric practice there are numerous common conditions which raise the question of whether a child's mental development is normal or abnormal. Every normal parent has a natural curiosity and interest in wanting to know whether his child is normal or not. There is all the more reason for his interest if there has been a previous unfortunate experience, such as the birth of a mentally or physically defective child, or if there has been some noxious influence in pregnancy, such as a virus infection or rhesus incompatibility. An odd facies or a peculiarity in the shape or size of the skull may raise the question of mental deficiency. One of the commonest conditions which raises doubts about a child's normality is retardation in one field of development, such as walking, talking or sphincter control. When a child suffers from epilepsy or physical defects, such as hypothyroidism, it is particularly important to assess his development. When he shows unusually bad and unco-operative behaviour one needs to assess his intelligence in order to decide whether the basic trouble is mental deficiency. When a child is examined for the purposes of adoption it is vital to be able to express an opinion as to the likelihood that he is mentally normal, for it is a tragedy if he turns out to be mentally defective. All too often babies are passed for adoption without any developmental examination at all. A great deal of anxiety and unhappiness is caused by an incorrect diagnosis of mental deficiency—a diagnosis which is often too lightly made.

For practical purposes one does not want to know whether an infant will at school age have an intelligence quotient of 100 or 105. That can be only of academic interest. What one does want to know is whether a child is likely to be of average intelligence or not. It would certainly be of very great interest if one could predict the future intelligence more accurately, but it might not be of advantage to the child. Routine intelligence testing of any kind is undesirable because much more reliance is apt to be placed on the findings than the accuracy of the tests warrants. They may very well cause totally unnecessary anxiety in the minds of parents.

The question of whether prediction of any kind is possible or not is discussed in the next chapter.

CHAPTER 15

IS PREDICTION POSSIBLE?

The Prediction of Intelligence

There is a difference of opinion as to whether developmental studies in the first 3 years have any predictive value. It would seem reasonable to suppose that if careful detailed observations were made of the course of development of a sufficiently large number of babies, record being made of the age at which various skills were learned, it should be possible to establish some relationship between records so obtained and their subsequent progress through childhood. Though it is impossible to say what is "normal," there is no difficulty in defining the "average," and it should be easy to determine the sequence and rate of growth in the average child and to note the frequency with which deviations from the usual growth pattern occur as a result of known or unknown factors. Having determined the developmental pattern of average children, it should be possible to determine whether an individual child has developed as far as the average one of his age, taking into account all factors which might have affected his development. By making further examinations at intervals in order to assess his rate of development, and by taking into account all possible factors in the child and his environment which might affect the future course of his development, one ought to be able to make a reasonable prediction of his future progress provided that one knows the frequency of abnormal growth patterns. Arnold Gesell and his staff at the Yale Clinic of Child Development have made such studies for 40 years or more, and they are convinced that such prediction is in fact possible.

In 1930 Gesell[143] wrote that 10,000 infants had been examined by his staff, most of them at repeated intervals. Many thousands more have been examined since. By following them up into later childhood he was able to determine what reliance could be placed on the developmental examination in the first 3 years for the prediction of future development. He established norms by selecting children born of a homogeneous group of apparently normal parents, chosen with the aid of a careful socio-economic survey. All children were excluded who had a history of birth injury or other disease. He followed the children up in later years in order to make sure that no abnormal children had been included.[145] The examination of the children was a very full one and included every aspect of their behaviour, including the development of locomotion, manipulation, feeding, play and social behaviour, the development of speech and of sphincter control. He pointed out that with the aid of "norms" so established one can determine how far an individual child has developed in relation to his age. He said "attained growth is an indicator of past growth processes and a foreteller of growth yet to be achieved." He emphasized the "lawfulness" of growth, the constancy of the sequence of development, pointing out that "where there is lawfulness there is potential prediction."* Having completed the developmental examination, he then considered all the environmental factors and relevant personality traits which might have affected his development in order that a fair assessment can be made.

It is obvious to anyone that the great majority of infants do conform with their norms at various ages, and that on following them up they turn out to be normal children. It is equally obvious that when infants lag seriously behind in all fields of development they grow up to be mentally defective, unless there is an associated serious physical handicap. When one goes back on the history of mentally defective children, such as Mongols, there is always † a history of lateness in achieving the various skills described by Gesell, while in going back on the history of normal children there is no such retardation. It is obvious to all that the mentally defective child throughout his first 3 years shows defective interest and concentration in his surroundings. He is late not only in the more obvious aspects of development, such as locomotion and manipulation, but also in dropping the practice of mouthing objects and in ceasing to slobber. In infancy he shows a persistence of primitive reflexes, such as the reciprocal kick, long after the normal child has lost them.

It would indeed be surprising if some children did not show unusual patterns of development. These deviations are responsible for much of the difficulty of developmental diagnosis, but they are rare. Gesell and his co-workers [143] have collected together some of these unusual patterns. They should be studied by all who are interested in the diagnosis and prediction of "normality." He described some children who were low average in infancy and yet high in later childhood: children who showed a progressive retardation of developmental rate after being "normal" for the first few weeks; children who showed a temporary developmental arrest and then developed normally; and children who were advanced in infancy and merely average in later years. It is particularly important to draw attention to the occasional slow starter—the child who is rather backward at first and later does very well. Such exceptions are rare but always have to be remembered.

* "Psychology of Early Growth," p. 225.

† Unless the mental defect arose after a period of normal development, as a result of encephalitis, trauma or some degenerative disease.

Gesell drew particular attention to the various factors which affect the course of development. These are discussed below. He wrote that in some cases presenting unusual patterns, or with physical defects which alter the course of development, prognosis should be completely withheld. In others the prognosis can only be built up cautiously after repeated examinations. To use his words, "Diagnostic prudence is required at every turn."*

Elsewhere [143] he wrote: "So utterly unforeseen are the vicissitudes of life that common sense will deter one from attempting to forecast too precisely the developmental career even of a mediocre child."

Gesell considered that the prediction of mental superiority is a matter of considerable difficulty. One would have thought, in view of the retardation which occurs in all fields of development in mentally defective infants, that there would be corresponding acceleration above the average in children who are going to be mentally superior. Such in fact is not often the case. Gesell [142] wrote that such speeding up may be present in early infancy, presumably having begun *in utero*, and that the whole cycle of development is accelerated. Much more often, however, the scorable end products are not far in advance of the age norms in early infancy, the child's superior quality being manifested in the manner of the performance of the tests, in his alertness, in the intensification and diversification of behaviour, in the vividness and vitality of his reactions. "He exploits his physical surroundings in a more varied manner. He is more sensitive and responsive to his social environment." Elsewhere [149] he described the superior infant as being "poised, self-contained, discriminating, mature. The total output of behaviour for a day is more abundant, more complex, more subtle than that of a mediocre child." † He said that the acceleration becomes much more obvious in the second and third years, with the development of speech, comprehension and judgment. Gesell, like many others, said that consistent language acceleration before 2 years is one of the most frequent signs of superior intelligence. General motor ability and neuromuscular maturity are not nearly as often advanced. Some of these exceptional cases are described in detail in his "Biographies of Child Development." [143]

There have been few other studies of mental superiority in infancy. Hollingworth [196] found that "gifted children walk and talk earlier than unselected children do." The majority of the children with an I.Q. of above 150 walked or talked or both walked and talked at an earlier age than usual. A small minority of children showed nothing abnormal in that respect. Terman [413] found that gifted children "talked and walked" earlier than average children. Rand, Sweeney and Vincent [341a]

* "Psychology of Early Growth," p. 224.
† "Developmental Diagnosis," p. 312.

said : " It is safe to assume that children who talk unusually early are probably superior mentally ; that feeble-minded children are always late in talking ; but it is not to be assumed that all children who are late in talking are feeble minded." Osnato [324] went so far as to say that " the development of speech and intelligence go hand in hand and are interdependent to such an extent that they may to all intents and purposes be regarded as the same process." Abt, Adler and Bartelme [2] found a similar relationship between speech and intelligence.

There are many isolated examples in the literature of mentally superior children who walked or talked unusually early, but single cases prove little.

After the period of infancy, the gifted child is likely to show unusual imagination, notable powers of concentration, wide interests, a retentive memory, precocity in speech and rapid learning. He may show an unusual ability in describing things which he has seen, and in recounting incidents and events. He may show striking creative ability in his drawings. Many such children learn to read at the age of 3 or 4. Twenty per cent. of the gifted children in Terman's study [412, 413] learned to read before five ; 6 per cent. learned before four, and 2 per cent. before three years of age.

Only a few papers describe attempts to correlate developmental findings in infancy with subsequent intelligence. Hallowell [177a] found good correlation between Gesell tests on 86 children under 1 year and intelligence tests at the age of 3–4 years. Nelson and Richards [307] found good correlation between Gesell tests on 123 infants at 5–8 months of age, and Stanford Binet tests at the age of 3 years.

Some studies have expressed doubt whether any sort of prediction of intelligence is possible. Bayley [41a] conducted a very careful study of 61 infants, with 200 test situations, and followed up 49 of the children for 3 years. There was little correlation between the tests at the different ages. She concluded that " the tests measure different functions rather than a unit function of intelligence which extends throughout life. Development during the first 6–8 months is largely sensorimotor in nature, and the more truly adaptive behaviour is measured by the tests only after this period. There was no evidence for a general factor of intelligence during the first 3 years, but the findings indicate instead a series of developing functions or group of functions, each growing out of but not necessarily correlated with previously matured behaviour problems. The results indicate that the behaviour growth of the early months of infant development has little predictive relation to the later development of intelligence." Linfert and Hierholzer [256] and Furfey and Muehlenbein [138] found a similar lack of correlation between tests in infancy and intelligence 4 years later. Bowlby [55] said that : " Mental tests have no predictive value in the first eighteen months of life. Probably the best guide to the intelligence of the child is the intelligence of the parents, though for many reasons this can be no more than a rough guide."

Kirman [236] wrote that tests in infancy are of little use in diagnosing mental deficiency. Another paper [20] described the "Meagre value of Gesell rating of adaptive behaviour at 2 years as compared with Stanford Binet rating at 5 years."

It seems very likely that the reason for the negative findings in the above papers lies in the efforts to use nothing but objective tests of development. The tests used were largely sensorimotor in character, and as such would fail to observe the *way* in which tests were carried out, the alertness, the responsiveness and other features of child behaviour which Gesell considers to be so essential in the assessment of a child. Many of the most important features of behaviour are unscorable, and so find no place in large statistical studies such as those of Bayley. Gesell rightly emphasizes that developmental diagnosis is an individual matter, and that, having made the developmental examination, the diagnostician then has to balance up all the various factors which may have affected the development and which may affect it in the future. Studies such as Bayley's are impersonal and inevitably fail to take into consideration the factors affecting the individual. The same criticism applies to the tests described by Griffiths.[167] Simon and Bass [382] wrote a good discussion of the subject, and found good correlation in their own study.

As Gesell said, it is much more difficult to predict mental superiority than to predict mental deficiency. Hallowell [178] in re-examining 250 children 5 to 13 years after the initial study, found that the original low estimate on infant scales was confirmed in 90 per cent. of cases, while diagnosis of superior endowment was confirmed in only 50 per cent. Others have made similar observations.[408] It should be noted that Bayley's children [41a] were highly selected, the mean I.Q. when they were 9 years old being 134.

In my opinion it is unquestionably possible to diagnose mental deficiency in the first year of life. Diagnosis becomes progressively easier with the increasing age of the child and there is usually little difficulty by the age of 6 months. It is similarly possible to recognize normality of development, thanks to the work of Arnold Gesell. There are very strong indications of normality by 2 months of age or earlier, but by 6 months it is not usually difficult to decide that a child's development is within normal limits. In all cases diagnosis is on much surer grounds if the examination is repeated at an interval or intervals in order to assess the rate of development. By observing how far the child has developed in relation to his chronological age, and by taking into consideration all factors which might have affected his development, one can predict his future normality with reasonable certainty, bearing in mind that there are occasional rare examples of an abnormal course of development. The prediction of mental superiority is a matter of considerable difficulty in infancy, but the indications are usually there to be seen by the experienced. In the present state of our knowledge more accurate prediction of future intelligence is impossible.

The Prediction of Personality

It would be a matter of great interest if one could predict the future personality of a child when he is yet an infant. One feels that one can predict in infancy that a child will have average intelligence. But there remains the serious possibility, as a result of the bad family background which inevitably pertains in many children for whom adoption is desired, that he may have a particularly unpleasant character, for it is now almost universally accepted that personality and character are products partly of heredity and partly of environment. Very few agree with the "Behaviourists," who consider that character is entirely engendered by environment. Watson [440] wrote: "Give me a dozen healthy infants, well formed, and my own specified world to bring them up in and I'll guarantee to take any one at random and train him to become any type of specialist I might select—doctor, lawyer, artist, merchant, chief, and yes, even beggar man and thief, regardless of his talents, peculiarities, tendencies, abilities, vocations and race of his ancestors. There is no such thing as an inheritance of capacity, talents, temperament, mental constitution and character." It is undeniable that environment has a profound effect on character formation, but there can be no doubt that much of a child's basic character is inherited from his parents.

In view of the profound effect of environment on character formation it seems almost inevitable that character prediction during infancy is practically doomed to failure, though one might think that some of the basic personality patterns might be present in infancy and persist into later life, even though moulded and modified by later environment. The obvious personality characteristics in infancy are discussed elsewhere (p. 231). It is another matter to decide whether such personality patterns persist into later life in spite of the impact of environment. Glover,[155] in the Foreword to Middlemore's book on "The Nursing Couple," wrote: "We have every reason to assume that within a week or so of birth infants manifest in a primitive form all the various types of response which form the basis of adult characterology. The book gives the strongest support to the view that what happens at the breast can really affect the infant all through his life." Shirley [380] found individual differences in behaviour in the 25 babies studied in the first 24 hours of their life. She wrote:

"Each baby exhibits a characteristic pattern of personality trends that changes little with age."

The difficulty of furnishing scientific proof that personality traits can be predicted in infancy is obvious. The greatest difficulty of all is the fact that personality traits are unscorable. They cannot be converted into figures. It is not surprising that the number of studies on the subject which are worth quoting is extremely small. Arnold Gesell [124] attempted to assess 15 character traits in the first year of life and to determine whether there would be any correlation with an independent assessment by another observer at the age of 5 years. The traits which were recorded were energy output, motor demeanour, self-dependence, social responsiveness, family attachment, communicativeness, adaptivity, exploitation of environment, humour sense, emotional maladjustment, emotional expressiveness, reaction to success, reaction to restriction, readiness of smiling and readiness of crying. There was a high degree of correlation. Shirley [380] wrote three volumes of detailed observations on 25 children who were observed by her from birth until the second birthday. Neilon [306] saw 15 of these at the age of 17, 15 years after Shirley's description had been written. She prepared new character sketches without reference to the original ones. Independent judges were then asked to try to match Neilon's 15 sketches with 19 sketches by Shirley. Ten sketches of boys were successfully matched by 5 judges, and 5 sketches of girls were matched by 10 judges. It was therefore proved that some of the important personality traits manifest in the first 2 years were also manifest in adolescent life.

It is obvious that the prediction of character from the personality traits in infancy is one of great difficulty. It is true that most intelligent parents of more than one child have little doubt that they could detect differences in the personality of the second child from that of the first-born in the first few weeks of life, and that their original impressions were subsequently confirmed in later years. But it is one thing for parents with intimate knowledge of their own children to have an impression—which incidentally is probably correct—and another thing for an outside examiner with less knowledge of the child in question to furnish statistical proof that such prediction is possible. The most that one can hope to do is to predict the continuance into later life, whatever the environment, of certain outstanding inborn character traits, such as independence of character, determination, placidity, ready smiling and social responsiveness. One might certainly be guided by a study of the character of the parents, but it is likely to be very difficult to forecast which traits the child has inherited from each parent, unless both parents have in common certain outstanding personality characteristics.

For some reasons it is a good thing that personality prediction is so very difficult. From the point of view of adoption it would be a great pity if such prediction were possible. Parents who have been unable to have children themselves certainly have a right to want to know whether the child whom they are thinking of adopting is of normal intelligence or not, but they must not expect to know in detail what his personality will be like. All parents take a risk in having children, and do not even know whether they will be mentally normal or not. Those who are about to adopt children have to take a risk in the form of the child's future character. If they are not willing to take that risk they should not consider adoption. It is a serious tragedy for a child to be considered unsuitable for adoption, for it means that he is condemned to institutional life and the deprivation of a normal home life, with all that that means to his future. It is a good thing that he cannot be considered unsuitable for adoption on account of some possible future personality traits.

CHAPTER 16

THE NORMAL COURSE OF DEVELOPMENT

THE following is a brief account of the normal course of development in the first 3 years. It is inevitably based largely on the books and papers of Arnold Gesell, supplemented by those of Shirley,[380] Buhler [75, 76] and others, and by my own experience. For further information the reader should consult these works, and particularly Arnold Gesell's books, "Developmental Diagnosis," [149] "The First Five Years of Life," [146] "Infant and Child in the Culture of To-day," [147] "Feeding Behaviour of Infants" [144] and "Biographies of Child Development." [143]

The Principles of Development

The chief principles of development may be summarized as follows :

(1) Development is a continuous process from conception to maturity. Development must not be thought of in terms of mere milestones. Before any "milestone" is reached a child has to go through many preceding stages of development, and in developmental diagnosis one has to be thoroughly conversant with all these stages. Diagnosis does not consist so much of observing *what* a child does but *how* he does it. For example, in a 7-month-old child one has to observe not whether he can sit, but how he sits, and with what degree of maturity he does it. Statistical studies almost invariably miss this. They record the fact that a child can sit, but fail to record the maturity which he has reached.

(2) Development depends on the maturation of the nervous system. It has been shown by Tilney and Casamajor,[415] Hardcastle [182] and others that the acquisition of new skills depends on the myelination of the appropriate part of the nervous system. Until that has occurred no amount of practice can make a child learn the relevant skill. When practice is denied, the ability to perform the skill lies dormant, but the skill is very rapidly learnt as soon as an opportunity is given.

(3) The *sequence* of development is the same for all children, but the *rate* of development varies from child to child. For example, a child has to learn to sit before he can walk, but the age at which children learn to sit and walk varies considerably.

(4) Certain primitive reflexes anticipate corresponding voluntary movement and have to be lost before the voluntary movement develops. Examples are the walking reflex and the grasp reflex of the new-born period. Another is the reciprocal kick—the rhythmic kicking

of the legs, which disappears when walking begins. In mentally defective children these primitive reflexes are likely to persist beyond the usual age. It is common, for instance, to see a 2-year-old mentally defective child demonstrating the reciprocal kick.

(5) The direction of development is cephalocaudal. The first step in the development of locomotion, for instance, is the acquisition of head control, involving the neck muscles. Later the spinal muscles develop co-ordination so that the child is able to sit up with a straight back instead of a round one. The child can do much with his hands before he can use his legs. He can crawl, pulling himself forward with his arms, the legs trailing behind, before he can creep, a movement which involves the use of the legs.

(6) Generalized mass activity gives way to specific individual responses. The young baby, for example, shows pleasure by a massive general response. His eyes widen, his respirations increase, his legs kick and his arms move vigorously. The older child or adult shows his pleasure simply by facial expression or by appropriate words. The aimless movement of the arms and legs of the first 6 months are replaced by the specific movements of locomotion and manipulation.

The Full-term Baby at Birth

The infant sleeps for the greater part of the 24 hours. He yawns, sighs, hiccoughs, sneezes, coughs, stretches and salivates. He does not usually shed tears till he is about 4 weeks old. He can swallow and suck. He shows a variety of mouthing reflexes when the lips are touched. He roots around for food when his face touches his mother's breast or the palm of the hand ("the rooting reflex"). He shows the Moro reflex—a symmetrical abduction of the upper limbs when there is a sudden noise or when he is suddenly moved. The tonic neck reflex is seen in the new-born baby; when lying awake on a flat surface his head is turned to one side, with his arm extended to the same side. There is often flexion of the contralateral leg. He shows the grasp reflex; when a finger or other object is slipped into his palm his hand closes on it and he can often be lifted off the couch by the strength of his grasp. When his foot is pressed down on to a firm surface he steps out because of the so-called walking reflex.

The Loss of the Primitive Reflexes

The walking reflex usually disappears in 2 or 3 weeks. The grasp reflex disappears gradually and little trace of it can be found by about 3 months. The Moro reflex has largely disappeared by 3 or 4 months. The tonic neck reflex is rarely seen after about 4 months. The reciprocal kick disappears when walking begins, but is seen occasionally after that when the baby is particularly pleased or displeased.

The Development of Locomotion

The first step towards the development of locomotion is the development of head control—the ability to support the head in all positions of the body. The steps in this are observed in three situations : in ventral suspension, the prone position and in the supine position. (Figs. 36–62). Another essential to the development of locomotion is the reciprocal kick—the rhythmic kicking of the legs, which disappears before walking begins. Other stages in the development of locomotion can be observed in the sitting and standing positions. For the sake of continuity these positions are described separately. An attempt has been made to tabulate the more important milestones of development in Table IX (p. 192). The table enumerates the various new skills which are acquired at different ages.

Ventral Suspension

When the new-born baby is held above the couch in the prone position with the hand under the chest or abdomen (ventral suspension) the head drops down. There may be a very fleeting tensing of the neck muscles, but that is all. By about 4 weeks of age the momentary tensing of the neck muscles is more obvious and the baby is able to lift the head up a little for brief moments. By the age of 6 weeks he is able to hold the head in line with the plane of the body. By 8 weeks he can momentarily lift the head up beyond that plane, and by 12 weeks he can maintain that position. After this age there is no further point in testing a child's head control in this position. The position of ventral suspension is the most sensitive one for the testing of head control in the first 3 months.

Pulling the Child to the Sitting Position

An essential test for head control consists of placing the child in the supine position on a firm surface and then pulling him to the sitting position. When supported sitting the position and movements of the head are noted, together with the degree of roundness or straightness of the back. When the new-born baby is pulled to the sitting position there is complete head lag. In the sitting position there is uniform rounding of the back because of lack of strength in the spinal muscles and the head droops forward, though he lifts it up for a short distance momentarily. By 6 weeks of age the head lag is clearly not complete, for he lifts it up in the last part of the movement when being pulled up. By 8 weeks the head lag is less. The head still droops forward when he is held in the sitting position, but he can lift it up for seconds at a time. By 12 weeks the head lag is only slight. By 16 weeks there is only very slight head lag, in the very first part of the movement of pulling him up, and when supported in the sitting position he holds the head up for prolonged periods and looks round actively. When the trunk is swayed gently by the examiner the head sways with it or plunges forward, whereas by 20 weeks this is inhibited. By 16 weeks the curvature of the back is seen only in the lumbar region. By 20 weeks head control is almost complete. There is no head lag when he is pulled to the sitting position. At 24 weeks he lifts his head off the couch in the supine position as the examiner is about to pull him up, and he holds his arms out to the examiner to help him. He likes to be propped up in his pram and he can sit for a few minutes with a cushion for support in his high chair. He holds his trunk erect. By 28 weeks he spontaneously lifts his head off the couch as if asking to be pulled up, and he can sit with his hands forward for support. From this age onwards there is no point in using the test of pulling the child up to the sitting position unless he is retarded. One must observe, however, the maturity with which he sits. At 32 weeks he can sit for a few seconds without support, but it is not till 36 weeks that he can sit for 10 minutes unsupported. At this age he is still apt to overbalance by falling backwards or sideways when trying to reach for an object at his side. It is not till 40 weeks that he can pull himself up from the supine to the sitting position. He can go forward from the sitting to the prone position, and thence back to sitting. By 46 weeks he can lean over sideways and recover his balance, and by 48 weeks he can twist well round to pick up an object without overbalancing. By about 15 months he can seat himself in a chair, very often by the process of facing it, climbing on to it, standing up on it, turning round and then sitting down. By 18 or 21 months he can sit in it in the adult fashion.

The Prone Position

The new-born baby lies with his head turned to one side, with the pelvis high. He kneels, with the knees drawn up under his abdomen. By the age of 4 weeks he momentarily lifts his chin off the couch. The knees are not drawn up under the abdomen as much as before and the legs are intermittently kicked into extension. At 6 weeks he readily lifts his chin off the couch so that the plane of the face is at an angle of 45 degrees to it. By 8 weeks the child no longer kneels, for the legs are partly extended. At 10 weeks he frequently lifts the chin off the couch so that the plane of the face is at an angle of 45–90 degrees to the couch. At 12 weeks he holds his chin and shoulders off the couch for a long time, bearing the weight on the forearms. The legs are fully extended. At 16 weeks he often arches his back so that his weight rests on his abdomen and lower chest, the arms and legs being lifted off the couch. He holds his head and chest off the couch so that the plane of the face is at 90 degrees to it. At 24 weeks he bears his weight on his hands with extended arms, the chest and upper part of the abdomen being off the couch. He may roll from prone to supine. (It is usually a month later before he can roll from supine to prone.) He may assume the "frog" position, with the legs extended symmetrically in abduction, with the feet everted. At 28 weeks he bears the weight on one hand while he looks round for a toy. From 30 to 40 weeks he is making increasing efforts to crawl. He often progresses backwards in the process. He may progress across the room by rolling. At 40 weeks he is able to move forward, pulling himself by his hands. He lies on his abdomen and the legs trail behind. His legs begin to help, and at 44 weeks he creeps with the abdomen off the couch. From time to time one foot may be seen to be flat on the couch, in the form of a primitive step. At 1 year he may walk on hands and feet like a bear. Creeping may persist long after this date, but at any time from now onwards he may discard the creep position and walk.

Though most children creep before they walk, not all go through this stage. I suspect that most of those children who miss the creeping stage have not often been placed in the prone position for exercise.

The Standing Position

In the first 2 or 3 weeks the baby shows the walking reflex when his foot is pressed against the couch. His back is rounded and his head falls forward. By 8 weeks he holds his head up momentarily, but at 12 weeks for a long time. At 20 weeks he bears some weight on the legs, and at 24 weeks a large fraction of his weight, if his mother gives him a chance to try. He sags at knee and hip. At 28 weeks he can maintain full extension of knees and hip when supported, and he bounces in delight. Much depends on whether his mother gives him a chance to stand. Many mothers deliberately prevent their children from bearing weight on the legs for fear they will become bow-legged. At 36 weeks he stands holding on to furniture, but he has to be helped into that position. By 40 weeks he can pull himself up to the standing position. At first his feet get into the wrong position and he has many slips and falls in his efforts. He is likely to be unable to let himself down, and falls down with a bump or cries for help. At 44 weeks, while standing holding on to furniture, he lifts and replaces one foot. He finds it extremely difficult to pick up a toy from the floor in this position. At 48 weeks he walks sideways holding on to furniture ("cruising") and walks with two hands held.

By one year of age he walks with one hand held. He may continue to demand this support for as long as 5 or 6 months. The age at which he decides to walk without support now depends in part on his confidence and his dislike of spills. The average age at which children walk without support is about 15 months. Many workers give an earlier age (e.g. 13 months). Walking is delayed by an aberrant form of progression called shuffling or hitching on one buttock and one hand. At 13 months he is likely to stand alone for a few seconds. When he eventually walks without help he progresses on a wide base, with a high-stepping gait, with steps of varying length and in varying directions. He falls repeatedly. He tends to keep his elbows flexed, with his arms abducted from the shoulder. He can creep upstairs, but has no idea of the importance of gravity and is likely to lean back into space when halfway up. At 15 months he can get into the standing position without support, but he cannot throw a ball without falling and he cannot stop suddenly or go round corners. He falls suddenly on to his buttocks. By 16 or 18 months he can walk backwards as well as forwards. He can walk upstairs, two feet per step, holding on to the rail. He can run and pull a toy as he walks. He can throw a ball without falling. By 21 months he can pick an object up from the floor without falling. At 2 years he can go up and down stairs alone with two feet per step. He can kick a ball without falling. At 2½ he can walk on tip-toe and jump, but he cannot stand on one foot. At 3 he can walk upstairs with a foot to each step, but when coming down he places both feet on the same stair. He jumps off the bottom step. He can now stand for a few seconds only on one leg, but he cannot skip. Even at 3 he has much to learn and the development of locomotion is still incomplete.

Manipulation

The primitive grasp reflex disappears before true voluntary grasping begins. Before voluntary grasping can occur the tightly closed hands of the new-born have to open, and the eyes have to become co-ordinated with the hands. The grasp reflex disappears by about 3 months of age, and often very little trace of it can be seen at 8 weeks. At about 12 weeks, and sometimes sooner, the baby begins to pull at his dress with his hands, and when a rattle is placed in his hand he retains it for several moments. When a brightly coloured toy is placed in front of him, he shows his obvious desire to get it and excites, with rapid movements of the arms and legs and increased respiration rate. Gradually and imperceptibly, as he grows older, it will be noticed that his hands are beginning to go forward to reach the object. At first he grossly misjudges the distance, trying to get an object which is quite out of reach or overshooting the mark. He plays longer and longer with a rattle placed in his hand. He eventually touches a larger toy but cannot grasp it. From 12 to 16 weeks he characteristically watches his hands as he lies on his back. At 16 weeks his hands come together into the midline and he plays with them. He pulls his dress over his face. By 20 weeks he can grasp an object near his hand. He is ataxic in his approach, still overshooting the mark, but eventually he gets what he wants. He soon grasps everything within reach : his mother's hair, clothes, brooch, spoon, paper and anything else he sees. He takes everything to his mouth, for the mouth is at this time the chief organ of manipulation. He is able in the supine position to get his legs into full extension and he plays with his toes. He loves to splash in the bath and he crumples paper. His approach to objects is two-handed. He can only grasp large objects. When he holds a cube in the hand it is held in the palm, not between the fingers. In the early stages of development it is held on the ulnar side of the hand, and later on the radial side. It is not until about 40 weeks of age or more that he can hold it between finger and thumb. At 28 weeks he characteristically begins to transfer objects from one hand to the other. It is now noted that he is beginning to go for objects with one hand instead of two. He can feed himself well with a biscuit and he helps to hold the spoon when eating. Whereas at 24 weeks he drops a cube from his hand if another is offered, at 28 weeks he retains the first when the second cube is presented. At 36 weeks he brings the two cubes together, as if comparing the size, and bangs them on the table. As manipulation increases mouthing decreases, so that by a year few things are taken to the mouth. He can easily lean forward now to pick objects up. At 40 weeks he can bring his finger and thumb together and so pick up very small objects, such as a piece of string. His index finger protrudes as he goes for it. Release of objects begins at about this age. Up to this time he was able to grasp objects but he could not deliberately let them go. He soon discovers the joy of deliberately letting one thing after another drop on to the floor, particularly if there is someone to pick them up for him. At 44 weeks he will hold an object out to his mother and even put it into her hand, but he will not let it go. By 48 weeks he will release it into her hand, and soon thoroughly enjoys the give-and-take game. He also loves to put one object into another, and spends a happy half-hour merely putting one cube after another into a basket and taking them out again. He particularly enjoys this repetitive game and continues to do so for the next 2 years. At 13 months he can hold two 1-in. cubes in one hand. His release is so accurate that he can build a tower of two cubes, but it is 21 months before he can build a tower of five or six cubes, and 3 years before he can build a tower of nine or ten cubes. At 12 months, when feeding himself, he rotates the spoon when it is near his mouth, spilling the contents, but by 15–18 months he gets it into his mouth before the contents are dropped. At 18 months he can feed himself completely, managing a cup with only occasional slight spilling. He turns two or three pages of a book at a time, but by 24 months he can turn them over singly. From 15 or 18 months he has tried to put his gloves, socks or shoes on but not succeeded. At 24 months he can put them on. He can now pronate and supinate the wrist sufficiently to turn an easy door handle or unscrew a lid. He begins to draw with pencils. At $2\frac{1}{2}$ he can take his pants off and put them on and thread beads. He begins to fasten easily-placed buttons. At 3 he can dress and undress himself completely with some help with back buttons, and he can buckle his shoes. Many children can draw quite well at this age and can cut paper fairly accurately with scissors. They can paint quite well over a suitable design.

The Use of the Eyes and Ears

The new-born baby looks vaguely at objects and momentarily follows a large moving object with a flicker of the eyes. By 3 or 4 weeks he watches his mother's face intently as she speaks to him, and he will watch a toy which is brought into his line of vision, following it from one side nearly to the midline. At 6 weeks he is beginning to follow moving persons with his eyes. At 8 weeks he will follow a moving toy from the side to a point past the midline, and at 12 weeks he will follow it well over to the other side. At 8 weeks the eyes show convergence and focusing. His eye becomes quicker and quicker at catching sight of objects in front of him. By 12 weeks he turns his head in the direction of sound. He excites when he sees toys in front of him and from now on shows increasing efforts to grasp toys, until eventually at about 20 weeks his eyes and hands are sufficiently co-ordinated for him to grasp them voluntarily. Up to 16 weeks very small objects failed to catch his eye, but he can see them now though he cannot touch them. He watches his hands from 12 to 16 weeks as he lies on his back. He shows considerable excitement when he sees his feed being prepared and shows obvious interest in a strange room. At 6 months he adjusts his position to see objects—craning his neck, bending back or crouching to see what he wants to see. He cannot follow a rapidly moving object until he is nearly a year old. By 2 years he can see everything which the adult can see.

Some babies are unable to hear for a few days after birth. It can be shown, however,[351] that most new-born babies can hear if properly tested when awake and not actively feeding or crying. The characteristic response to a sudden noise in the first 2 months is the Moro reflex. By 3 months the baby turns his head towards the source of sound. At 32 weeks he responds to his name, and at 36 weeks he may imitate sounds made by his mother. Between 9 and 12 months he understands the meaning of several words, such as names of members of the family.

General Understanding

The whole of a child's development is so intimately bound up with the development of his understanding and with his intelligence that it is difficult to discuss the development of understanding separately.

Probably the first sign of the dawn of understanding in a baby is seen when his mother talks to him at the age of 3 or 4 weeks. He quiets, watches her intently, opening and closing his mouth, often bobbing his head backwards and forwards, obviously enjoying the conversation. At about 6 weeks he begins to smile, at first only once or twice a day, when his mother speaks to him, but more and more frequently and to more and more different stimuli as he grows older. In 3 or 4 weeks he vocalizes his pleasure when spoken to. By 10 weeks he has considerable interest in his surroundings, following moving persons with his eyes. At 12 weeks he may be quite reluctant to be left outside, much preferring to be in the kitchen where he can see some activity. His interest and exciting when he sees a brightly-coloured toy is an index of his understanding. He recognizes his mother at this age. He turns his head towards a sound. He may resist the nose swab of cotton wool by turning his head away when he sees it approach. (The reaction to cotton wool swabs from the age of 2–10 months is used by Charlotte Bühler in her developmental tests.) At 16 weeks he shows his understanding by opening his mouth for the feeding bottle or breast. He cries when his mother departs. His interest in his surroundings has increased and he shows obvious interest in a strange room. He tries hard to grasp objects. At 20 weeks he smiles at his own mirror image, and when he drops his rattle he looks to see where it has gone to. At 24 weeks in the supine position he stretches his arms out when he sees that his mother is about to pull him into the sitting position. When he drops his rattle he not only follows it with his eyes but tries to recover it. He smiles and vocalizes at his mirror image, and at 28 weeks he pats it. Any time after the age of 5 months he may begin to imitate such acts as chewing or protrusion of the tongue. From the age of about 24 weeks he shows his memory of foodstuffs by his strong reaction of like or dislike when he sees them. His interest in his surroundings is partly related to his personality, but most babies of this age are intensely interested in their surroundings and they bend their necks and twist round to see what is happening. He may try to establish contact with a stranger by coughing or making other noises. He enjoys the game of peep-bo with a towel or napkin over his head or over his mother's head. He responds to his name. At 32 weeks he reacts to the cotton-wool swab by grasping his mother's hand and pushing it away. He reaches persistently for toys out of reach. He responds to "No." At 36 weeks he tries to prevent his mother washing his face by putting his arm in front of it. The degree of concentration on his toys should be particularly noted from this age. Some children can only concentrate for a minute or two on a toy, while others play for prolonged periods with them. Such prolonged concentration and determination to reach a toy is a good sign of intelligence. At 40 weeks he may pull the clothes of a person to attract his attention. He learns to clap his hands and to wave bye-bye, laughing as he does it. He learns to repeat any performance laughed at, and if he finds that his audience laughs when he drops spoonfuls of food on to the carpet or smears it over his hair, he will repeat the act. He is beginning to release objects, and greatly enjoys the game of dropping bricks or other objects from his high chair for someone else to pick up. Any time after 9 months he will perform simple acts on request, such as sitting down or standing up. He enjoys the frequent repetition of nursery rhymes and may anticipate certain actions in the rhyme by bodily movement, thus well revealing his developing memory. At 44 weeks he will hand a toy to his mother, but at first he refuses to let it go when it has reached her hand. He soon learns to kiss on request. He shows considerable interest in the colour masses in pictures in his books, particularly when his mother describes them. He shows that he is beginning to understand quite a number of words, such as foot, shoe, sock, though he may be unable to say any. At 11 months, he is still enjoying the peep-bo game and now covers his own face up with a towel. He laughs at his mother when she pulls faces at him or puts some strange object on her head. At a year he begins to co-operate in dressing by holding his arm out for the sleeve of his coat, or the foot up for his shoe. He will go on a simple errand such as fetching his sock from the other end of the room. Speech has been developing in the last 3 months and he may now be able to say three or four words with meaning, though he understands the meaning of many more.

The development of understanding in the first year has been discussed in some detail, because it is in the first year that developmental diagnosis is regarded by many as particularly difficult. The various manifestations of understanding, and especially the baby's powers of concentration, persistence and interest in surroundings, are particularly important in such diagnosis. The further signs of developing intelligence after the first birthday are briefly summarized below.

In the second year his increasing understanding is shown by his greater and greater understanding of what is said to him and his ability to execute simple requests. It is shown by his increasing interest in books and his ability to point out objects in them on request. It is shown by his imitation of his mother in sweeping, washing and doing odd jobs about the house. The girl's play with her doll is well worth observing. The play becomes more and more complex as she grows older. From 18 months to 2 years it is apt to be fairly simple and include "potting," napkin changing and washing. From $2\frac{1}{2}$ to 3 years it is much more complex and her imaginativeness should be noted. It is observed in her play with boxes, bricks and other toys. The child may arrange complicated situations with her dolls and spend long periods dressing them and undressing them.

The tests commonly used for the investigation of a child's intelligence between the ages of 1 and 3 years are tabulated in Table IX, and there is no need to repeat them all here. From 18 months onwards the child enjoys playing with pencil and paper, and his memory is well shown by his ability to draw, though other factors play a part. By $2\frac{1}{2}$ years he can tackle simple jigsaw puzzles (e.g. those made of four or five pieces) and enjoys matching wools of various colours, and cards with pictures on them. His ability to match such cards and pictures is a good index of his intelligence. His memory is tested by his ability to repeat digits. He knows his full name by $2\frac{1}{2}$, and at this age he is first likely to note anatomical differences between the sexes. By 3 he is constantly asking questions, shows great interest in his surroundings and knows various nursery rhymes.

Pleasure and Displeasure

The first sign of pleasure is the quieting of the new-born baby when he is placed in a warm bath or when he is cuddled by his mother. When he is fed his crying stops, and he shows his pleasure by the splaying of his toes and their alternate flexion and extension. As he grows older he shows more and more pleasure at being picked up by his mother and at being spoken to. By 6 weeks he smiles at her as she speaks to him, and in 3 or 4 weeks vocalizes his pleasure. In the third month he emits squeals of delight. By about 16 weeks he shows his delight by a massive general response—by his rapid panting respirations, widening of the palpebral fissure and rapid movements of the arms and legs. He laughs aloud. He thoroughly enjoys playing with the rattle which is placed in his hand and soon he is able to grasp objects himself (by 20 or 24 weeks). Thereafter he takes particular pleasure in the newly-acquired skills—manipulation, sitting, standing and walking. After 20 weeks he is constantly using his hands, banging bricks, grasping everything which comes within his reach. He smiles when pulled to the sitting position and dislikes lying down. When he is able to stand he enjoys standing and dislikes sitting. When he is able to walk he wants to be helped to walk all day long. After 5 months he enjoys simple games such as peep-bo (see section above on General Understanding), and from now onwards he takes increasing pleasure in any simple game. At 4 or 5 months he becomes ticklish, and soon he laughs at the mere prospect of being tickled when the finger is approaching. At 6 months he smiles when he sees a dog or another baby, and often smiles at every stranger he sees. After a year he delights still more in his newly found skills of manipulation and he enjoys domestic mimicry, imitating his mother in her housework. He enjoys his books, toys and his friends. Much can be learnt from the simple observation of a child's behaviour with his toys and from his response to various stimuli. In general the nature of the stimuli which produce pleasure depends on his developmental level.

A baby can show his displeasure before he can show his pleasure, but as he matures he shows less displeasure and more pleasure. The causes of crying are discussed elsewhere and will not be discussed here.

Feeding Behaviour

For details of the development of feeding behaviour in children the reader is referred to the book by Gesell and Ilg.[144] The new-born baby frequently gags and chokes. He hiccoughs when his stomach is distended by a good feed. He cannot usually approximate his lips tightly to the areola of the breast, so that milk leaks out as he sucks and he swallows air. As he grows older he approximates his lips much more tightly, so that there is no leakage and practically no air swallowing. The older baby therefore has much less trouble with wind than the younger one. He cannot take solids at this age, for they initiate sucking movements with elevation of the posterior part of the tongue, so that the food is ejected. He can manage semi-solids by the age of 4 months. He begins to chew at about 6 months and so can manage true solids. At this age he can approximate his lips well to the rim of a cup, and his eyes are so well co-ordinated with his hands that he can feed himself with a biscuit or crust. From the age of 5 months almost everything which the baby picks up is taken to the mouth, and this persists until he is really adept with his hands, when mouthing largely ceases.

Most babies make some attempt to help to feed themselves at about 6 months by helping to hold the bottle, cup or spoon. This should be encouraged. They can manage a biscuit, crust or toast at this age, and by 9–12 months they can manage by one means or another largely to feed themselves. They are apt to put their fingers into the food and to play with the food with their hands. They tend deliberately to drop items of food from the high chair on to the floor, particularly if this causes laughter. They smear it over their faces and often into the hair. They may even invert the dish on to the head. Anna Freud[110] says: "It is an error to ascribe this messing of the young child to lack of skill. The child's actions in this respect are deliberate and intentional. They are motivated by the pleasure of smearing, an anal-erotic activity transferred from the excrements to the foodstuffs which are similar to the former in consistency, colour and temperature."

I prefer to regard the messing as a sign of the child's inco-ordination, with a natural desire to feel the consistency of foods, together with a desire for attention. He is much more likely to make a mess with food which he does not like than with that which he enjoys. When he is first given the cup without help he is apt to let go as soon as he has drunk what he wants. Later he tends to bang it down on to the table. The age at which children learn to manage a cup with practically no spilling varies tremendously. It is greatly influenced by the factor of practice. If he is given a chance early he is likely to manage it early. Gesell and Ilg [144] say that the typical age at which self-management of a cup occurs is 65 weeks. Some need help to the end of the second year. There is no doubt, however, that many children manage a cup very well by 12 months. Without having performed any statistical study, I would have thought that most children who are given a chance as soon as they are ready to feed themselves can do so quite efficiently, managing a cup as well, between the age of 15 and 18 months. This is rather earlier than the age given by Gesell. Similar remarks apply to the age at which a child learns to use a spoon. Gesell says that spilling from a spoon is marked at 15 months, moderate at 18 months and tends to disappear by the close of the second year. Again without statistical study, I feel that most children who are given a chance early can manage a spoon with a minimum of spilling by 15–18 months. Earlier than this they are very apt to rotate the spoon just before it reaches the mouth, spilling the contents. This rotation may persist as a habit, and have to be checked accordingly. By the age of 2½–3 years most children can manage a knife and fork with help in cutting such hard articles of food as toast. It is a good thing to let the child use a knife and fork as soon as he is developmentally ready instead of a spoon. At about this age he should be encouraged to use an ordinary plate instead of a child's plate with a high rim.

Many make the mistake of expecting perfect table manners in the 2- or 3-year-old. It is a mistake to be too strict at mealtimes and to make mealtimes a misery. Gentle loving advice is altogether desirable, but constant remonstrances do nothing but harm. The child will slowly but surely learn by imitating his parents. The parents should see that their own manners leave nothing to be desired.

The frequency of demands for food decreases with age. Between the fourth and ninth day many babies demand up to twelve or thirteen feeds in the 24 hours, including two at night. Aldrich and Hewitt [11] showed that at 1 month of age 61 per cent. of a large number of babies observed by them at Rochester preferred a three-hourly feed, and 26 per cent. a four-hourly feed. By 7–9 months the majority of babies want four feeds a day. By the age of 1 year 91 per cent. wanted three meals a day. Some babies as early as 2 or 3 months, however, only demand three feeds in the 24 hours. The great majority of babies drop the night feed by the age of 10 weeks.

Speech

The earliest manifestations of developing speech are in the throaty sounds of the 4-week-old baby and the vowel sounds—ah, eh, uh—of the 8-week-old child. By the age of 12–16 weeks a baby will have a long conversation in his own way with the mother, responding to her overtures by prolonged "speech." At about 20 weeks he begins to use guttural sounds and say "Ah goo." At 28 weeks he says "Ba," "Da," "Ka" and sounds like "mm" when he is crying. At 32 weeks he begins to combine syllables, saying "Baba," "Dada," "Kaka." Not until about 44 weeks does he say one word with meaning, saying "Dada" more in his father's presence than when he is not there. The average child says about three words with meaning by about a year. Between 15 and 18 months jargoning begins, the child speaking in a language of his own. By 21–24 months children put two or three words together into sentences. At 24 months they use pronouns—I, me, you. By the age of 3 the child has an extensive vocabulary and talks incessantly throughout the day.

Handedness

In many children handedness is not finally established until the age of 4 years. In infancy the direction of the tonic neck reflex gives an indication of future handedness; in fourteen out of nineteen babies observed by Gesell[150] the ultimate handedness was successfully predicted in this way. During the first year there are commonly shifts in handedness, and there is frequently a stage of bilaterality at about 18 months. A good review of the subject was given by Bakwin.[35]

Ambidexterity in older children may be associated with speech and reading difficulties. If by the age of 3 or 4 there is ambidexterity, no harm will be done by gently training the child to use predominantly one or other hand, preferably the right. Once established, no attempt should be made to change the laterality.

It is said that approximately 6·6 per cent. of male adults and 3·8 per cent. of female adults are left handed. There is an unduly high proportion of sinistrality in geniuses and criminals (Bakwin). A left-handed child may adopt mirror writing and reverse letters more than normal children. Leonardo da Vinci was left handed or ambidextrous and was in the habit of writing in a mirror image with his left hand.[328] Lewis Carroll was left handed, and stammering prevented him from preaching. It is doubtful, however, whether the incidence of stuttering is higher in left-handed than in right-handed children. There is a tendency now to doubt the role of handedness in the genesis of stuttering.

The problem of crossed laterality was reviewed by Pearce.[329] Normally the laterality of the dominant hand corresponds with that of the foot, ear and eye. When there is an irregular dominance, the term crossed laterality is used. It is associated with a higher than usual incidence of speech and reading difficulties, and with other behaviour problems partly connected with these difficulties.

Sphincter Control

The development of sphincter control and other aspects of psychological development are discussed elsewhere (p. 277).

Summary

Table IX gives a summary of the principal milestones of development.

For convenience the table has been divided into six columns. This is in many ways purely artificial, for there is inevitably some overlapping. Some skills which are included in the column entitled "Manipulation" could very well be included under the column entitled "General Understanding," and *vice versa*, largely because general understanding is required for so many manipulative feats.

The table does not set out to give a list of all the child's skills at the various ages listed. This would involve a great deal of repetition. The age at which a child learns to smile, for instance, is given as 6 weeks, but this is not mentioned under all the subsequent age headings, it being assumed that all "normal" children over the age of 6 weeks are able to smile. The table is intended solely to give the ages at which average children first acquire the skills described. In using the table in the assessment of an individual child of a given age, therefore, one has to determine how far he has developed in comparison with average children. In other words it may be found that a 40-week-old infant has only developed as far as the average 28-week-old child.

The sequence of development in locomotion and manipulation is shown in Figs. 14–68 in the form of sketches. These were chosen partly because they are patterns which are readily observed by anyone and partly because of their importance as being particularly characteristic for the age.

Most children will reach these milestones sooner or later than the ages given. The ages are only useful for helping to form a picture of the development as a whole.

STANDING POSITION

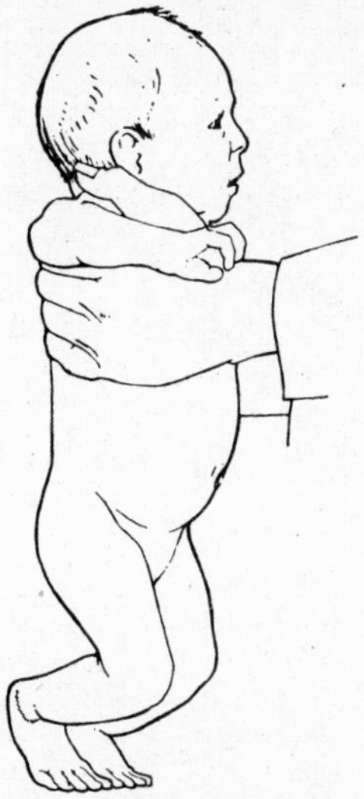

FIG. 14. 12 weeks : Bears small fraction of weight.

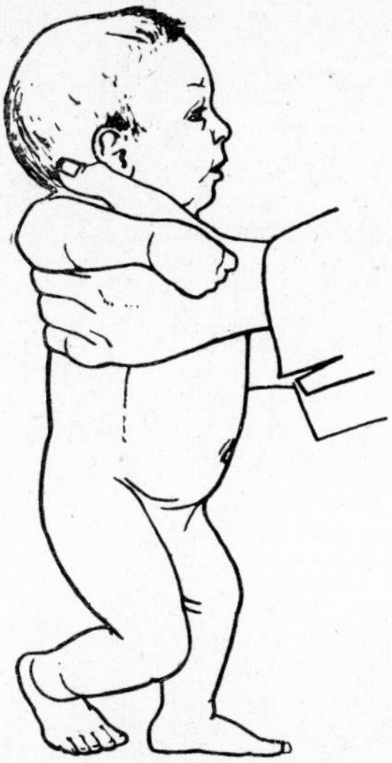

FIG. 15. 16 weeks : Fair fraction of weight. Sags a lot at hip and knee.

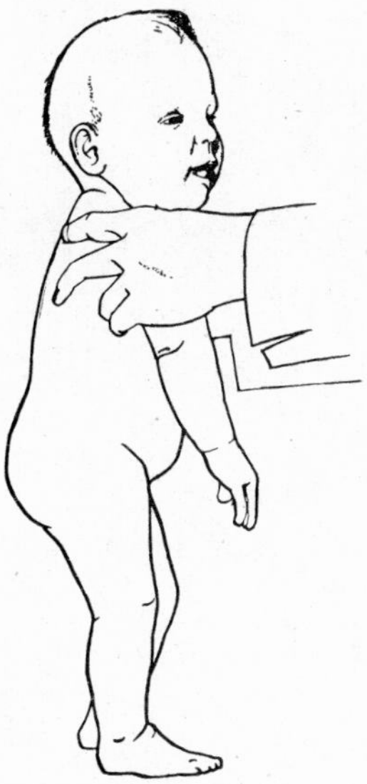

FIG. 16. 24 weeks : Bears large fraction of weight. Sags a little at hip and knee.

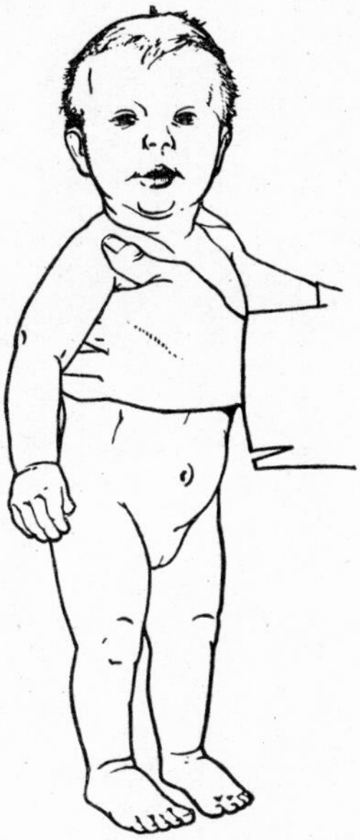

FIG. 17. 28 weeks : Maintains extension of hip and knee when supported.

STANDING POSITION

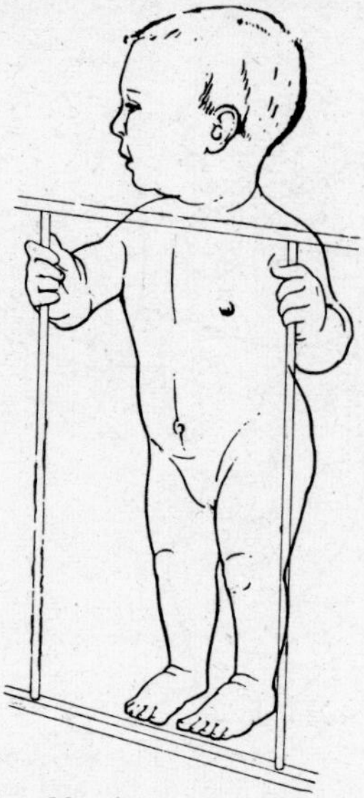

Fig. 18. 36 weeks : Stands, holding on to furniture.

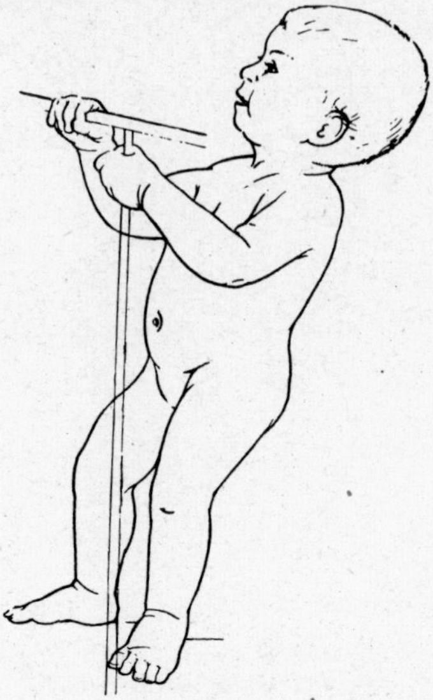

Fig. 19. 40 weeks : Pulls self up to stand.

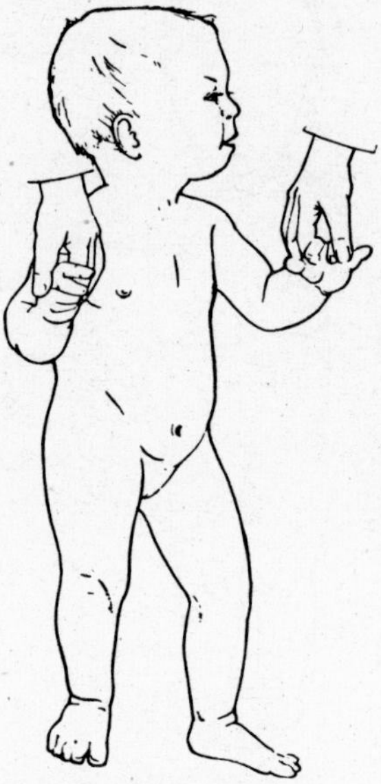

Fig. 20. 48 weeks : Walks, two hands held.

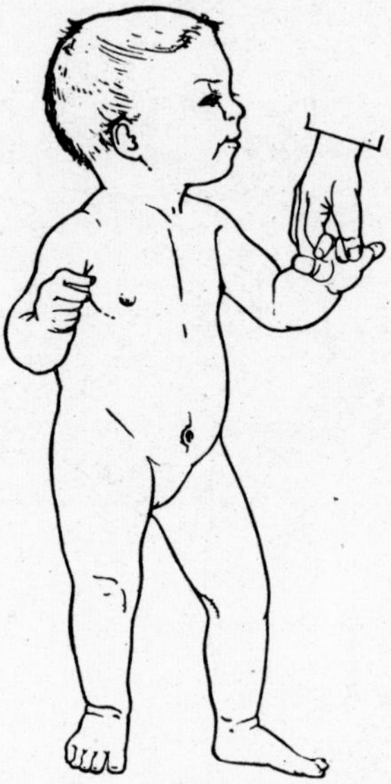

Fig. 21. 52 weeks : Walks, one hand held.

STANDING POSITION

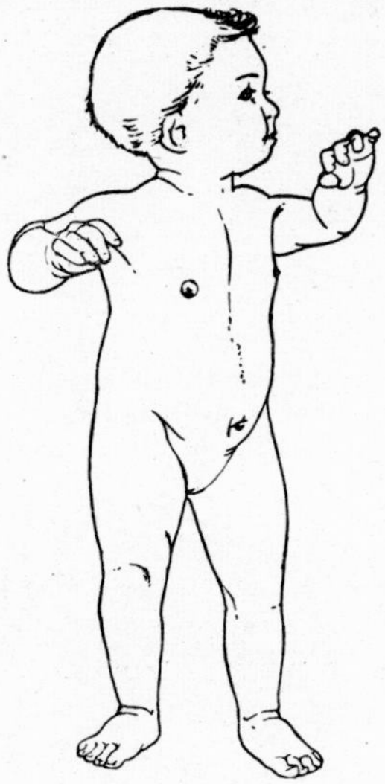

FIG. 22 (*left*). 13–15 months : Stands alone. Walks without support, elbows flexed, arms abducted, broad base.

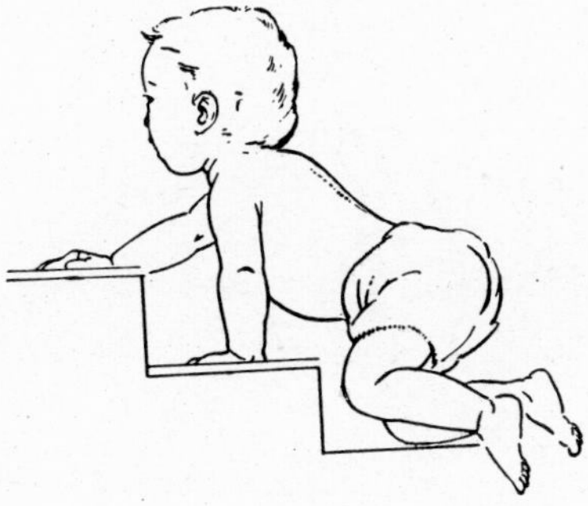

FIG. 23 (*above*). 15 months : Creeps upstairs.

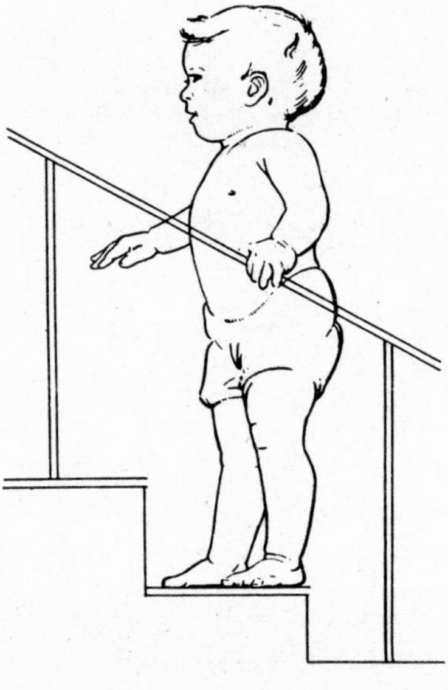

FIG. 24 (*left*). 18 months : Climbs stair unaided, holding rail. 2 feet per step.

STANDING POSITION

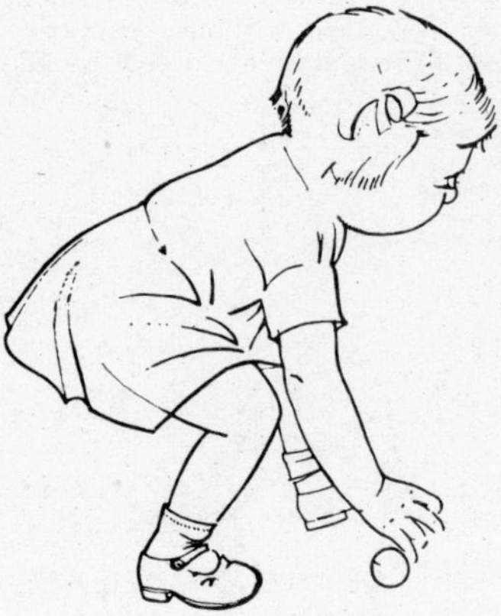

FIG. 25 (*left*). 21 months : Picks object up from floor without falling.

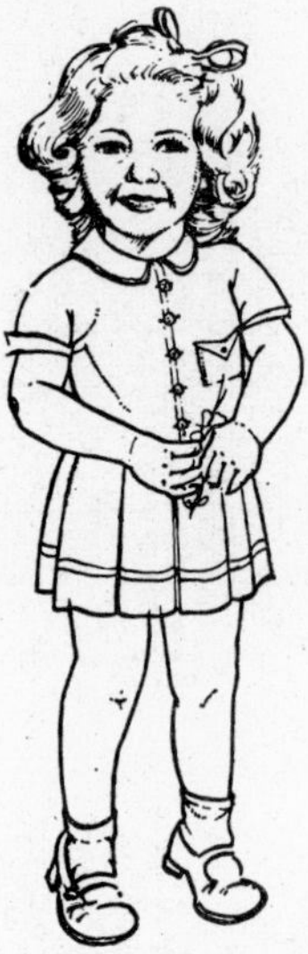

FIG. 26. $2\frac{1}{2}$ years : Stands on tiptoe.

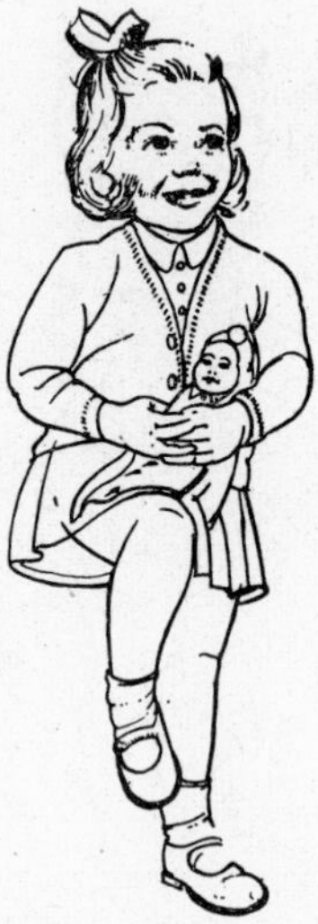

FIG. 27. 3 years : Stands on one foot for a few seconds.

SITTING POSITION

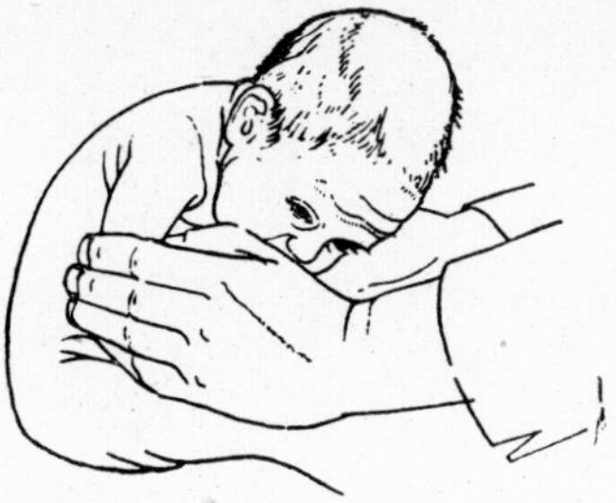

FIG. 28 (*left*). New-born : Uniformly rounded back.

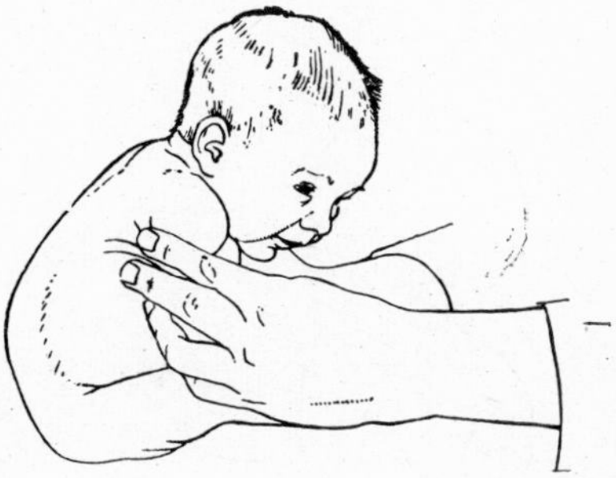

FIG. 29 (*right*). 4 weeks : Rounded back. Head held up momentarily.

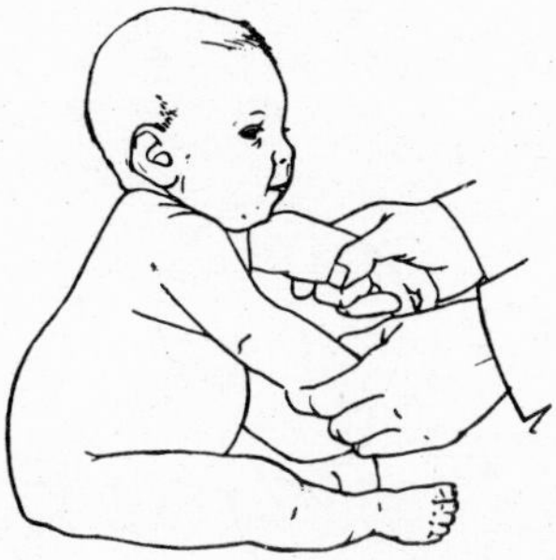

FIG. 30 (*left*). 16 weeks : Held sitting. Curvature only in lumbar region.

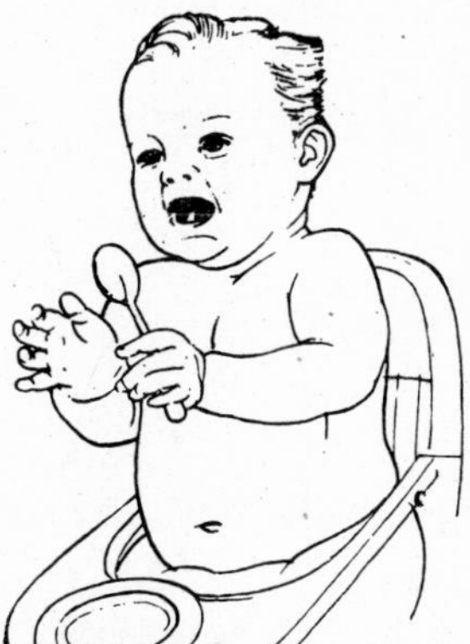

FIG. 31 (*right*). 24 weeks : Sits in high chair, propped.

SITTING POSITION

FIG. 32 (*right*). 28 weeks : Sits, hands forward for support.

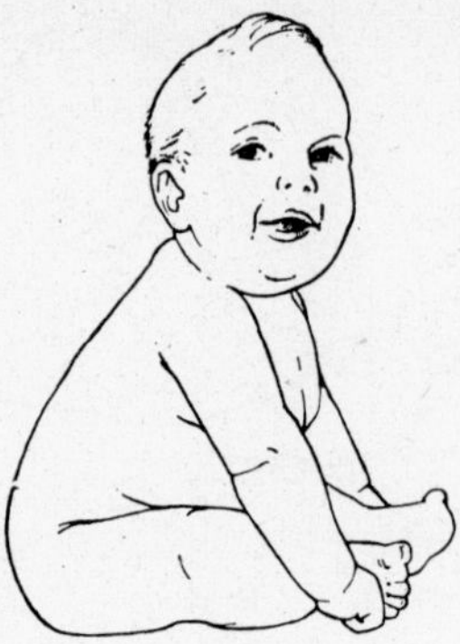

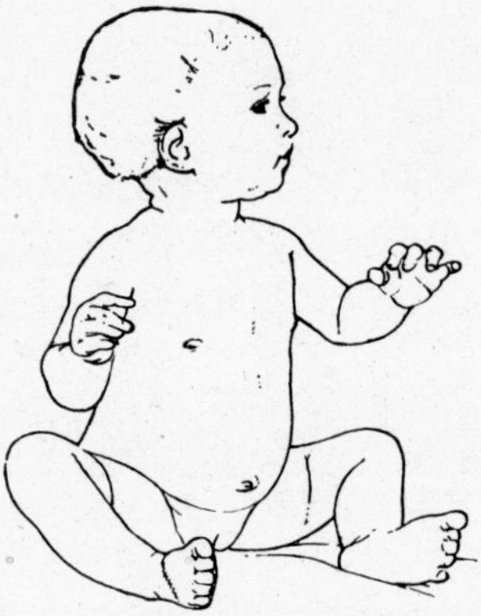

FIG. 33 (*left*). 32 weeks : Sits, no support.

FIG. 34 (*right*). 36 weeks : Leans forward to recover toy.

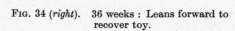

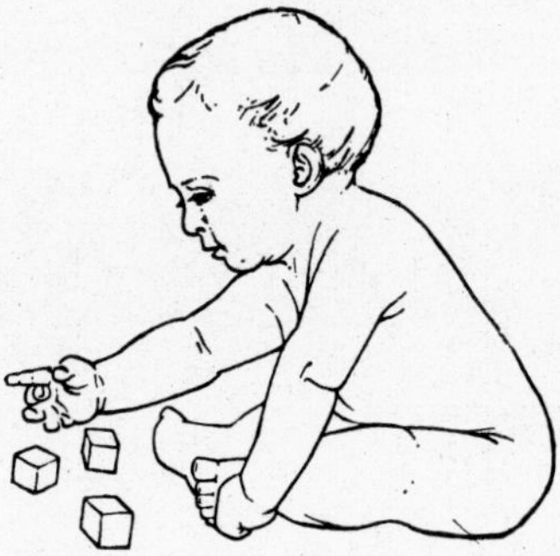

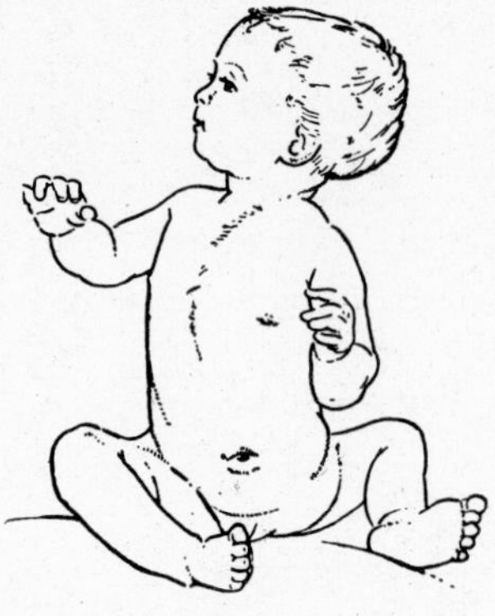

FIG. 35 (*left*). 48 weeks : Pivots.

VENTRAL SUSPENSION

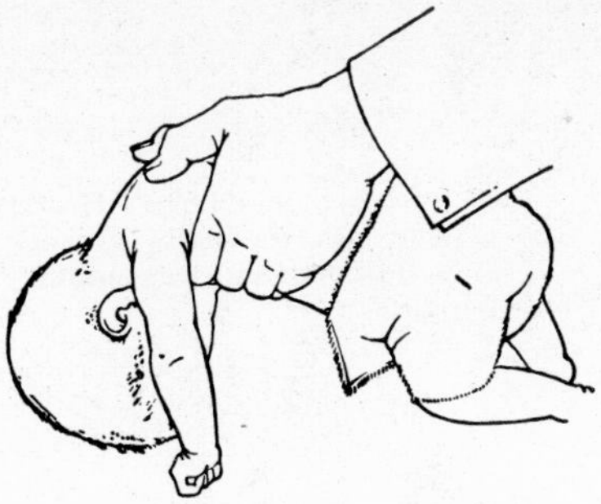

Fig. 36 (*left*). New-born : Complete head lag. Head drops.

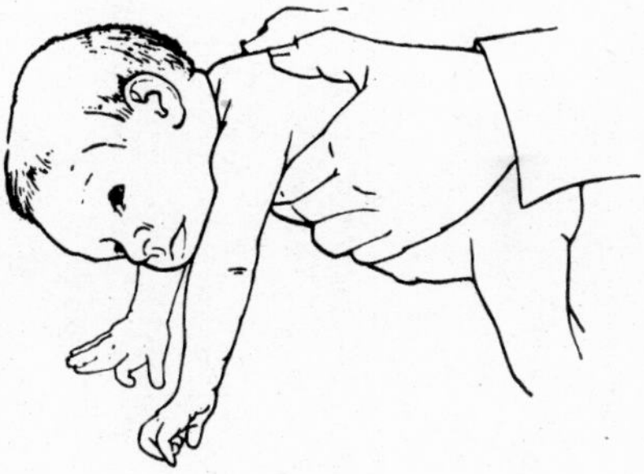

Fig. 37 (*right*). 6 weeks : Head in line with abdomen.

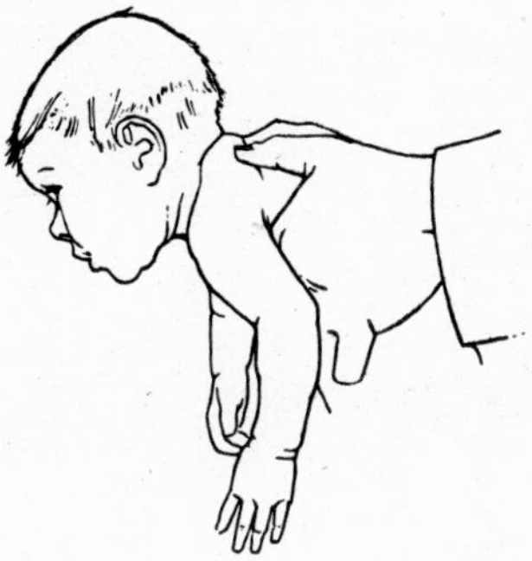

Fig. 38 (*left*). 8 weeks : Head slightly beyond plane of trunk.

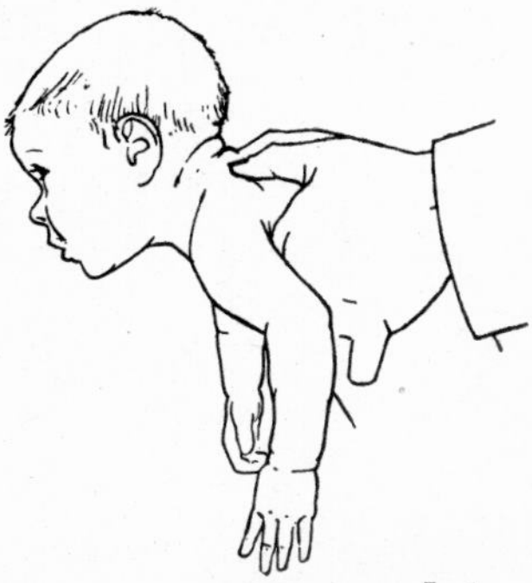

Fig. 39 (*right*). 12 weeks : Plane of head well beyond plane of trunk.

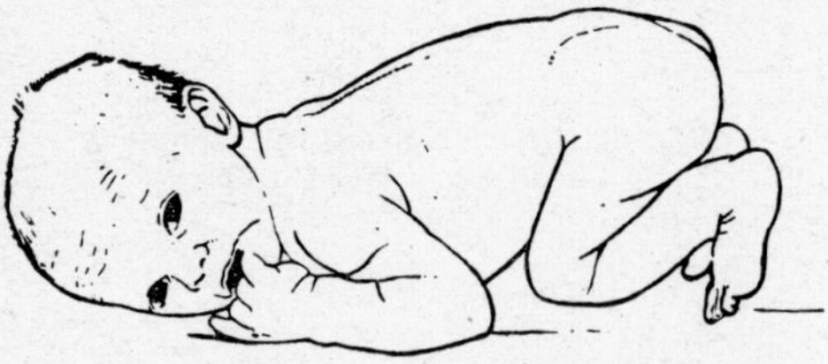

FIG. 40 (*left*). New-born : Head to side. Pelvis high. Knees and hips flexed, legs under trunk.

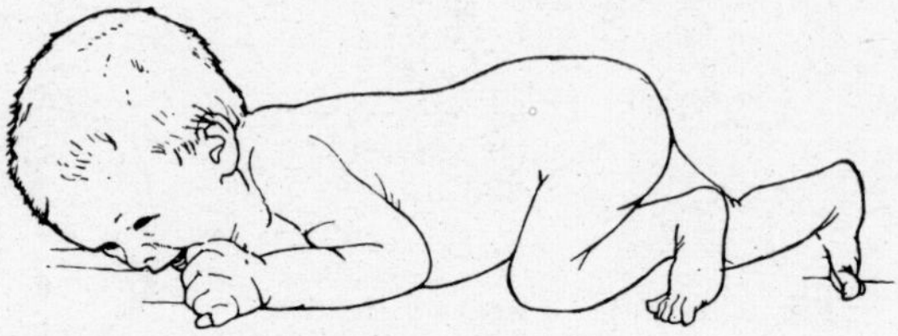

FIG. 41. 4 weeks : Chin just off couch. One leg partly extended. Other flexed.

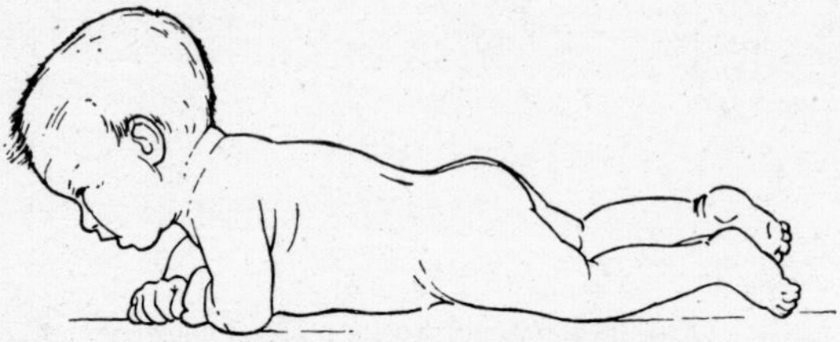

FIG. 42. 8 weeks : Plane of face at angle of 45° from couch. Legs largely extended.

FIG. 43 (*right*). 16 weeks : Plane of face at angle of 45°–90° from couch. Legs well extended.

Weight on forearms. Chin and front part of chest off couch.

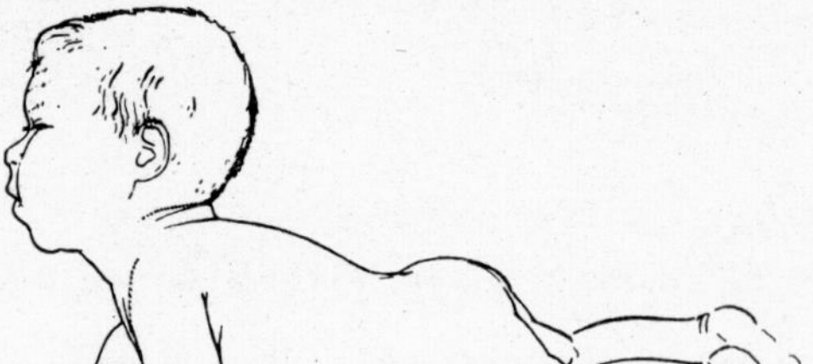

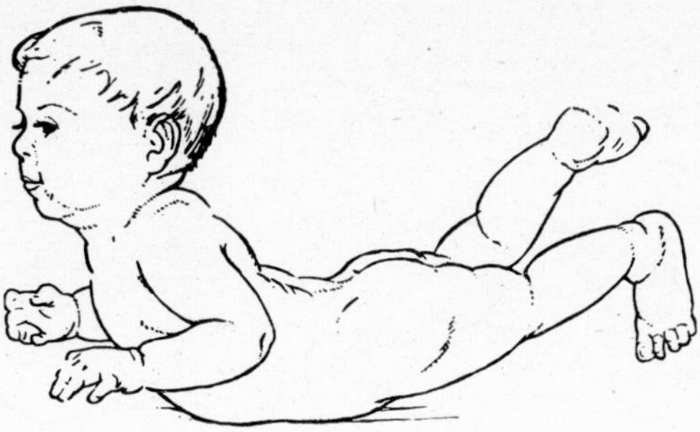

FIG. 44 (*left*). 16 weeks : Swimming.

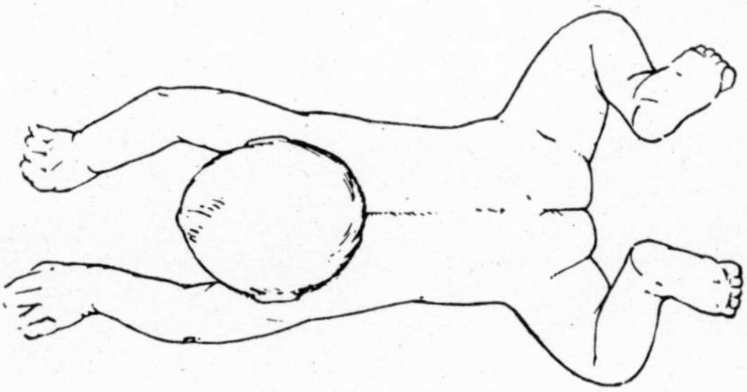

FIG. 45 (*right*). 24 weeks : Frogging.

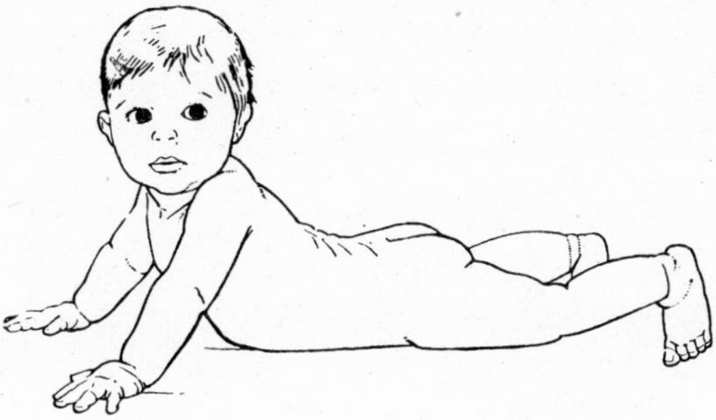

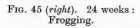

FIG. 46 (*left*). 24 weeks : Weight on hands with extended arms. Chest and upper part of abdomen off couch.

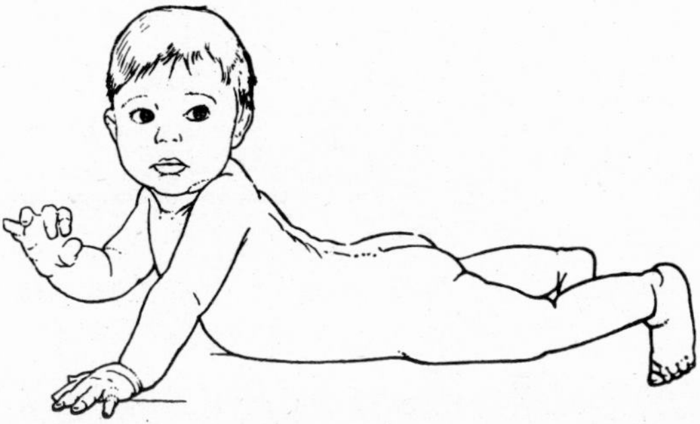

FIG. 47 (*right*). 28 weeks : Weight on one hand.

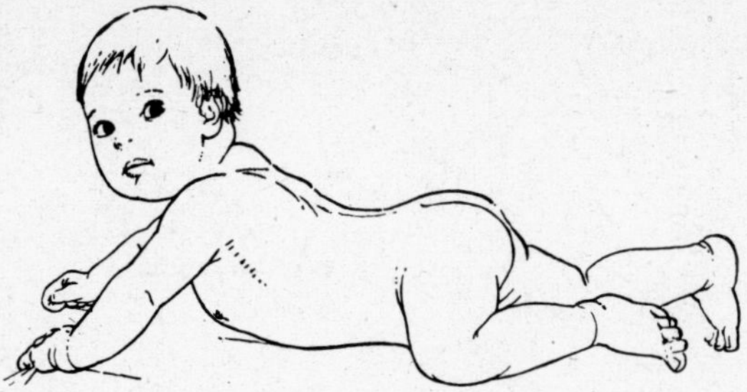

FIG. 48 (*left*). 36 weeks: Crawl. Child pulls self forward on abdomen by hand.

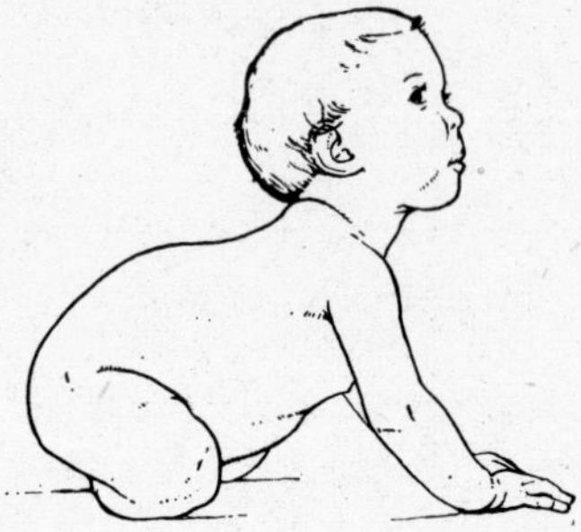

FIG. 49 (*right*). 40 weeks: Creeps. Trunk off couch.

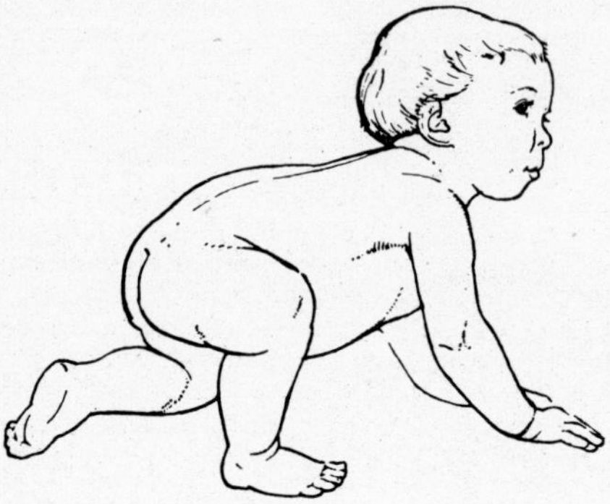

FIG. 50 (*left*). 44 weeks: Creeps. One foot flat on couch, early step.

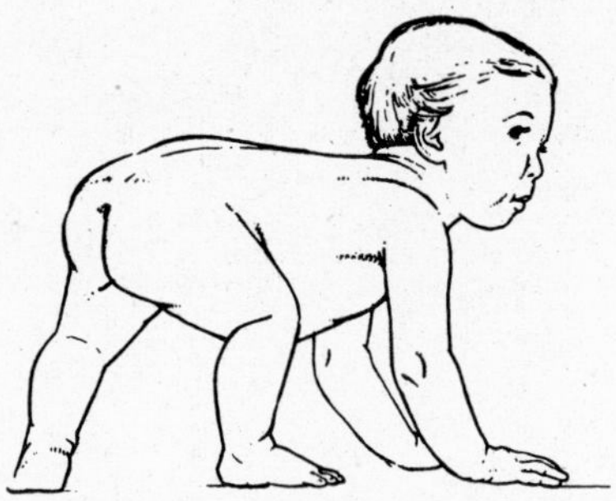

FIG. 51 (*right*). 1 year: All fours.

PULLING TO THE SITTING POSITION

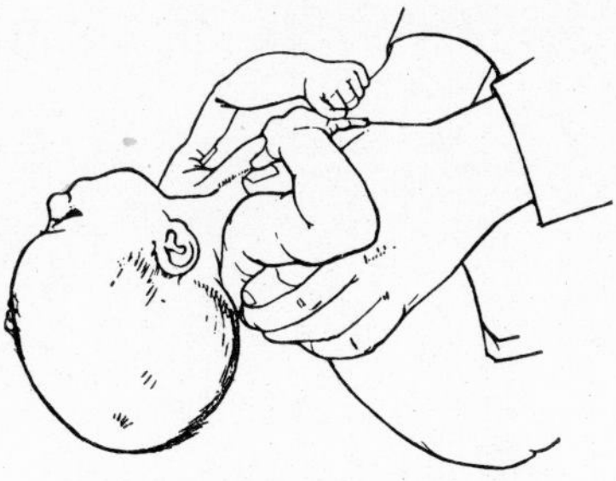

FIG. 52. New-born : Complete head lag.

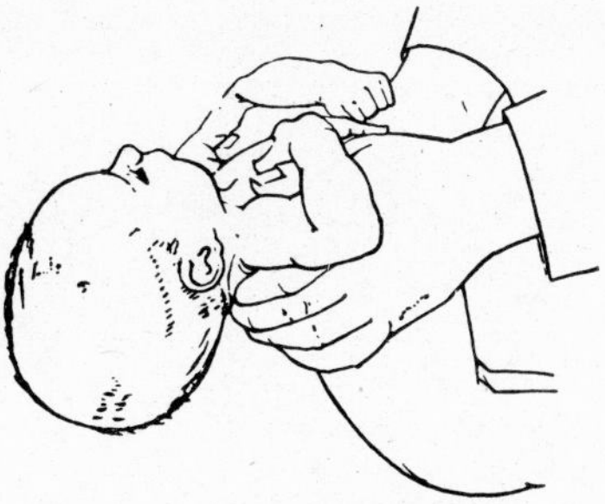

FIG. 53. 6 weeks : Not quite complete lag.

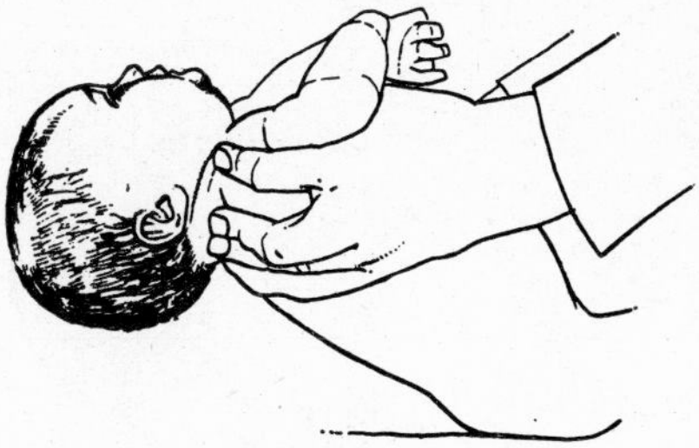

FIG. 54. 12 weeks : Only slight lag.

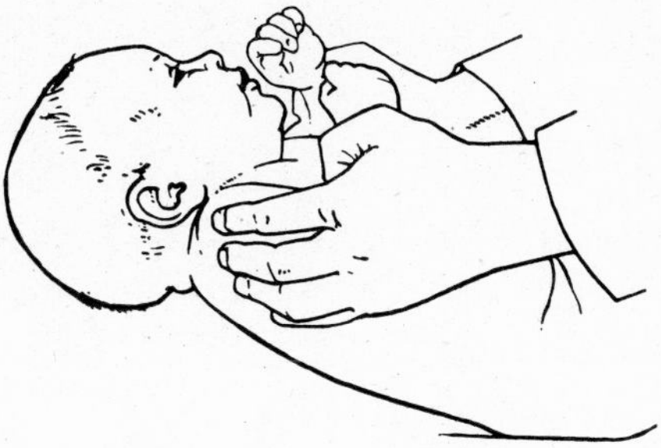

FIG. 55. 20 weeks : No head lag.

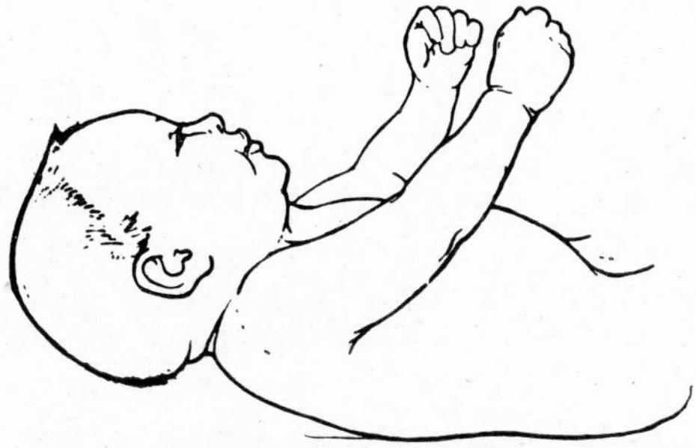

FIG. 56. 24 weeks : Lifts head off when about to be pulled up.

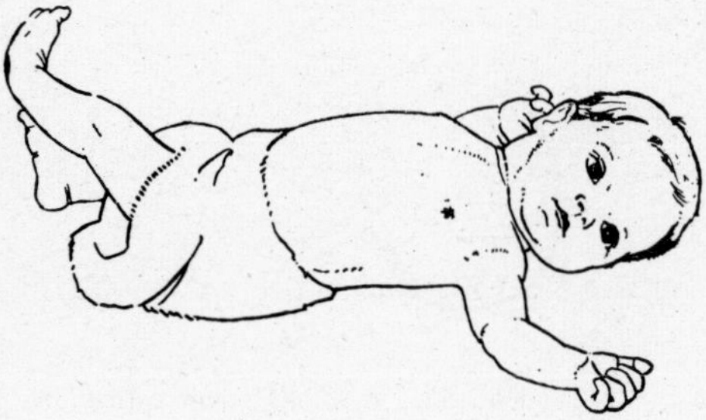

Fig. 57 (*left*). New-born : Tonic neck reflex.

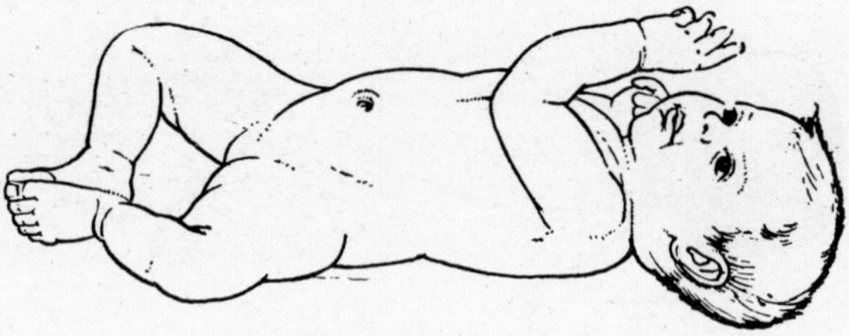

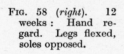

Fig. 58 (*right*). 12 weeks : Hand regard. Legs flexed, soles opposed.

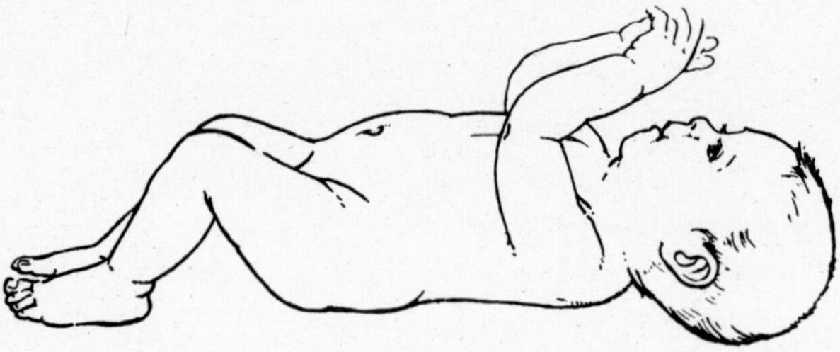

Fig. 59. 16 weeks : Head central. Plays with hands. Soles of feet on couch.

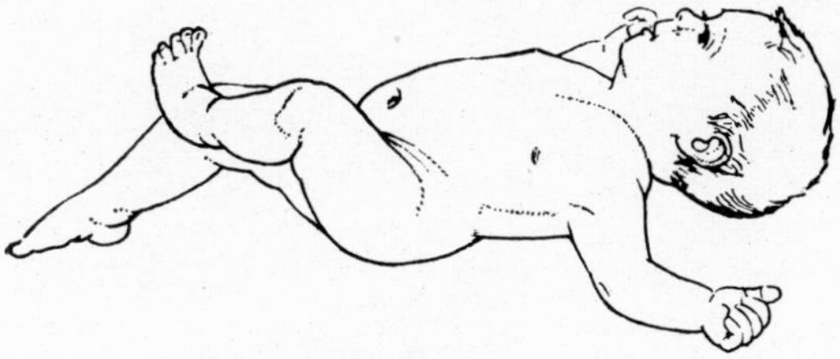

FIG. 60. 20 weeks : Foot on knee.

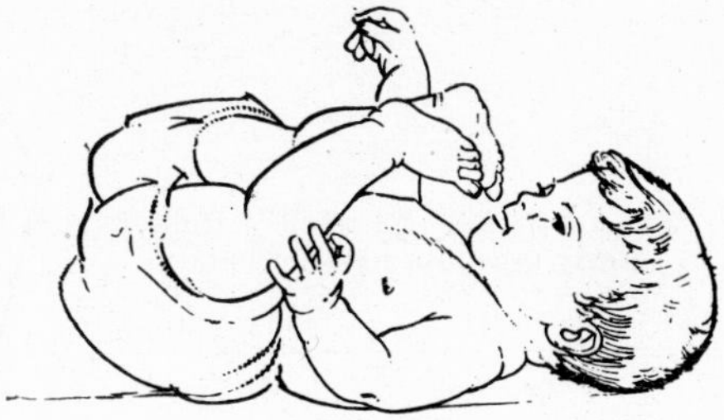

FIG. 61. 24 weeks : Grasps feet. Feet to mouth.

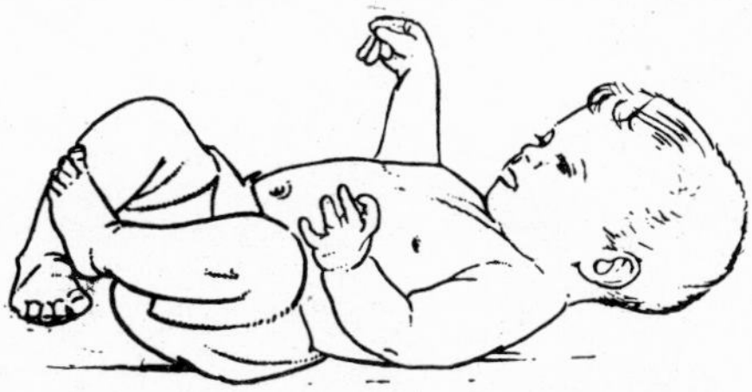

FIG. 62. 28 weeks : Spontaneously lifts head up.

MANIPULATION

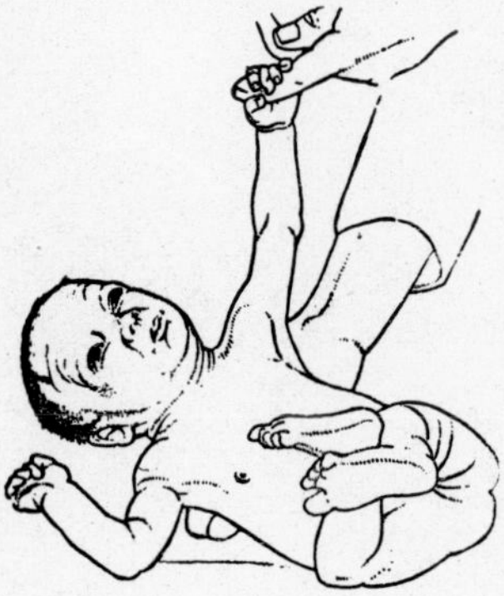

FIG. 63 (*left*). New-born : Grasp reflex.

FIG. 64 (*right*). 24 weeks : Cube. Early grasp, in palm of hand.

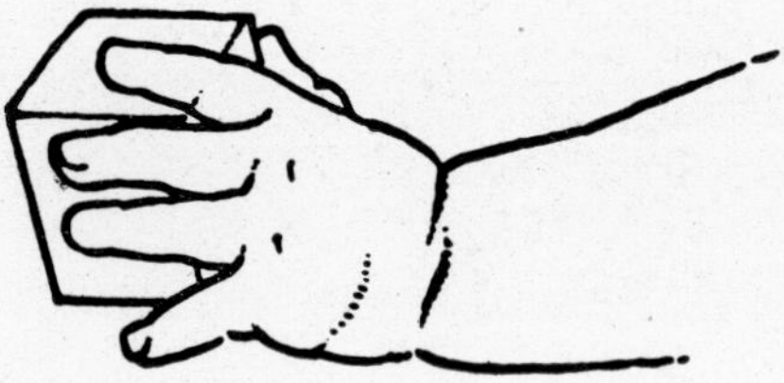

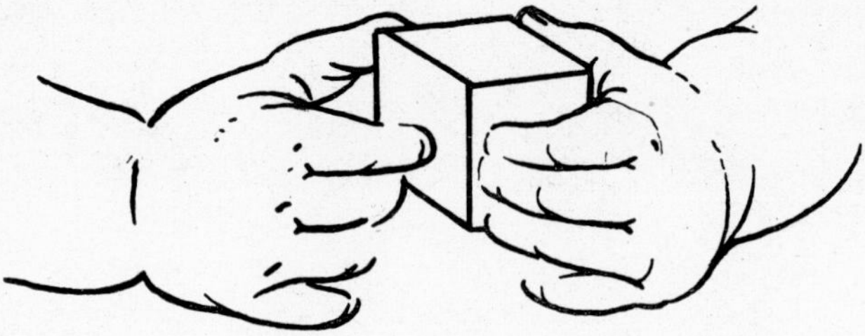

FIG. 65. 28 weeks : Transferring of object from hand to hand.

MANIPULATION

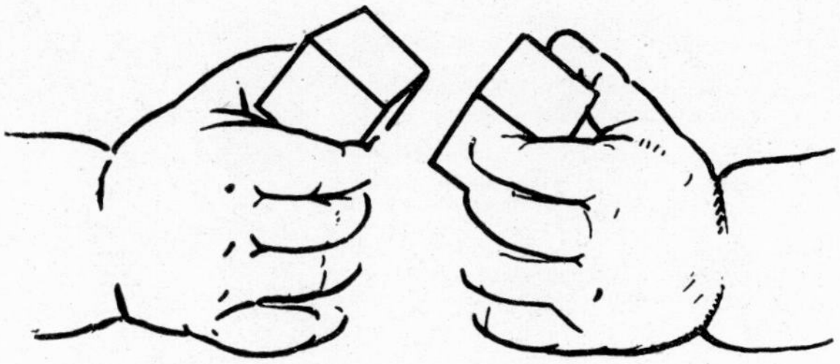

FIG. 66. 40 weeks : Matching of cubes.

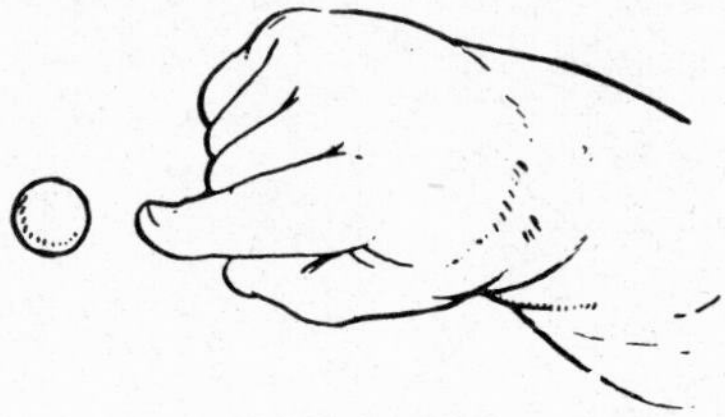

FIG. 67. 40 weeks : Index finger approach to object.

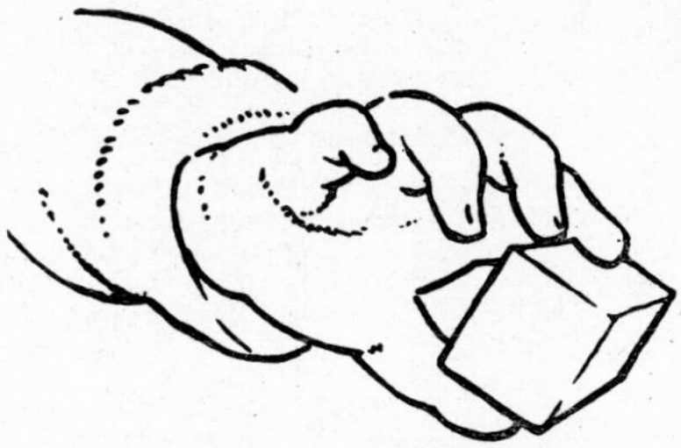

FIG. 68. 1 year : Mature grasp, between finger and thumb.

TABLE

Summary of Normal Development in the First

Age *	Gross Motor	Manipulation
4 weeks . .	Held in sitting position—may hold head up momentarily. Held in prone position with hand under abdomen, momentary tensing of neck muscles should be noted. Prone—momentarily holds chin off couch. Pull to sit—almost complete head lag.	
6 weeks . .	Held in prone position with hand under abdomen—the head is held momentarily in line with the body. Prone—readily lifts chin off couch so that plane of face is at angle of 45 degrees to couch. Pull to sit from supine—head lag not quite complete.	
8 weeks . .	Held in sitting position—head is held up but recurrently bobs forward. Held in prone position with hand under abdomen—holds head up so that its plane is in line with that of the body. Prone—head no longer mainly turned to one side as in earlier weeks. Recurrently lifts chin off couch so that plane of face is at angle of 45 degrees to couch. Held in standing position—is able to hold head up more than momentarily.	
12 weeks .	Prone—holds chin and shoulders off couch prolongedly, so that plane of face is at angle of 45–90 degrees from couch. Bears weight on forearms. Pull to sit from supine—only moderate head lag. Held in prone position with hand under abdomen—holds head up so that its plane is beyond that of the body.	Pulls at his dress. No more grasp reflex. Holds rattle voluntarily when it is placed in his hand ; retains it more than a moment. Hands no longer tightly closed as in previous weeks, but mostly open. Desire to grasp objects seen (see next column).
16 weeks .	Held in sitting position—holds head well up constantly. He looks actively around, but head still wobbles if examiner causes sudden movement of trunk. Curvature of back now only in lumbar region as compared with rounded back of earlier weeks. Prone—holds head and chest off couch so that plane of face is at 90 degrees to couch. Weight still on forearms. Pull to sit—only slight head lag in beginning of movement. Supine—head no longer rotated to one side as in earlier weeks.	Hands come together and he plays with his hands. He pulls his dress over his face in play. Approaches object with hands, but overshoots the mark and fails to reach it. Plays with rattle prolongedly when it is placed in his hand, and he shakes it.
20 weeks	Full head control. Held in sitting position—head stable when body is mildly rocked by examiner. Pull to sit—no head lag.	Now able to grasp objects deliberately. He plays with his toys, splashes in the bath and crumples paper. (From this time onwards one must note the maturity of the grasp, the ease with which he is able to secure objects, the security with which he holds them and the size of the object which he is able to grasp. He cannot bring finger and thumb together to grasp a small object of the size of a thin piece of string till he is about 9 months old.)
24 weeks .	Prone—weight borne on hands with extended arms, the chest and upper part of abdomen therefore being off the couch. Pull to sit—head lifted off couch when about to be pulled up. Hands are held out to be lifted. Sits (supported) in high chair for a few minutes. Rolls from prone to supine. Held in standing position—bears large fraction of weight.	He grasps his feet. Holds bottle. Supine—may take toes to mouth. If he has one cube in hand he drops it when second one is offered.

* For mature babies; due allowance

IX

Three Years (based largely on Gesell)

General Understanding	Speech	Sphincter Control	Miscellaneous
Watches the mother when she talks to him. Opens and closes mouth as she speaks, bobs his head, quiets. (In next two weeks or so, before smiling begins, note the duration and intensity of this reaction in assessing a child.) Supine position—regards dangling toy when it is brought into his line of vision and will follow it, but less than 90 degrees.			
Smiles momentarily when talked to by mother. (Smiling henceforward becomes more and more frequent. The frequency of smiling and the ease with which it is elicited should be noted.) Supine—looks at dangling toy when it is in midline; follows it to midline when it is moved from the side. Beginning to follow moving persons with eyes.			
Supine—follows dangling toy from side to point past midline. (Always note the promptness with which child sees the ring. At this age he does not usually see it immediately.)			Eyes show fixation, convergence, focusing.
Supine—follows dangling toy from one side to the other (180 degrees). Catches sight of it immediately. Not only smiles when spoken to but vocalizes with pleasure. Squeals of pleasure heard. (From now onwards it is essential to note the child's interest in what he sees. One must also note the obvious desire to grasp objects. This desire can be observed long before he can voluntarily go for them and get them. In another month his hands go forward for the object, but he misjudges the distance. By 5 months he can get the object.)			Supine — characteristically watches movements of own hands.
General understanding becoming much more obvious. Excites when he sees toys. Shows considerable interest when he sees breast or bottle. Shows interest in strange room. Laughs aloud. Vocalizes pleasure when pulled to sitting position. Likes to be propped up in sitting position. Turns head towards a sound.			
Smiles at image of self in mirror. When he drops his rattle he looks to see where it has gone to.			
Smiles and vocalizes at his mirror image. When he drops the rattle he tries to recover it. May "blow bubbles" or protrude tongue in imitation of adult. May show fear of strangers and be "coy." Laughs when head is hidden in towel in peep-bo game. Beginning to show likes and dislikes of foods.			

to be made for prematurity.

TABLE

Summary of Normal Development

Age *	Gross Motor	Manipulation
28 weeks .	Prone—bears weight on one hand. Sits with hands forward for support. Rolls from supine to prone. Standing position—can maintain extension of hip and knees for short period when supported. He bounces with pleasure. (Previously he sagged at hip and knees.) Supine—spontaneously lifts head off couch.	If he has one cube in hand he retains it when second cube is offered. Transfers objects from one hand to the other. Bangs objects on the table. Now goes for objects with one hand instead of two, as he did previously. Takes all objects to mouth. Feeds self with biscuit. Loves to play with paper.
32 weeks .	Readily bears whole weight on legs when supported. Sits for a few moments unsupported.	
36 weeks .	Stands holding on to furniture. Sits steadily for 10 minutes. Leans forward and recovers balance. (Cannot lean sideways.) Prone—in trying to crawl may progress backwards. May progress by rolling.	Can pick up small object such as currant between finger and thumb. When he has two cubes he brings them together as if making visual comparison between them.
40 weeks .	Pulls self to standing position. Pulls self to sitting position. Goes forward from sitting to prone, and from prone to sitting. Sits steadily without risk of falling over (except for occasional accident). Crawls, pulling self forward with hands, abdomen on couch.	Goes for objects with index finger. Beginning to release objects, letting them go deliberately instead of accidentally as before.
44 weeks .	Prone—creeps (abdomen off couch). When standing holding on he lifts and replaces one foot. Sitting—can lean over sideways.	Will place object into examiner's hand on request, but will not release it.
48 weeks .	Walks sideways, holding on to furniture. Walks with two hands held. Sitting—can turn round to pick up object.	Rolls ball towards examiner. Gives and takes toy in play, releasing object into examiner's hand.
1 year . .	Walks with one hand held. Prone—walks on hands and feet like a bear. May shuffle on buttocks and hand.	
13 months .	Stands alone for a moment.	Can hold two cubes in one hand. Makes line or marks with pencil.
15 months .	Can get into standing position without support. Creeps upstairs. Walks without help with broad-base, high-stepping gait and steps of unequal length and direction. (The maturity of the gait must be noted from now onwards.)	Builds tower of two cubes. (This requires some accuracy in release.) Constantly throwing objects on to floor. Takes off shoes.

* For mature babies; due allowance

IX—*continued*

in the First Three Years—continued

General Understanding	Speech	Sphincter Control	Miscellaneous
Pats image of self in mirror. Responds to name. Tries to establish contact with person by cough or other noise. May imitate movement, such as tongue protrusion.	Says "Da," "Ba," "Ka."		Feeds well from cup. Chews and so can take solids.
Reaches persistently for toys out of reach. Responds to "No."	Combines syllables, "Da-da," "Ba-ba."		
Puts arms in front of face to try to prevent mother washing his face. (From this age onwards note excitement when certain liked foodstuffs are seen. Note particularly degree and maintenance of concentration in getting objects and in playing with toys.)			
May pull clothes of another to attract attention. Plays "Patacake" (clapping hands). Waves bye-bye. Pats the doll. (From this age the understanding of words should be observed. The child can understand the meaning of perhaps a dozen words by the age of a year, though he is only able to say two or three words at that age. At 9 months he may respond to such questions as "Where is Daddy?" "Where is the cow?")			Slobbering and mouthing beginning to decrease.
Covers own face with towel in peep-bo game. Drops objects deliberately in order that they will be picked up. Beginning to put objects in and out of containers. (The maturity of the release behaviour and the manipulative skill must be noted as he plays with his toys).	Says one word with meaning.		
Repeats performance laughed at. Now likes repetitive play, putting one cube after another into basket, etc. Anticipates with bodily movement when nursery rhyme being told. Shows interest when shown simple pictures in book. (This interest should be carefully noted from now onwards.)			
Holds arm out for sleeve or holds foot up for sock in dressing. May understand meaning of "Where is your book?" "Where is your shoe?" May kiss on request. (Such evidence of developing memory is important and must be noted.)	Says two or three words with meaning.		Apt to be shy. Very little mouthing of objects. Little slobbering except during concentration on an especially interesting toy.
May kiss mirror image.			
Asks for objects by pointing. Pats pictures and may kiss pictures of animals. Negativism beginning. Feeds self, managing cup.	Jargon.	Tells mother that he has wet pants. (First sign of sphincter control.)	

to be made for prematurity.

TABLE

Summary of Normal Development

Age *	Gross Motor	Manipulation
18 months .	Climbs stairs unaided, holding rail. Runs. Seldom falls. Jumps. No longer broad-base and high-stepping gait when walking. Seats self in chair, often by process of climbing up, standing, turning round and sitting down. Pulls toy as he walks. Throws ball without falling, as previously.	Builds tower of three cubes. Manages spoon without rotating it near mouth as previously. Turns pages of book two or three at a time. Scribbles spontaneously. Takes off gloves, socks. Unzips fasteners.
21 months .	Walks backwards in imitation. Picks up object from floor without falling. Walks upstairs, two feet per step.	Builds tower of five or six cubes.
2 years . .	Goes up and down stairs alone, two feet per step.	Builds tower of six or seven cubes. Turns pages of book singly. Turns door knobs, unscrews lid. Puts on shoes, socks, pants. Washes and dries hands.
2½ years .	Jumps with both feet. Walks on tiptoe when asked.	Builds tower of eight cubes. Holds pencil in hand instead of in fist.
3 years . .	Goes upstairs one foot per step, and downstairs two feet per step. (Goes downstairs with one foot per step at 4 years.) Jumps off bottom step. Stands on one foot for a few seconds. Rides tricycle.	Builds tower of nine cubes. Dresses and undresses self if helped with buttons, and advised occasionally about back and front and the right foot for the shoe. Unbuttons front buttons. Can be trusted to carry china and so to help to set the table.

* For mature babies; due allowance to be made for prematurity.
† Two cards, showing dog, cup, house, shoe, flag, clock, star, leaf, basket, book.
‡ Penny, shoe, pencil, knife, ball.
§ "Take it to mother," "Put it on the chair," "Bring it to me," "Put it on the table."
|| Copying a circle implies copying a representation of a circle on a card given by the

IX—*continued*

in the First Three Years—continued

General Understanding	Speech	Sphincter Control	Miscellaneous
Points to picture of car or dog in book. Picture Card.† Points correctly to one when asked "Where is the . . .?" Simple objects.‡ Names one. Points to nose, eye, hair on request. Copies mother in her domestic work—e.g. sweeping the floor, dusting. Carries out two simple orders.§		Clean and dry with only occasional accident.	Dawdling in feeding.
Pulls people to show them objects. Knows four parts of the body. Picture Card.† Points correctly to two when asked "Where is the . . . ?" Simple orders.§ Obeys three.	Joins two words together. Repeats things said. Asks for drink, toilet, food.		Sleeping difficulties common. Sleep rituals beginning.
Imitates train with cubes, without adding chimney. Imitates vertical stroke with pencil. Knows two common objects.‡ Obeys four simple orders.§ Parallel play—watches others play and plays near them, without playing with them. Picture Cards.† Names three when asked "What is this ?" Identifies five when asked "Where is the . . . ?" (Much can be learnt by noting the maturity of the play and the imaginativeness shown.)	Uses words : I, me, you. Talks incessantly.	Dry at night if lifted out late in evening.	
Imitates train with cubes, adding chimney. Imitates vertical and horizontal stroke with pencil. Repeats two digits (one out of three trials)—e.g. asked to say "Eight—six." Picture Cards.† Names five objects when asked "What is this?" Identifies seven when asked "Where is the . . . ?" Common objects.‡ Names three. Beginning to take interest in sex organs. Peak of negativism. Gives full name. Helps to put things away.		Attends to toilet without help, except for wiping. Climbs on to lavatory seat.	Colour sense beginning.
Copies circle with pencil,‖ imitates cross (copies cross at 3½, square at 4, diamond at 5). Constantly asking questions. Knows own sex. Picture Card.† Names eight when asked "What is this . . . ?" (Names ten at 3½ years.) Repeats three digits (one out of three trials). (Repeats four digits in one out of three trials at 4½.) Obeys two requests when asked "Put the ball under the chair, at the side of the chair, behind the chair, on the chair." (Obeys four at 4 years.) Knows some nursery rhymes. May count up to 10. Now joins children in play. Dresses and undresses doll. Beginning to draw objects spontaneously (e.g. a man), or on request. Cubes. Imitates building bridge of three cubes.			

examiner. When a child "imitates" a circle he draws one after seeing the examiner do it.

CHAPTER 17

GENERAL FACTORS WHICH AFFECT THE COURSE OF DEVELOPMENT

THE factor which affects the rate of development more than any other is the intelligence of the child. This has already been discussed.

The following additional factors have always to be borne in mind when an assessment of a child is being made :

Premature Delivery

It is obvious that if a baby is born prematurely, due allowance must be made in comparing his development with that of average children. If, for instance, he was born 2 months prematurely, he has missed 2 months' development *in utero*, and so he must be expected to achieve various skills 2 months later than full-term infants. A corresponding allowance has to be made in the case of post-mature infants.

The Environment

Development depends on the maturation of the nervous system. It cannot be accelerated by training and practice until the nervous system is ready, and then the acceleration is only slight. It can be considerably retarded by lack of practice when the nervous system is ready for a particular skill. Owing to the fact, however, that the nervous system continues to mature throughout the period of deprivation of practice, there is a very rapid progress as soon as practice is allowed, so that in a short time the child catches up to the average. Weiss [446] points out that the butterfly inside the pupal case is unable to move because of lack of space. After breaking the case it immediately frees itself by well-co-ordinated movements, creeps out of its envelope, spreads its crumpled wings and flies off as soon as they have dried without ever having had a chance of learning and practising the various performances. The Dennises [106] performed a particularly cruel experiment on a pair of twin girls whom they obtained at the age of 5 weeks. They reared them with an absolute minimum of stimulation and of practice until the age of 14 months. The children were not allowed to see each other. They were removed from the crib only for the purpose of feeding or washing. No one spoke to the twins or made any kind of overture to them. They were given no opportunity to sit, stand or practise other skills. Neither twin was able to sit alone at a year of age and neither could bear any weight on the legs, but after 4 days of practice they could sit and bear their weight on the legs. Swaddling is still practised in Albania and amongst certain American Indians.[166] Greenacre[166] and Bühler[76] showed that within a few hours of their release infants who had been bound down and kept immobile for a year could do as much with the hands and legs as average children. Bühler remarks that they appear to pass through a series of stages in a matter of hours for which normal children require several months.

Gesell,[149] Bowlby[55] and many others have discussed the profound effect which institutional life has on the rate of development. Children who are brought up from earliest infancy in institutions are frequently not given opportunities to sit when they are ready for it, to stand holding on when they are ready to do so and to walk with help when they have reached that stage, simply because no one really has time to give to them. As a result they are retarded in sitting, walking and other skills. There is also retardation in physical, intellectual and social development. Even by the age of 2 or 3 months babies in such institutions are found to vocalize less than normal babies. By 4 months there is considerable retardation. Bowlby wrote that the developmental quotient falls from about 65 for those who have been in institutions for 2–6 months to 50 for those who have been in them for over a year. The retardation is least marked in locomotion and most marked in speech. Sphincter control is acquired late, because there is no individualization of training, all children, irrespective of their needs, merely being taken to the toilet at set times. Bowlby therefore emphasized the importance of early adoption, before the harmful effects of institutional life are fully experienced. The progressive nature of the retardation is important in the assessment of suitability for adoption, for when one finds that a child so separated from his mother is retarded, it is wrong to ask to see the child again for assessment after a further period in the institution, for in that case further retardation will have occurred. The correct line to take is to try to have the child placed into a good foster-home as soon as possible and then assess him after 2 or 3 months in such a home. If his retardation was merely due to institutional life and emotional deprivation, it will rapidly disappear as soon as he gets into a good home. If there is still significant retardation after such a trial period, the prognosis for future intelligence is poor. Every effort is now being made in institutions to reduce the damaging effect of institutional life on the child's development.

Minor degrees of emotional deprivation and of restriction of opportunities to learn commonly occur in the home. Some mothers seem to be unable to hear the cries of their baby in the pram outside the house. He cries for hours on account of sheer boredom and inability to see what is going on and to practise his new skills. Full-time employment by the mother is apt to lead to this neglect of children when they most need their mothers. Some mothers deliberately keep their children off their feet for fear that they will develop knock-knee or rickets. They prevent them from sitting for fear the spine will be weakened. Severe illnesses have a similarly retarding effect. It must be remembered, however, that when practice is given, the recovery is very rapid. It is inevitable that a child who is never given a chance to learn to feed himself or to dress himself will be late in learning those skills. A child who is given no chance to use a toilet when he asks to do so will inevitably be late in acquiring sphincter control. One commonly sees a 6- or 7-year-old child in an out-patient clinic who is dressed and undressed by his mother, because he has never been given the opportunity to learn to do it himself.

The same kind of deprivation may be responsible for lateness in speaking. Some mothers fail to talk to their children. They fail to point out the names of objects and to show them pictures in books. As a result their children are late in learning the meaning of words, and so they are later than others in learning to speak.

Wellman * went so far as to say that intelligence depends entirely on environment. Wellman thought that normal children can be made feeble-minded, and feeble-minded children geniuses, if the environment is suitable. Few, however, would agree with this extreme view.

The factor of practice is of vital importance in development. Due allowance must always be made for it in the assessment of a child. It affects almost all fields of development, and failure to allow for it may lead to considerable errors.

Familial Factors

It is well known that intelligence is in large part genetically determined. Bowlby [55] went so far as to say that the intelligence of the parents is probably the best guide to the intelligence of the child, though he admits that this is only a rough guide. One difficulty is that there is a tendency for the intelligence of children from one generation to another to revert to the average. Terman and Oden,[412] in a long-term follow up of 1,528 children with an I.Q. of 140 or more, found that the mean I.Q. of 384 offspring was 127·7. Nevertheless the number of offspring with an 1.Q of 150 or more was 28 times greater than that of unselected children. On the other hand, Skodak [386] tested the intelligence of 16 children whose mothers were feeble-minded, with an average I.Q. of 66·4. The average I.Q. of the children was 116·4, ranging from 95 to 131, and therefore within normal limits. Fairbank [125] made a very similar observation with a much larger

* Quoted by Arlitt.[22]

number of children. In each case there is a tendency for the level of intelligence to revert to the average.

The familial factor is often prominent in individual fields of development. In some families the development of locomotion, speech or sphincter control may be unusually early or unusually late, the development in all the other fields of development being average.

Sex

Girls tend to learn to walk, speak and to acquire sphincter control earlier than boys.

Normal Variations

There are great normal variations in the rate of development. These variations concern primarily individual fields of development, though the rare abnormal patterns of development, such as that of the slow starter, have been mentioned elsewhere. Particular emphasis has been placed on the fact that most children will pass the various "milestones" of development earlier or later than the average figures given. It is impossible to give the range of "normality" because it is impossible to define "normality" in development. As a rough guide, however, I have set down below some of the variations in the ages at which various milestones are passed by children who turn out to be perfectly "normal" in later years. It would be quite wrong to suggest that any child who fell outside these ranges (on the wrong side of them) was mentally defective or otherwise abnormal, but it stands to reason that the further away from the average a child's development is the less likely it is to be "normal."

Smiling. The earliest age at which I have myself seen a child smile in response to social overture was 6 days. From that day onwards the smiling in this child became more and more frequent. Very few normal full-term babies have reached 8 weeks of age without having begun to smile.

Grasping. Voluntary grasping may occur as early as $3\frac{1}{2}$ months. It is commonly not seen till the age of 6 months.

Locomotion. Few normal children are unable to sit without help by the age of 8 months. I have, however, seen a child who was unable to sit without help until 19 months, or to walk without help till 30 months. He had no detectable physical disability, and he was followed up till the age of 5 years, when his I.Q. was 110. It is quite common to see a normal child who cannot walk without help until the age of 17 or 18 months. On the other hand I have seen children sitting without support on the floor at 5 months. I saw a child roll from supine to prone at the age of 18 weeks, creep at 22 weeks, pull himself to the standing position at 25 weeks, walk holding on to furniture at 6 months, and walk well with two hands held at the same age. He walked unaided at 8½ months. He was in no way advanced in any other field of development, and at the age of 5 his I.Q. was 88.

Speech. The normal variations in speech are very considerable. Gesell and his co-workers [146] wrote that the first word is usually spoken with meaning any time between 9 and 15 months. They found that the normal 2-year-old may have only a few words in his vocabulary or well over 2,000. Speech in some is acquired unusually early and there are many recorded instances of precocious speech. Barlow, for instance,[41] described a child who could talk perfectly at 4 months and read at 1 year. It is recorded that Thomas Carlyle, hitherto unable to say a single word, at the age of 10 months heard a fellow baby crying and suddenly said, "What ails thee, Jock ?" and from that time onward spoke in sentences. Retardation in speech is extremely common ; some of the causes of this are discussed on p. 205, but in many children there is no discoverable cause. It is common for no word to be spoken till the age of 15 months, and for a child normal in every other respect to be saying nothing but single words at the age of 2½ years. One has certainly heard of otherwise normal children who could not be said to be able to "talk" till the age of 4 or 5 years, but such children should always be fully investigated for the various factors mentioned on p. 206, and especially for high-tone deafness.

Sphincter Control. There are great individual variations in the age at which this is acquired. In many children the early "conditioning" may be replaced gradually and unnoticeably by voluntary control, so that they are dry by day from 6 months or so onwards without anything but an occasional accident. Apart altogether from mismanagement, which is discussed on p. 280, some children do not acquire control by day till 2½ or 3 years and are still unreliable by night at the age of 3½ years. In all other respects they are entirely normal.

It is worth emphasizing again that no child is mentally retarded who is backward in a single field of development and normal in all other fields. The mentally retarded child is backward in all fields of development, except sometimes in sphincter control, though often more so in some (especially speech) than in others (especially locomotion). As far as I know the only exception to this rule is the child who acquires the mental defect as the result of encephalitis, a vascular catastrophe or a demyelinating disease, after a period of normal development. It is obvious that in such a child the milestones may have been passed at the ordinary times. Other exceptions to the rule are excessively rare and can for practical purposes be ignored.

Personality

The personality of a child may have a considerable bearing on the age at which he learns various skills. Some babies are much more independent than others, and therefore much more determined to practise new skills, such as feeding themselves or attending to their own toilet needs. Lack of confidence will retard walking. Some children have a much greater desire than others to speak, and the age at which speech is acquired is therefore influenced by this.

The great part played by personality in the later progress of the child is responsible for the comparative failure of many efforts to predict a child's future progress. Developmental tests may with reasonable certainty enable one to predict average intelligence, but the prediction of personality is a matter of extreme difficulty (p. 159). A man with only moderate intelligence but the right sort of personality is quite likely to do better in life, given equal opportunities, than a man with a high degree of intelligence with an unpleasant personality. The personality factor is the source of the greatest difficulty in the assessment of a child for the purposes of adoption. It is inevitable that a child will have inherited personality characteristics from his parents, and it is almost impossible, particularly without knowledge of the parents, to know how these will affect his future.

Physical Handicaps

Cerebral palsy may affect almost all fields of development and cause severe general retardation. Other handicaps such as deafness and blindness have a considerable influence on the rate of development. This is not the place to discuss the early diagnosis of these conditions. They are discussed in detail by Gesell and Amatruda.[149]

Lulls and Spurts

Shirley [380] and others have pointed out that when one skill is being actively learned another skill tends to go into abeyance. When, for instance, a child is actively learning to grasp objects vocalization may decrease. It then reappears, only to decrease when sitting is being perfected. There is often a lull in the development of speech at the time that a child is learning to walk. The child seems to make no progress at all for some months, and then suddenly, for no apparent reason, he makes very rapid headway. I have seen a child who at 15 months was well below the average in speech, while at 18 months he was far above the average. It seems as if in some children two major skills cannot be learnt at the same time. During the decreased activity in the one skill, however, the nervous system is maturing, and when the activity reappears it is found that surprisingly extensive progress is suddenly made.

CHAPTER 18

RETARDATION IN SINGLE FIELDS OF DEVELOPMENT AND FACTORS RESPONSIBLE

Sitting

THE age at which a child learns to sit is affected by all the general factors mentioned in the preceding chapter. The role of practice is particularly important. If a mother has kept the baby lying flat all day he will inevitably be retarded in learning to sit. Hypotonia for any reason, such as rickets, postpones the date at which the child is able to sit alone. Due allowance must always be made for premature delivery.

It is interesting to note that children who are brought up in institutions sometimes learn to creep before they learn to sit. This is presumably because they are able to creep without help, but they need help in learning to sit and there is little time for the attendants to help them in this way.

Walking

Any of the general factors already mentioned may delay walking. Anything which keeps a child off his feet, whether illness, mismanagement or institutional life, will retard walking. Some babies become so adept at creeping that they do not bother to learn to walk. Many babies learn an aberrant form of progression called shuffling or hitching, progressing by means of buttock and hand, often at considerable speed. This retards walking, largely because the movements involved in shuffling do not naturally lead to walking.

The personality of the child has an important bearing on the age at which a child walks without help. Some babies are very cautious and are unwilling to walk without support when ready for it, even though that support consists only of the mother's finger. It is not unusual to see a child who has been walking with one hand held for 4 or 5 months because of such lack of confidence. When he does walk without support he walks well, because his nervous system has been maturing throughout, and within a day or two of first taking off without support he is walking a great deal with only an occasional fall. A cautious child like this is apt to be badly disturbed by falls, and he may refuse to try to walk for several days after a bad bump. Falls are apt to occur as a result of slipperiness of the soles of shoes, and for this reason the soles of shoes for children of this age should have a non-skid surface.

Walking is severely delayed by hypotonia, due to rickets, pink disease and other conditions, and by hypertonia due to cerebral palsy. Congenital dislocation of the hip does not delay walking. Familial factors are important. In some families children walk particularly early, at 8 or 9 months of age, while in others they walk later than the average, at 17 or 18 months, and yet the children are " normal " in every other respect. It is likely that there is a genetic factor which governs the rate of myelination of parts of the nervous system, and so the age at which the relevant skills are learned.

Sphincter Control

Sphincter control may be seriously delayed by mismanagement of " training " in the form of compelling the child to sit on the toilet when he is trying to get off, and punishing him for " accidents." This is discussed on p. 280. It is delayed in children in institutions which are apt to have rigid routines that involve placing all the children on the toilet at definite times every day. This inevitably fails to take into account the needs of the individual, and control is likely to be months later in such children than in others. A similar failure to help children when they are learning to control the sphincters is found in some homes. In private homes, however, excessive attempts to " train children " are far commoner than neglect to " train " them at all.

In more than half of all cases of serious delay in the acquisition of control of the bladder, there is a family history of the same complaint.

The single passage of a hard stool which causes pain may lead to withholding of stools, and so to constipation with diarrhœa and incontinence (p. 281). Structural changes in the urethra may delay the acquisition of control of the bladder for years (p. 283). Personality factors operate here as in other fields of development. Some children acquire control with little emotional disturbance. Others, particularly the more sensitive and determined types, are apt to experience phases of resistance and so are delayed in the acquisition of control.

Manipulation

The way in which children are delayed in learning to feed and dress themselves has already been described.

Play behaviour is greatly modified by the parental management. Some parents fail to give their children toys suitable for their age, and in particular they fail to give them constructive toys at a time when they are ready for them and enjoy them. It is inevitable that such children will be less advanced than others who have had more opportunities to use their fingers.

Speech

By lateness in the development of speech I do not mean lateness in learning to speak distinctly. Dyslalia, or the substitution of letters, leading to indistinctness of speech, though it often occurs in children who have learnt to speak late, by no means always does so. By lateness in developing speech I mean lateness in beginning to say single words with meaning, and subsequently in putting two or three words together.

The commonest cause of lateness in the development of speech is a low level of intelligence. A mentally backward child is late in all fields of development (except occasionally in sphincter control), and he is usually more retarded in speech than in motor and manipulative development. It is essential to reiterate, however, that one should never even suspect mental retardation in a child who is late merely in one field of development, like speech, and who is normal in other fields. The understanding of words is of much greater importance in assessing a child's intelligence than his ability to say them. I saw a 15-month-old child who could readily point out 200 common objects in picture books, when asked "Where is the . . . ?" (drum, cup, soldier, etc.), though he could only say four or five words himself. Einstein caused considerable anxiety in his parents because he was unable to speak at the age of 4. Many other highly intelligent children have been late in learning to talk. The factors responsible are obscure.

Familial factors are very commonly concerned with speech development. When a child is late in learning to speak, and yet there are other indications that his intelligence is normal, one more often than not finds that there is a family history of similar lateness in speech development. Karlin and Kennedy [228] suggested that speech, like other skills, depends on myelination of the appropriate part of the nervous system, and that this is related to familial factors.

Deafness is a most important condition which must always be borne in mind in these children. The child who is deaf in both ears in infancy does not learn to speak without special training. An excellent account of the early diagnosis of deafness is given by Gesell.[149] Amongst other features he mentioned the child's general indifference to sound, his lessened vocalizations and sound play, his yelling and screaming in his efforts to express pleasure, annoyance and needs. The child shows exaggerated alertness to gesture and movement, preoccupation with things rather than persons and an inquiring, confused or thwarted expression. Of all these symptoms the lessened vocalizations and sound play are probably the most important.

When a child is partially deaf in both ears, he may learn the sounds which he can see made—b, f, w but not the g, l, r. He tends to substitute other letters—d for g, y for l, w for r.

High-frequency deafness is a very important cause of lateness in speaking. It is well discussed by Orton [323] and others. The defect in hearing involves pitches which are used in human speech, normally those between 512 and 2,048 double vibrations per second, while the child may be able to distinguish sounds of the 256 or 512 double-vibration tuning forks, responding to the low-frequency whispers, clicks and clapping of the hands that are commonly used as hearing tests. He can hear the passing car and banging door and will listen to the radio, so that his parents are loth to consider the possibility that he is deaf. Such children are either late in learning to speak or, more commonly, speak badly owing to the omission of certain high-pitched sounds such as consonants, and particularly the s and f, which they do not hear in the speech of others.

Only experts can test for hearing, particularly for high-tone deafness, in infants and small children. The tests which can be used were discussed by Beebe [42] and by Dix and Hallpike.[112, 113] The latter workers use a peep-show technique which gives good results long before a standard audiometer can be used.

Attention has already been drawn to the fact that the development of speech, including the early vocalization of the infant, goes into abeyance when motor skills, such as walking, are being learnt. A child may appear to make no progress at all in speech for some weeks or months and then quite suddenly speak a great deal.

It has been said that delay in the establishment of handedness is associated with delay in learning to speak, but I am doubtful whether this is true. I am also uncertain whether the so-called " congenital word deafness " (" congenital auditory imperception ") exists or not.

When a child is brought up in an institution, he may not be given opportunities to learn speech because attendants have not sufficient time to talk to him. It is fashionable to say that some children are late in learning to speak because their parents do not talk to them sufficiently, or because they do everything for them so that they do not bother to speak. I do not believe that there is any truth in these ideas. I do not believe that any child fails to speak because he is " lazy." It is very wrong to instruct a parent of a late speaker not to do things for the child unless he speaks, on the grounds that he is being lazy. I have seen this cause the most troublesome behaviour problems. The child does not speak because he cannot, and it is sheer cruelty to refuse to attend to his needs in an effort to make him talk.

The psychological background of late speakers was fully reviewed by Eisenson.[120] He concluded that there is a higher incidence of maladjustment in the parents, especially the mothers, of late speakers than there is in parents of children who speak at the usual time. There was a greater emotional instability in those parents, more perfectionism, restrictiveness and over-protectiveness. The home environment tended to be characterized by confusion, tension and lack of organization.

Obviously this did not apply to all cases : but it did apply to the group of late speakers as a whole.

Eisenson suggested that parental rejection, taking the form of continuous disapproval and criticism of speech as well as of other forms of behaviour, may cause a child to stop talking or to talk less. He wrote that a child's speech may regress when a new sibling arrives. In my opinion the idea that jealousy is a common cause of lateness in speech is overdone. I have never seen such a case. All children are jealous, and lateness in speech is common. It is not easy to relate one to the other. Lateness in speech is never due to tongue tie (p. 117). In cerebral palsy lateness in speech is very common ; it may be due to one or more of the following factors—a low level of intelligence, inco-ordination or spasticity of the muscles of the tongue, and partial deafness.

It must be admitted that in many cases the reason for lateness in speech is not clear.

Dyslalia. The commonest form of dyslalia is the lisp, due to protrusion of the tongue between the teeth when the letter s is being used. In the great majority of children it disappears without treatment. Other forms of dyslalia should only be treated by a speech therapist if they persist past the fourth birthday. They should be treated then, so that the child's speech will be normal by the time he starts school.

"Nasal speech," involving the substitution of b for m, may be due to postnasal obstruction by adenoids. The speech returns to normal a few weeks after their removal. The distinctness of speech is often temporarily disturbed by coryza.

Tongue tie may cause difficulty in the pronunciation of certain letters (p. 117). Severe malocclusion may be a cause of indistinct speech. As speech is learnt by imitation, it is obvious that defective speech may be learnt from others.

The problem of stuttering is discussed elsewhere (p. 315).

Conclusion

It will be seen that there are many factors other than the intelligence of the child which affect the course of development. Some of those factors affect practically all fields of development, while others affect isolated skills only. All these factors must be considered in the assessment of every child. *Developmental diagnosis is a personal individual problem, in that no prediction can be made until all the various factors which may have affected the development and which may affect it in the future are duly assessed.* It is for this reason that some large-scale statistical studies have failed to demonstrate correlation between observations in infancy and subsequent intelligence tests. They were impersonal, failing to consider the children as individuals.

No diagnosis of mental deficiency must ever be made or suspected on account of retardation in a single field of development. If such a diagnosis is made, it will be wrong.

The Treatment of Isolated Retardation

When a child is retarded in a single field of development, such as locomotion, speech or sphincter control, there is usually nothing to be done about it, unless there is an underlying cause which is treatable, such as lack of practice in the case of locomotion, deafness in the case of speech or parental mismanagement in the case of sphincter control. It has already been explained that development depends on the maturation of the nervous system, and therefore that no amount of practice and teaching will enable a child to learn skills unless the nervous system is ready for them. The physiotherapist, therefore, cannot help to make a child walk unless there is an associated mechanical difficulty, such as hypotonia or spasticity. The speech therapist cannot help in teaching a child to talk unless there is an underlying cause of the retardation, such as deafness, and the nervous system is otherwise ready for the acquisition of speech.

CHAPTER 19

DEVELOPMENTAL DIAGNOSIS

The Developmental History

It is often said that it is a waste of time to take a history of past development because it is so unreliable. I disagree strongly with this opinion. It is obvious, of course, that some parents when questioned know very little about the skills which their children have developed and when they developed them. Of all the hundreds of parents whom I have interrogated concerning their children's development, probably the least knowledgeable were a doctor and his medically-qualified wife. Many parents are not only non-observant but have a bad memory, and therefore cannot remember when skills were learned. This is particularly liable to be the case in large families. Nevertheless it is always the task of a doctor in taking a history to assess the story which he is given. In taking a developmental history the doctor assesses the mother's veracity and memory. He decides by the way she replies whether the answer was made up on the spur of the moment or whether it was likely to be a true one. When in doubt he comes back to the point at issue and asks the question in a different way in order to see whether the replies tally. He knows quite well that parents of a retarded child are often unwilling to allow themselves to believe what they know is the truth—that the child is backward. They try to make themselves believe that his development and his understanding are normal. It is the duty of the examiner to observe this attitude and so to assess the weight which can be placed on the story given. Many mothers, having forgotten when their child acquired various skills, fabricate their replies, basing their answers on the age at which they know these skills are usually acquired instead of on what they can remember of their own child. It is the duty of the examiner to read the mother's mind and decide how much reliance can be placed on her story.

The developmental history is of particular importance if the child, on examination, is unco-operative on account of shyness or for other reasons. Objective examination of the child is always necessary, but in some children such an examination can be very difficult. It must also be borne in mind that even when a child is fully co-operative, it is likely to be quite impossible even for the most skilful of examiners to obtain a really full picture of the child's behaviour and achievements. An observant mother sees a great deal more of her child's skills by living with him and watching his day-to-day progress than an examiner who only sees him for half an hour in the strange surroundings of a consulting room on perhaps two or three occasions, or even less. In my opinion a full, careful developmental history is of vital importance in the establishment of a developmental diagnosis.

The *first* essential in taking the history is to ensure that the parents and the examiner each know exactly what the other means. For this reason it is quite impossible for the examiner to take a developmental history of any value unless he is thoroughly conversant with the normal development of infants. The following are some important examples of milestones the interpretation of which shows the importance of accuracy in history taking.

Smiling. Some mothers interpret facial grimaces due to wind as smiling. It is always necessary, therefore, when a mother refers to the age at which smiling began, to ask her what it was that made the child smile. The first smiles are always in response to social overture, when the mother talks to her baby. If the mother says that the smiles were in response to other stimuli or not in response to any stimulus at all, the story should be disregarded.

It is, in fact, extremely difficult to say when a child first smiles. Smiling is not a thing which suddenly happens for the first time. There is a gradual, almost imperceptible advance from the intent regard and mouthing of the 4-week-old baby to his smile when he is 6 weeks old.

"*Taking notice.*" This is very difficult to define, and unless a definition is made it is of little value to ask a mother when her baby first began to "take notice." A child of 2 or 3 weeks very often "takes notice" in the sense that when the mother talks to him, when he is in a good temper, he watches her face intently. From that age onwards he takes more and more notice until at about 12 weeks he is seen to turn his head from side to side to follow his mother about the room, and at about 16 weeks he turns his head towards a sound.

"*Holding the head up.*" It is common to read in a "scientific" paper that a baby "held his head up" at such and such an age. Without accurate definition such a statement means nothing. At 2 weeks of age a baby, when held in the sitting position or in ventral suspension (with the hand under the abdomen), may momentarily hold the head up. It is obvious that the further a child is propped up the easier it is for him to "hold the head up." It is not until the age of 28 weeks that the average child can lift his head off the couch when he is lying supine.

Grasping. Every new-born baby shows the grasp reflex, and this must be distinguished from the voluntary grasp of later weeks. At 12 weeks or sooner a baby will hold a rattle when it is placed in his hand, but this achievement precedes by 8 weeks or more the age at which he can go for an object and grasp it when it is placed near his hand, and probably by 3 or 4 weeks more the age at which he can grasp an object placed within reach at a distance from his hand. It is 9 months before a child can pick up a small object of the size of a currant between finger and thumb. It will be seen, therefore, that it is of little value to ask a mother when the child was " able to grasp objects " without being more precise in one's question.

Sitting. A child can be held in the sitting position immediately after birth. By about 5 months he can sit up well in a pram when propped up, but it is not until about 6 months that he can sit for a few seconds in the pram without support, and 7 months that he can sit unsupported for a few seconds on a hard surface. At about 6 months he can probably sit with his hands forward for support. It is not until about 9 months that he is reasonably secure in the sitting position. It is not enough, therefore, merely to ask a mother when her child was first able to " sit."

Self-feeding. Whereas a child of 6 months can hold a biscuit and feed himself with it, it is not until 15–18 months that an average child can feed himself with a spoon and manage a cup without help. He has to go through numerous intervening stages of trying to load the spoon, of succeeding in loading the spoon but not getting it anywhere near his mouth, and later of getting it near the mouth but rotating it and therefore spilling the contents just before it enters the mouth. With the cup he has to go through the stages of helping to hold it, of suddenly letting go when he is drinking or has had what he wants, of spilling most of the contents, until finally he can pick it up, drink and replace it with only occasional accidents. It would clearly be futile merely to ask a mother " when he was able to feed himself " without more accurate definition.

Speech. It is still regrettably common to find in a medical journal that a child " first spoke at 12 months." This means in itself practically nothing. It is common to be told by a mother that her child began to say words at 6 months. On further questioning it is found that the child was making the sounds " mm," " mum " when crying or annoyed. Later on the proud father hears the baby combine syllables—" baba," " da-da-da "—at about 32 weeks and calls this a word. All children go through this stage. It is not till 10 or 11 months of age that the average baby begins to say one word *with meaning.* In the case of " da-da " he shows that he means " daddy " by saying it more when his father is present than when he is not there. By the age 21–24 months the average child combines two words for the first time.

It is, in fact, very difficult to decide when a child says his first word and to decide how many words he can say at a given age, chiefly because of the difficulty in defining what is meant by a word. It is not usually the case that a child one day is unable to say a word, while he can on the next day. The evolution of speech is a much more gradual process. The baby may say " g," denoting " girl," a few weeks before he says " gir " and finally " girl." He may " moo " when he sees a cow and make primitive barking noises when he sees a dog, or else on seeing the dog he says " g," and later " og," before finally he can say " dog." He may make a sound like " tebba," meaning " teddy bear," months before he can say " teddy bear " properly. It is a hopeless undertaking to count the number of " words " he really can say. Of much greater importance than the number of words he is able to say is the number of words which he can understand.

Walking. There are still many papers which make the bald statement that a child first " walked " at a given age. Without accurate definition this is of little value. The child of 8 or 9 months may walk after a fashion with two hands held, but it is not till 13–15 months that he can walk without support for a few steps. It has already been pointed out that a cautious child may walk with one finger held for some months before daring to walk without support. This can be elicited by careful history taking.

Helping to Dress. The first sign of helping to dress is holding the arm out for the armhole or holding the foot out for a sock. Even in one's own child it is by no means easy to say when this begins. The mother might well interpret the question as meaning helping to pull the sock on or to push the hand through the sleeve. Once more the question must be precise.

Sphincter Control. This, like all other skills, is learnt gradually and it is essential to be precise in one's questions. Points of value are the age at which a child first begins to point out the fact that he has wet his napkin, the age at which he begins to tell the mother that he is about to pass urine, the age at which he can first do without a napkin by day, and later by night, with only an occasional " accident." It is not enough to ask when a child was first " clean."

The *second* essential in taking the developmental history is to cover, as far as possible, all fields of development—locomotion, manipulation, play and social behaviour, memory, the mode of display of pleasure and displeasure, feeding behaviour, sphincter control and speech. The history should include the general understanding, the degree of concentration shown on toys and books, the response to such stimuli as the repetition of nursery rhymes, the appearance of food, the methods of drawing attention and the other items listed in the table, which need not be repeated here.

It is also useful to ask the mother how the child in question compares with his siblings or with neighbours' children in the various fields of development. A simple question about the progress of these children in school gives an idea whether they are likely to be reasonably normal.

The *third* essential is a careful inquiry about the various factors which are known to affect the course of development, such as the amount of practice which the mother has given the child, the sort of toys he has, the history of illnesses and other factors. Some of the relevant particulars about the child's personality should also be elicited.

In my opinion the developmental history is an essential part of the developmental diagnosis. It enables the doctor to assess the rate of development and to determine whether there has been any change in the rate, such as that which occurs with the advent of a degenerative disease of the nervous system, or with a sudden spurt of development which is seen when a child is taken out of an institution and placed in a good foster-home. It enables him to determine whether there are any environmental or other factors which may affect his development. It enables him to obtain the family history. If the developmental history tallies with the findings on examination it helps to confirm the accuracy of one's findings. If it does not tally, one has to decide whether the mother's story is correct, or whether for some reason the child's true abilities have not been revealed by the examination. In either case it would be essential to see the child again in order to check one's findings.

The Developmental Examination

For research purposes the examination must be performed in exactly the manner prescribed by the originators of the tests, with the exact equipment specified, for otherwise the norms laid down are not strictly applicable. The nearer one adheres to the method of examination described by the authors of the tests the more accurate will be the results. For details of these methods the reader should consult the works of Arnold Gesell (particularly his " Developmental Diagnosis " and " The First Five Years of Life "). Charlotte Bühler described further tests in her book, " The First Year of Life," along with other tests based on those of Gesell. Cattell's tests [86] are also based on those of Gesell. Her book has the merit of giving good simple descriptions of the tests, but they do not sufficiently cover all the fields of development. For ordinary purposes extreme accuracy is not needed, and hence in the section to follow no rigid methods of performing the tests are given. It is for the specialist, to whom are referred the specially difficult cases, to employ accurate tests in order that valid comparisons can be made at subsequent examinations.

The first essential in the developmental examination is to secure the full co-operation of the child. At Gesell's clinic care was always taken to determine beforehand the infant's normal playtime, and the developmental examination was timed accordingly. It is almost useless to test a small child when he is tired or hungry. I usually prefer to have the mother present during the examination, but she must be asked not to interfere with the tests by trying to "help." Much can sometimes be learned of the mother's attitude to the child, and the child, especially the toddler, is apt to be more co-operative when she is present.

In the first 2 months the baby is best examined in the first place in his mother's arms. The mother should be asked to talk to him, so that the responsiveness, the intentness of his regard and, after the age of 6 weeks, his smiling and even vocalizations can be noted. He is then held in ventral suspension with the hand under the abdomen, so that head control can be observed, and thereafter placed in the supine position. Here his posture is watched. The younger child always lies with the head turned to one side and at frequent intervals shows the tonic neck reflex. The dangling ring or rattle is brought up to the midline about a foot away from his head and then, if necessary, moved into his line of vision. When he catches sight of it, it is moved slowly towards the midline or beyond in order to observe how far he will follow it with his eyes. During this test the hand is observed. In the new-born the hand is clenched. It gradually opens as he grows older. The baby is then pulled into the sitting position so that the extent of the head lag can be seen. In the sitting position momentary elevation of the head is noted. The position of the head, as an index of head control, is also seen in the supported standing position.

Between 2 and 4 months it is again wise to observe the child first in his mother's arms. The interest which he shows in his surroundings, his smiling and his vocalizations are noted. By the age of 3–4 months he may show an obvious desire to grasp a toy when it is held in front of him : he excites, both arms move, he watches the toy intently, but in the earlier weeks of the period he does not go for it. Later he moves both hands out for it but completely misjudges the distance and does not contact it. This can readily be observed as he sits on his mother's knee. A rattle is placed in his hand. By about 3 months of age he will hold it and soon wave it deliberately. He is then held in ventral suspension in order to observe head control, and then placed on his back and tested with the rattle or dangling ring, so that his eye following can be estimated. In the latter part of the period his hands come together in the midline and he may pull at his dress. The hand regard, characteristic of the 12–18-week-old baby, should be looked for. He is pulled to the sitting position in order to test for head lag, and in the sitting position the degree of roundness of the back is noted. The head should be held well up at this age, but in the earlier weeks it tends to bob forwards. If it is held up by the baby, the trunk should be gently rocked so that one can observe whether the head is held steadily even if the baby is moved. Head control is also tested in the standing position, in which he bears a small fraction of his weight. He is placed in the prone position so that head control and the posture of the lower limbs can be seen. From this age onwards it is particularly important not to begin with the supine or prone position, because it is so often disliked by babies and crying then results.

From 4 to 8 months the interest shown by the baby, his alertness and responsiveness are noted before the examination proper begins. He is offered a cube in the supported sitting position and the maturity of the grasp is observed. In the latter part of the period he is offered a second cube so that one can see whether he drops the first on seeing the second. He is offered a small pellet or a thin piece of string in the latter part of the period, in order to test for finger-thumb apposition. Head control and the other necessary preliminaries to locomotion are tested in the sitting, prone and standing positions. In the supine and prone positions the posture of his lower is limbs noted. He is allowed to see himself in a mirror so that the response can be seen. After about 6 months of age he should transfer objects from one hand to another, and the maturity of this act is assessed. After 6 months he goes for objects with one hand instead of two. In the latter part of the period he is likely to try hard to crawl without success. The maturity of his rolling is observed. His vocalizations are carefully listened for.

From the age of 8 months to a year the child is first tested in the sitting position, and then standing. Even at this age he may dislike the prone position. The development of locomotion and manipulation is observed, particular emphasis throughout being placed on *how* the acts are performed and with what degree of maturity he does them. The most careful observation is needed to observe such characteristic behaviour as the nature of the grasp, the index finger approach to objects, the beginning of release and the understanding of the meaning of words.

After the age of a year it is particularly important to secure the child's co-operation. When he first enters the room he should be allowed to wander about as he wishes and to play with toys which have been placed there for the purpose. No apparent notice is taken of him, but he is closely watched, for much can be observed from his behaviour. When he is old enough to understand, his confidence can often quickly be gained by taking notice of his shoes and clothes and by talking about his dolls or toys.

In this age group it is particularly important to maintain the child's interests in the tests. The tests therefore must be done rapidly and not repeated more than is absolutely necessary. There is not usually much difficulty in testing the infant under a year, but it can be very difficult to get a determined child in the negativistic stage to co-operate. He is very distractable, very active and easily bored. He is given a picture-book at the outset and much can be noticed by the interest which he shows in the pictures and his ability to point out familiar objects. In order to maintain interest it is as well to try roughly to alternate the more interesting tests with the less interesting ones. The more interesting ones include the cubes and pictures. The less interesting ones include verbal tests, such as the repetition of digits. As soon as boredom seems to be impending a rapid change is made to more interesting tests. The method must be elastic so that changes like this can be made if necessary. The child is never told that he has made a mistake. The word " no " is never used. Nothing but encouragement is given.

Fallacies and Difficulties in Developmental Diagnosis

A developmental diagnosis must never be made on clinical impression. It can only be based on a careful history and thorough examination. Mental superiority is often wrongly diagnosed in a 2- or 3-year-old child because of charm of manner, absence of shyness and good looks. An infant is apt to be called mentally defective because of a peculiar facies, an unusually large or small head, or because of asymmetry of the skull—all conditions which are perfectly compatible with normal mental development. Unusually bad behaviour in a child may lead the unwary to diagnose mental deficiency. Shyness and failure to co-operate in tests for any reason must never lead one to a wrong conclusion about a child's mental development. Some children at about the age of 3 may regard some of the tests as silly and so fail to co-operate. Failure to present the tests quickly enough and to maintain interest in the tests will lead to a fallacious result.

Many mistakes are made as a result of attaching too much importance to an unusual performance in one particular field. Mental superiority can never be diagnosed on the basis of advancement in one particular field of development, with the sole possible exception of early speech. Mental deficiency can *never* be diagnosed on account of retardation in any one skill, such as locomotion, speech or sphincter control. It can largely, however, be eliminated by the normal or unusually early development of speech—provided that the mental retardation did not develop after speech had been learnt. It can certainly not be eliminated by the early acquisition of sphincter control, which is sometimes learnt relatively early in mentally defective children—earlier, in some cases, than in some children of superior intelligence.

It is very easy to be misled by lulls which occur in some fields of development. I once saw an intelligent child who at the age of 11 months was thought to be rather backward compared with a sibling in feeding himself. Suddenly one day he decided to use the spoon himself, and it was immediately noted that he was in fact considerably advanced in the skill, for there was minimal rotation and spilling. It was clear that, owing to progressive maturation of the nervous system, he was well able to manipulate a spoon although he had had no practice in the art. The common lulls which occur in speech development have been discussed elsewhere. When a 12–18-month-old child is unable to walk without help it is essential to note the degree of maturity with which he walks when supported, in order that one can decide whether the factor which is preventing him from walking alone is merely his personality. It may even be observed that although he cannot walk alone he can stand alone and pick an object up from the floor without support, or that he can get up into the standing position without holding on to anything—performances which normally *follow* the ability to walk unaided instead of preceding it. The factor concerned in this behaviour is merely lack of confidence, which is not related to his intelligence.

It is always wrong to conduct a developmental examination in an epileptic child when he is in a confusional state after a major convulsion, or when he is under the influence of sedative drugs.

In the actual performance of the test other mistakes can be made. Head control cannot be properly tested when the child is very sleepy or when crying. One can easily be misled into thinking that there is excessive head lag when one pulls the child into the sitting position from lying on his back. In the prone position babies are often rather cross and may fail to lift the head up as far as they are able to do. A child may refuse to sit without support during the examination if he has a wet or soiled napkin while, in fact, he is normally able to do so.

Very serious mistakes are made in developmental diagnosis if the various factors which affect the course of development are not properly considered, and if the normal variations which occur are not borne in mind. It is for these reasons that it is so rarely desirable to assess the "intelligence quotient" in terms of a single figure in a pre-school child. Such a figure cannot take into account the various factors and variations which the trained observer knows to be of importance. Some of the tests used, for instance, in the 2–3-year-old child depend on the acquisition of speech. But a child may be of normal or superior intelligence and yet be unusually late in learning to speak. Norms of development, used in the assessment of the I.Q., will miss this and lead to the child being given an unduly low score simply because he cannot speak. Simple observation might well show that the child's understanding of words, as shown by his ability to identify objects and to carry out simple acts on request, is considerably advanced and indicates mental superiority. In the same way a child might be given a low score in other fields of development, such as sphincter control, while in fact his lateness in acquiring sphincter control was due to nothing more than parental mismanagement and bore no relationship to his intelligence. Serious fallacies, therefore, would arise if one were to attempt to calculate the I.Q. merely by converting each observation in the developmental examination into a figure, adding all the figures up, and taking the average.

Attention has already been drawn to the occasional slow starter, who is somewhat backward for some weeks or months in infancy and then shows a normal or superior performance later. The occasional occurrence of encephalitis, vascular catastrophes or demyelinating diseases must also be borne in mind. If their possibility is forgotten, undue reliance on previous milestones of development may lead one to make the mistake of saying that a child is mentally normal whereas actually he is mentally defective. In these cases his general behaviour, destructiveness, lack of concentration, hyperkinesis and general disinterestedness in the surroundings reveal the underlying mental deficiency, even though in other fields of development he is within normal limits. *In any doubtful case with any unusual features the developmental examination should be repeated after an interval, an opinion being in the meantime withheld in order that the rate of development can be observed.*

The rate of the appearance of teeth and the closing of the fontanelle are of no value as milestones of development.

The great difficulty in developmental diagnosis lies in the fact that some of the most important items—the alertness, the rapidity with which acts are performed, the degree of concentration and of understanding, and the interest shown by the child—are unscorable. One can only form an impression of those features. Tests which are entirely sensorimotor, covering locomotion and manipulation only, inevitably miss very important aspects of development. It is unfortunate that the least useful skills for the assessment of a child happen to be the easiest to study and to record.

Another difficulty is the fact that the tests do not include the personality of the child. Though one thinks that one can predict the child's intelligence with reasonable likelihood of being right, it is extremely difficult to predict his personality.

This is not the place to discuss the various physical handicaps, such as cerebral palsy, which retard development in children who are mentally normal. A good review of these conditions, under the name of "pseudo-feeblemindedness," was given by Bakwin.[36]

Section IV
BEHAVIOUR PROBLEMS

INTRODUCTION

ALL normal children have behaviour problems. It is wrong to think that children with these problems are in any way abnormal, naughty, nervous or maladjusted. Many of the problems are merely part and parcel of the normal development of the child. Wisely managed they are short-lived. Improperly managed they may become exaggerated, last for years and become moulded into the character which a man will carry with him for the rest of his life.

Problem children are children with problems. These problems are related to mismanagement by their parents, to lack of loving home life, to the character which they have inherited and to their level of intelligence. The cause of much of the mismanagement lies in the parents' character, in their unhappy childhood, in the excessive domination or lack of discipline, over-protection or spoiling, from which they suffered. Yet no parents are perfect. It is not, however, the occasional mistakes, the occasional outbursts of temper and loss of patience which harm the child, but long-continued harmful attitudes, the withholding of love and the fear of spoiling.

Much of the mismanagement is due to ignorance. Parents cannot be blamed for it. They receive conflicting advice from parents, friends, doctors, magazines and books. There are still many books which advocate rigidity of method without any deviation to suit the needs of the individual. They frighten mothers about the dire results of spoiling children, about the dreadful results of failure to " train " them in strictly regular sleeping, eating and bowel habits. They cause parents to depart from all the dictates of common sense. Other books, such as those of Gesell,[144, 149] Aldrich,[7] Kanner,[227] Shirley [379] and Spock,[396] advocated a more natural common-sense approach to child management, but they are known to far too few.

Some practitioners and pædiatricians evince little interest in behaviour problems and fail to give the parents the advice which they need. They regard the mother's complaint of her child's poor appetite or sleep problems as a nuisance or of no importance. Their interest lies more in disease than in the problems of the normal child. All too often the mother is merely told that " It's his nerves," " It is just naughtiness," " He just wants a good smacking," " He is just spoilt,"

" He will grow out of it "—all statements which give the mother no help at all.

Very often the child does not grow out of his behaviour problems. It is commonly believed that the psychological problems of the adult—the anxiety states, the aggressiveness, the marital unhappiness—have their origin in early life. The seeds of personality disorders and of social problems, of juvenile delinquency, divorce, illegitimacy, selfishness, dishonesty and war, are very often sown in the first 3 years of life.

It is estimated [411] that of every 100 children born in Great Britain, eight will have a nervous breakdown, and three will spend some part of their lives in a mental hospital. It would be interesting to know how many of these psychological troubles of later life could be prevented by wise management in childhood. Bad management in childhood, and in particular emotional deprivation, is likely to effect the next generation. An adult who was deprived of love in his own childhood is liable to be unable to give or receive affection, and so his children will suffer too.

It happens far too often that the parents are given advice which is manifestly unsound, in that it completely ignores the child's fundamental needs, which are the cause of the problem. I was asked to see an older child on account of disobedience. A fortnight previously the mother had taken her to see a psychiatrist. His advice, given in the girl's presence, was that she should be thrashed into obedience. The girl, as one would expect, was a very great deal worse when the advice was carried into effect and was then brought to me. The psychiatrist had completely failed to recognize the fact that the cause of the disobedience was insecurity and a great yearning for love, which the mother had never given her. The mother herself had had an unhappy childhood and had been handed over as an infant to a relative to be brought up. A child of 7 was referred to me because of fæcal incontinence with gross constipation of 5 years' duration. The boy had been repeatedly taken to his doctor, who had always reassured the mother by saying, " It's just his nerves. He will grow out of it." A child of 3 was brought up on account of food refusal. A doctor had told the mother to lock her out of the house if she refused to eat her dinner. Such stories could be duplicated by every pædiatrician.

Parents hardly ever blame themselves for the problems of their offspring. Yet, whether the problems are the result of inherited character or the effect of environment, the parents are ultimately responsible for the problems which arise. They have to be brought to understand the child's basic needs and the way in which their attitudes and beliefs have come into conflict with them.

It should be remembered that difficult parents, parents for instance who are determined, short tempered and irritable, are likely to beget difficult children. Placid, easy-going parents are likely to beget placid easy-going children.

It is wrong to term a child "maladjusted." It is the parents who are maladjusted to the child's emotional needs.

Problems are rarely isolated ones. If there is one behaviour problem there is usually another. It is useless to treat the symptom—the thumb sucking, the masturbation, the sleep refusal—without treating the cause, which is so often the underlying mismanagement. In my opinion the treatment of behaviour problems depends simply on a thorough knowledge of the normal, a careful detailed history and on common sense.

In every case a full detailed history of the whole management of the child must be taken—often not only from the mother but also from the father. When children are old enough to understand (from the age of 2 onwards) the history should not be taken in their presence, and their case should not be discussed in their hearing. Above all things, the aim must be to help the parents rather than to criticize them, to be sympathetic with them and to understand their point of view, rather than to condemn them for their mismanagement. It is useless to rant at mothers who have done their best and yet by their mismanagement caused behaviour problems. It does not help a mother in the least merely to be told that she is over-anxious or worrying about nothing.

It is inevitable that there should be differences of opinion about the management of children and about the prevention and treatment of behaviour problems. It is because of these differences of opinion that in the pages to follow particular emphasis has been laid on the basic causes of the problems, so that the reasons for the management recommended can be fully understood. Fundamentally, behaviour problems arise from a conflict between certain trends in the development of the normal child and the ideas and attitudes of his parents. These developmental trends, which are inevitably bound up with the child's fundamental needs and the parental attitudes with which they come into conflict, are discussed in the pages to follow. Thereafter the specific behaviour problems are discussed in detail.

CHAPTER 20

RELEVANT FEATURES OF THE PSYCHOLOGICAL DEVELOPMENT OF THE CHILD

The Need for Love and Security

It is not unusual to find that the crying of a day-old baby stops not when he is fed or when his napkin is changed, but when he is picked up and cuddled. From this day onwards there is an increasing demand for love and security. By 3 or 4 weeks of age the baby's manifestations of pleasure when he is picked up and talked to are obvious to all. His respirations slow, the mouth opens and closes, his head bobs backwards and forwards, while he watches his mother's face intently. Two or 3 weeks later he begins to smile, and shortly after to vocalize his pleasure. His demands to be picked up tend to increase as he grows older and he becomes reluctant to let the mother out of his sight. When he learns to sit and use his hands to play with toys he may become temporarily less demanding, and more willing to watch his mother depart without crying. At 9 months he may begin to fuss when he sees his mother picking up another baby or his older brother.

The child has an even greater need for love and security after the first year. He becomes increasingly dependent on his parents and increasingly demanding for their presence. He is learning things and seeing things which he has never seen before. He has nightmares and he is frightened by the unknown—by cars, dogs and noises, and he expects his parents to protect him. His demands for love and security are particularly great when he is ill, tired or in pain, as from a fall or from teething. He always needs to be assured of his parents' love. He constantly wants the feeling that he is wanted, that he is a person and has a place in the home. He needs love, above all, when he is cross, irritable or lachrymose, and when he is behaving badly and has been in trouble. He needs love most when he is least lovable.

As Vining wrote,[427] children appreciate love from the facial expression, the tone of voice, the patience, gentleness and understanding with which they are treated, from what the parents say to him and how they say it. To quote Vining : "In so far that the parents apply the forcing method in their endeavour to obtain obedience, and in so far that they make use of the heavy hand, the biting tongue and the frozen face, then so much the more does such a régime produce rebellion, negativism, unhappiness and a feeling of insecurity. I believe that if parents would cut out such words as 'naughty,' 'dirty,' 'disobedient,' 'bad,' 'I do not love you,' and in their place use 'good,' 'helpful,' 'brave,' 'I love you,' 'thank you,' even if the situation does not always deserve it, that the result would be the disappearance of many of these common behaviour problems. The more we give children courage, confidence, affection, and the more we lift them up and give them freedom, instead of keeping them down and suppressing them, the more they will respond. What children need more than anything, and what to a very large extent determines their behaviour and makes it easy and possible for parents to bring about normal behaviour, is love and affection."

Unfortunately some parents seem to be unable to give this sort of love. Bowlby,[55] in his excellent monograph on the effect of emotional deprivation in the first years of life, said that one of the outstanding consequences of such deprivation is the inability to give or receive love in later life. Many parents think that love consists of giving the child everything he wants and buying him expensive presents. One often hears parents say: "We can't make it out. We have given him everything that he wanted, everything that money could buy." But they did not give him love. It takes a great deal more to make a child happy than to give "him everything that he wants." There is a big difference between feeling love and showing it.

His feeling of security is disturbed by prolonged separation from either parent. He may be disturbed, for instance, when placed in a nursery every day so that his mother can work in industry, or when she consistently leaves him for a large part of the day so that she can go out and enjoy herself, or when she leaves the child in charge of a "nanny" because she cannot be bothered to bring him up herself or because she thinks that it is fashionable. No harm is done by an occasional short holiday away from the child. Repeated separations from the child cause insecurity. He is gravely disturbed by stupid threats about exchanges—selling him if he is not a good boy, or of giving his baby sister away.

He is disturbed by removing from one house to another. He is upset by changes of "nannies." His feeling of security is disturbed when a new baby arrives, for then he fears the loss of the love which he has enjoyed so long without competition from another. Every effort should be made at this time to give him a constant feeling of certainty that he is wanted and loved just as much as he ever was.

He is upset by criticisms and constant scoldings. I heard a father say to his boy, who was feeling shy: "Look intelligent. Close your mouth. Stop looking like a congenital idiot." A mother brought her 9-year-old child up on account of a behaviour problem, and said to me in front of her: "She is very backward compared with her sisters. She has always been a great disappointment to us." Another mother said in front of her problem child : " He will soon be going away to school, thank goodness." The child does not interpret this sort of remark to mean that he is loved and wanted. He needs to feel that his parents are not critical of him, that they love him for what he is, and that they are interested in what he says and does.

Every parent hopes that his child will grow up to love him. Parents must remember that future relationship will depend on the love, tolerance and understanding shown to him in the early years.

It is always wrong to ridicule a child or to draw unfavourable comparisons between him and his siblings or friends. They are apt to promote bad feeling between child and child, and they lead to jealousy and insecurity. The devastating effect of favouritism is described elsewhere (p. 239).

The Desire to Practise New Skills

Babies and small children take a great pride in practising the new skills which they have learnt or which they are in the process of learning. When a baby can sit, either propped up (at 4–6 months) or without support (from 7 months), he wants to sit, and dislikes lying down. When he is older, he delights in standing holding on to furniture (8–12 months), creeping (9 months), walking with two hands held (from 10 months) and then with one hand (at a year), and later without support (13–15 months). When he can grasp objects (5 months) he wants to have toys to play with, and soon to help in feeding himself by helping to hold the cup and spoon.

Meanwhile he takes great pride in other manipulative skills—playing with bricks (from 6 months), releasing objects into containers (from 10 or 11 months), threading beads and using blunt scissors (at about $2\frac{1}{2}$). He enjoys looking at books from about 9 months, beginning with linen or cardboard varieties. He learns to dress himself, beginning at 10–12 months, when he holds his arm out for a sleeve, and progressively improving until at 3 years he can dress and undress himself completely if he is helped with the back buttons and advised occasionally about putting the right shoe on the right foot and not putting clothes on back to front. The sight of a 2-year-old child being fed by his mother, or of a 5–7-year-old child being dressed and undressed by her, is all too common and a sad reflection on his upbringing.

The child takes pride in many other skills. They satisfy his ego and give him a feeling of responsibility and independence in the house. When he is learning sphincter control he should be given responsibility to look after himself as soon as he is ready for it. By the age of 2–3 years he is likely to be able to attend to his own needs, provided that he has some help with his pants and that he is wiped. Many mothers make the mistake of retaining entire responsibility for their children, so that they are delayed in learning to be clean.

An important principle of upbringing is the encouragement of a child to practise new skills when he enjoys doing so. He should be allowed to practise them even though he makes a mess or has an occasional accident, and even though it takes the mother twice as long to do a job with his " help " as without it. Probably the chief reason why children are not allowed to dress themselves at about the age of three is that they take a long time to do it and the mother can dress the child herself in half the time. Failure, however, to encourage him to learn new skills when he is ready and anxious to learn them leads to discouragement, dependence instead of independence and lack of initiative, and when the mother later decides that he is old enough to do things for himself he has lost interest and refuses.

The Ego and Negativism

The development of the ego and of resistance begins insidiously. The age at which its first manifestations appear depends largely on the intelligence and personality of the child. Many babies of 5 or 6 months have strong likes and dislikes and are very firm in their refusal of disliked foods. Many of the common weaning problems are bound up with the development of the ego. One reason for advocating the early giving of solids is that the longer they are delayed the more difficult it becomes to persuade the baby to take them.

The baby's desire and determination to practise new skills may become obvious at 6 months. I have seen babies of 6–9 months who consistently refused all food and suffered a serious loss of weight because they were being denied the right of helping to hold the cup or spoon. As the baby grows older he insists more and more on being allowed to practise his new skills, and interference with this desirable trait is the cause of many tears.

From the age of 10 months or so he repeats performances which are laughed at. From this age onwards he shows an ever-increasing determination to be recognised as a person, and he adopts an ever-widening variety of methods of asserting himself. If he discovers any way of drawing attention to himself and putting himself in the centre of the stage, he will repeat the performance (see Attention-seeking Devices, p. 318).

The child passes through a normal stage of aggressiveness in the transition from the dependence of infancy to the independence of later childhood. He becomes a domineering determined fellow. He wants his own way like his parents and sees no reason for being refused it. In the first 2 years at least he is utterly self-centred. It is only in the third and fourth years that the very earliest signs of unselfishness appear. It takes him many months to realize that, important as he is, he is not the only one that matters. He talks incessantly to himself, makes a tremendous noise, and is completely oblivious to the feelings of others. It is wrong to try to break his character. His determination will stand him in good stead in later life. He will learn unselfishness in time. His love of praise, the assertion of his personality, is perfectly normal. It should be utilized in his training. Nothing helps him more than judicious praise and encouragement to be independent.

Negativism is a characteristic feature of the normal child from 18 months to 3 years or more. Children at this age are nonconformists. They seem to take a delight in doing the opposite of what they are asked to do. When the mother wants her child to go out he decides to stay in. When she wants to go upstairs he wants to go down. When she turns to the left he wants to turn to the right. If an attempt is made to make him hurry in eating, clearing his toys away or dressing, he will dawdle. If he discovers that his mother is most anxious for him to eat a particular food, and that his refusal will create a scene, he will certainly refuse it. If he finds that he can cause consternation by withholding a bowel movement or refusing to empty the bladder, he will hold it in, even though it causes him some discomfort to do so. If he finds that refusal to go to bed, to lie down or to sleep results in a fuss and enables him to get his own way and stay up longer, or cause his mother to stay in his bedroom and play games with him, then he will refuse and continue to be difficult until he finds that this method is no longer successful in giving him power over his environment. In short, he has emerged from the stage of being a little angel, and has become a little devil. His mother doesn't know what has got into him. It is because of the development of the ego and of negativism that it is always wrong to have a fight with a child over anything, for in a fight the child always wins. For the same reason any attempt to force him to do something against his will, unless it is really essential, is always undesirable. It is for the same reason that any display of anxiety over any habit or trick which he learns will almost certainly result in the continuance of the practice, for it enables him to assert his personality and to show his power.

There are other reasons for his resistance. Resistance is not always so much the child's revolt against authority as a desire to continue doing what he wants to do. He has no sense of time. A clock means nothing to him, except as a toy. He sees no reason why he should stop playing the game which he is enjoying so much, and he completely fails to see why his parents want him to stop. Very often the parents themselves have an inadequate reason for their insistence. If they have a reason, if they want to take him out or if his meal is ready, he fails to understand why he should hurry.

Arnold Gesell [148] has another explanation for negativism. Referring to the $2\frac{1}{2}$-year-old child, he says : " He has not yet learned to make a distinction between two opposites ; every pathway is a two-way street for him ; life is charged with double alternatives. He is both so inexperienced and immature that he does not make a clear-cut differentiation between yes and no, come and go, give and take, grasp and release, push and pull. His interest in these double alternatives is so evenly balanced that he goes from one extreme to the other. He is confused, confusing and contradictory. He is not sure of himself. What he wills to do he cannot, what he can do he will not."

It is very difficult to draw the line between normal and abnormal negativism. It is greatly exaggerated by hunger, fatigue, insecurity and jealousy. It is exaggerated by excessive sternness, by perfectionism, by constant criticism, and by attempts to push him beyond his developmental level. It must be remembered that it is not all environmental in origin. It is developmental and some show it more than others, for it depends largely on the child's inherited personality.

Habit Formation

It is difficult to define a habit and to distinguish it from reflex action, association and conditioning. Aldrich[6a] described an interesting test for hearing in new-born babies. He had an invisible bell rung every half hour, day and night, and at the same time scratched the foot with a pin, thus causing the baby to draw the leg up and cry. By mid-morning of the second day the child drew the leg up when the bell was rung without the foot being scratched. A child of 3 or 4 weeks may quieten when the bib is being tied on prior to the breast feed. From a month or two of age babies may be " conditioned " to pass urine in the chamber when regularly placed on it. It is uncertain whether any of these examples bear any relationship to the intelligence of the child.

Habit formation may arise as a result of evening colic in the first 3 months (see p. 60), which makes it necessary to pick the baby up and cuddle him at a time when he would otherwise have been in bed. Spock [398] drew attention to the sleep problems which may result, and I can confirm his observations. In a similar way the baby who is constantly being picked up when he is not in need comes to expect to be picked up whenever he is awake. As he grows older habit formation becomes more and more rapid. Any repeated departure from routine in the direction favoured by the child soon leads to habit formation. In an illness the mother may sleep in the child's room, or for the first time keep the light on throughout the night. On holiday the child may have to share a bedroom with the parents. Return to the original routine is difficult.

Habit formation is largely due to a desire to satisfy a primitive instinct. That instinct may be a desire for love or attention. If the result does not accord with the dictates of society, or with the mother's convenience or with her opinions as to what is best for the child, it is called a bad habit. The creation of good habits was the aim of the old rigid ideas of infant feeding, of bowel training and sleep management. The establishment of a routine of good habits is eminently desirable and rigid methods work well with many children, but not with all. In some children they have the opposite of the effect desired, for in children who have particularly well-marked primitive instincts of desire for love or desire for power they cause conflict between parent and child and lead to troublesome disturbances of behaviour. Attempts to break a bad habit cause similar conflict. If in the attempt to break the habit a great deal of anxiety is shown, if the child finds that by his behaviour he can attract attention, if he overhears his mother discussing his problems with her friends, the habit will continue as an attention-seeking device.

An important factor in habit formation is the child's natural imitativeness. Another is his intelligence and memory. It would be natural to assume that the highly intelligent child, who learns rapidly and has a greater understanding than others of his age, should develop habits good and bad quicker than the less intelligent ones.

Imitativeness

The earliest sign of imitativeness is seen at 5 or 6 months of age, when the baby may imitate the adult in putting out the tongue, chewing or making razzing noises. In the next 3 or 4 months the baby learns to imitate the mother in playing simple games—peep-bo, patacake—and in waving bye-bye. He learns to speak. Between 2 and 3 years domestic mimicry is a characteristic feature of development. The child copies the mother in sweeping the floor, washing and drying objects, in baking and in many other household occupations. A girl dresses and undresses her doll, places it on the chamber and changes the napkin. Between 18 months and 3 years children are especially apt to imitate the mannerisms and attention-seeking devices of their playmates.

It is inevitable that children should imitate their parents. The importance of example is obvious. Attempts to inculcate good manners, good habits and kindness to others are doomed to failure unless the parents set the example. If the parents fail to reply to their child when he speaks to them and if they constantly interrupt his conversations, if they are rude and impolite with him, they cannot expect him to be anything else. If they show bad temper and irritability, use bad language and are unloving, dishonest and selfish, they cannot expect their child to be any different. When the divorce rate is 30,000 per year, what one might call the "friction rate"—the frequency with which the mother and father quarrel—must be a very great deal higher. Domestic friction has a serious effect on the mind of the growing child.

The importance of example is in part related to his developing memory and understanding. At the age of a year the memory span may be one of several weeks. By the age of 3 it may be one of many months. Parents should not make the mistake of thinking that a child's memory is short-lived. His understanding is apt to be underestimated. It is far in advance of his powers of speech. They fail to realize this and so fail to realize the importance of a good example.

Sensitiveness to Atmosphere and Surroundings

The effect of maternal nervousness on the sucking of the new-born baby was described by Middlemore.[293] The baby of a thyrotoxic mother is particularly liable to show feeding and sleeping problems at a result of the mother's nervousness. Escalona[123] commented: "It has always been known that infants respond best to calm, secure, warm persons, that they are more irritable and tense under the management of tense, nervous and insecure persons." I have seen a baby burst into tears on several occasions between the age of 6 and 9 months when a mishap befell his sister or friends, or when he thought that his sister was being hurt by rough play. A child between 1 and 3 years of age readily cries when he sees his mother cry, without knowing what is troubling her. It is easy to understand that domestic friction, particularly if there is obvious resultant unhappiness or violence, may have a considerable psychological effect on the child.

At 4 or 5 months of age the baby may show interest in a room in which he has not been before, and he may refuse to sleep in a strange bedroom.

Imagination

Most children after the age of 15 months or so develop a vivid imagination. There are great individual differences. In general, the greater the intelligence the greater is the imagination. Between 15 and 18 months it begins to appear in his doll play. Between 2 and 3 he has imaginary playmates behind the sofa. He tells tall stories and plays highly imaginative games with his friends. His imagination may lead to the development of fears—fear of the dark, of noises and of animals.

Suggestibility

Likes, dislikes and fears are readily suggested to a child. Dislike of certain foodstuffs is suggested by chance remarks made by adults.

Fears of animals, motor cars and thunder are suggested in a similar way. In a child who is liable to motion sickness, vomiting is readily suggested by unwise conversation in front of him. Gruesome tales and stories about ghosts, giants, devils and suchlike may terrify the small child and lead to serious sleep disturbance.

The Intelligence of the Child

Behaviour problems may arise in a child with a lower than average intelligence for a variety of reasons. He is likely to be a slow learner, and if his training is related to his age instead of to his level of development, too much will be expected of him, so that he becomes thwarted, negative and insecure. It is not easy to appeal to him, to explain to him what sort of behaviour is expected and to get him to understand the reason for restrictions which are necessary for him. Speech is late in developing and he feels thwarted by his inability to express himself.

Superior intelligence may be a problem in later years.[196] It is probable that habit formation is quicker in the more intelligent child. He is likely to learn attention-seeking devices more quickly, because of his greater appreciation of the reaction of his parents. His greater imaginativeness may lead to fears of various kinds. Under-estimation of intelligence causes parents to be careless about speaking in front of him. It may lead them to be too slow in teaching him skills and responsibilities for which he is ready on account of his superior mental endowment.

Personality Differences

Full realization of the great differences in the personality of children is fundamental for an understanding of behaviour problems. Personality traits may be obvious in the new-born period. One baby takes the breast without difficulty. Another is irritable, sucks for a minute and screams and is difficult to manage. Some are much more intolerant of hunger than others. Some are much more active. Irwin [216] recorded the activity of 73 normal new-born babies by means of a mechanical device, and showed that the activity of the most active one was 290 times greater than that of the least active one. The active babies, with rapid movements of the arms and legs, tend to posset excessively. The slow, placid babies present fewer feeding problems.

There are great differences in sleep requirements. Some babies even at 4 or 5 months of age are asleep for the major part of the day. Others at that age only have two or three short daytime naps. The active, determined baby discards the midday nap months or even years before his placid brother. Some are willing to lie outside in the pram all day long with no one to talk to and nothing to see. They have little interest in their surroundings. Others at 3 months, or even sooner, refuse to be left outside. They want to see what is going on, they are intensely curious and are perfectly content lying in the pram in the kitchen, where the mother is busy with her household duties.

Some are placid, quiet babies who cry little even when they are tired. Others are active, determined ones who cry a great deal until given the attention which they demand, and are difficult to keep quiet when tired, hungry or bored.

Some babies present no problem at weaning time. They take what comes, with only mild likes and dislikes. They do not bother to try to feed themselves and would rather do without than have to help. Others have strong likes and dislikes; they spit the cod-liver oil out, they become greatly excited when they see a food which they like. They would rather starve than be denied the right of helping themselves.

There are great differences in social responsiveness. Some smile readily and are easily amused. Some love company, while others do not care so much. Some prefer cuddling to toys, others toys to cuddling. There are great differences in the demand for and giving of love.

After the first year the differences in the degree of determination, negativism and independence become more marked. Some will not tolerate the play pen for more than a week or two. For others it is a useful commodity for months. Some are willing to be wheeled about in a pram when they are 3 years old. Others will have nothing more to do with it when they are not yet 2. Some are extremely insistent on practising their new skills and on "helping" the mother; others care much less and are more willing to have things done for them. Children differ widely in the amount of caution which they show. Some show fear a great deal more than others. They differ in imagination, sensitiveness to criticism, in concentration, in distractibility and in their demands for love and security. Some are born to lead, others to be led. Some boys are born to excel at rugger, others at the violin. Some girls are born to be nurses, some to be soldiers in Korea.

Rigid standardized methods of child management fail to take these individual differences into account. They work well for the average child but not for the child who is different from the average. It is for this reason, as well as for the differences in intelligence, that child management should be elastic and adaptable to the needs of the individual.

There is no doubt that differences in the personality of children are an important cause of behaviour problems. Trouble arises in a family when the first-born has a placid, easy-going disposition and the next is an active, determined independent child. The mother naturally tries to adopt the same methods of upbringing with the second child as those which she used successfully with the first, and it does not work. The child objects. Food-forcing, sleep-forcing and bowel-forcing methods are apt to result. It is most important that parents should understand that personality differences are almost inevitable in a family, and management should accordingly be elastic.

Annoying Characteristics of the Developing Child

Any parent could say a great deal about this subject, yet it is surprising how little sympathy many doctors show with mothers who are faced with behaviour problems. Mothers have to tolerate not only the dreadful social circumstances, such as overcrowding and poverty, in which they have to bring up their children, but they have to live with their children all through the day, with their annoying characteristics, which irritate and tire. They cannot get out in the evening. Holidays are out of the question. It is one thing for the father to see the children for an hour each evening, and another for the mother to have them for the whole of the day and never to be able to get away from them.

In the first 6 months, if the baby is of the active wide-awake type, his frequent demands for attention and his ready crying when the mother is tired and busy may get on top of her. After this age the baby should be learning to feed himself. He makes a dreadful mess with his food, dropping much of it on the floor and spilling milk on the carpet. He gets hold of some paper when her back is turned, tears it up into numerous pieces and eats some of it. After 9 months he is mobile and constantly creeping or walking into mischief. He has an insatiable desire to learn and wants to know what happens when he pulls the lamp flex or the table cover. The coal bucket and rubbish tin are fascinating. An open bookshelf or a cupboard carelessly left open keep him occupied for a long time. By the age of a year he may object to the play pen and refuse to stay in it. He may push it round the room or creep under it, the better to get into mischief. He possets on the new carpet.

His activity is greater after the first birthday. He gets into constant trouble, hitting the window with hard objects, playing with the coal bucket, pulling at the table cover or upsetting the clothes-horse. He loves casting games and throws one thing after another on to the floor. He is on the go all day long and will not sit still for a minute. He is constantly fighting his elder brother. He leaves a litter of toys all over the floor for the mother to fall over. He delights in noise and loves the drum which an unkind friend gave him, beating it for hours on end. He likes repetitive play, making the same noise, performing the same action over and over again till his mother is distraught. He never modulates his voice, and when he learns to talk he never stops talking for one minute. He constantly wants help in practising his new skills. He tends to cling to his mother instead of playing alone with his toys as she would like him to do. He totally fails to understand that she is tired, irritable, worried or feeling poorly.

By the age of 2 he is well into the resistant stage. He does the opposite of what he is asked to do, or else takes no notice of what she says and appears to be deaf. Of all the annoying tricks, dawdling can be one of the most trying. He takes a dreadful time to eat his dinner, to get ready for going out or to put his toys away, and any attempt to hurry him makes him worse. If sent to get ready or to fetch an item of clothing, he finds an interesting toy half-way to his destination and forgets what he has been sent for. He tries various attention-seeking devices—turning the gas tap on, constantly repeating the same noise which he finds gets on his mother's nerves, and even throws temper tantrums. She feels thwarted when she finds that she cannot make him do what she wants him to do. She cannot even obtain emotional release by smacking him, because it only makes him worse. When she finally gets him to bed he refuses to lie down. She cannot even leave him to cry it out because he has learnt to make himself sick if left to cry. She cannot reason with him because he is not old enough to understand. When she has a fight with him, he always wins. He sleeps badly and next day he is tired and even more resistive than usual. He wails and nothing pleases him. It rains all day ; she cannot take him outside, and he is bored and intolerable. Where there is more than one child, the constant fighting, bickering, shouting and shrieking, aggravated by boredom, gets her down.

She wants to clean him up to take him out, but he runs away when she calls him, and the more angry she becomes the more difficult it is to catch him. When she has tidied him up she turns her back for two minutes to get dressed herself, and he gets into the coal bucket, vomits over his clothes or soils his pants. When they eventually reach her friends, before whom she wants to show him off, he is on his worst possible behaviour. She has friends into her house, and just before their arrival he empties the whole contents of his playbox with a crash on to the floor.

Between 2 and $3\frac{1}{2}$ he begins to ask questions, and soon asks them all day long. She cannot answer many of them, but he insists on an answer. Each answer leads to another question. He asks : "Why is it to-day ?" "When will it be to-morrow ?" "Why is it not to-morrow now ?" "What is a soul ?" He asks her to "draw a difference," "draw an appetite," and repeatedly asks her why she cannot do it.

This picture is not exaggerated. Most mothers could add a great deal to it. The mother says that the child is getting on her nerves, has got right on top of her. She feels that she would love to run miles away. She becomes cross and irritable and tactless. The child then becomes worse. Many mothers have several small children ; some of them have twins ; and sometimes one of them is a mentally defective child of the hyperkinetic type.

Behaviour problems must be treated against this background. Far too little sympathy is shown with the mother. It is very easy to criticize her when she has lost her temper with the child. Ogden Nash* apparently knew something about it when he wrote the following lines :

> " Oh, sweet be his slumber and moist his middle.
> My dreams, I fear, are infanticiddle.
> A fig for embryo Lohengrins.
> I'll open all of his safety pins.
> I'll pepper his powder and salt his bottle,
> And give him readings from Aristotle.
> Sand for his spinach I'll gladly bring,
> And Tabasco sauce for his teething ring,
> And an elegant elegant alligator,
> To play with in his perambulator."

* Ogden Nash (1943). " Song to be sung by the Father of Infant Female Children," in " The Face is Familiar," London. J. M. Dent & Sons.

CHAPTER 21

PARENTAL ATTITUDES AND MANAGEMENT

The Fear of Spoiling

MANY mothers seem to be haunted by the fear of "spoiling" their children. It is a strange paradox that it is to these mothers that most spoilt children belong.

A child is not spoilt by being loved. A mother never harms her baby by giving him all the love that he demands. She should not hesitate to pick him up when he cries for company. His demands may be frequent at first, but if satisfied they usually rapidly decrease. If he cries because of colic, pain from teething, fatigue or other reasons, he should be picked up and loved. As Spock[396] wrote in his book, "A baby who gets extra attention when he is uncomfortable is usually perfectly willing to do without it when he feels well." A baby is spoilt more by a mother arguing with him than agreeing with him. It is surprising how many mothers turn a completely deaf ear to the crying of their child. They seem to be completely unperturbed by it. It may be very convenient for the mother to leave the baby outside in the pram all day, however much he cries. It may well, however, lead to behaviour problems later. According to Aldrich,[7] "Most spoiled children are those who as babies never had essential gratifications owing to a mistaken attempt to fit them into a rigid régime. The spoiled child who has missed satisfaction as a baby adopts the efficient technique of whining and temper tantrums to get what he wants." He adds : "The mechanism of spoiling is the neglect of needs rather than over-indulgence. Adults often present the behaviour problem instead of babies. It is negativism to fail to respond to a child's basic needs.

Twenty-five years' experience has taught me that responsive adults breed responsive babies, and that rigid disciplinarians of babies at this age breed spoiled, unhappy children with no confidence in themselves or their parents."

Children certainly can be spoilt, and frequently are. The baby is spoilt by the mother who will never leave him alone when he is not wanting attention. Escalona[123] described "immature narcissistic personalities who love their babies to death." "They have a continuous desire to touch the baby, to move it about, to play with it, to kiss it and hug it. The baby is never left in peace for a minute, and becomes tense and irritable." Grandmothers are particularly liable to spoil their grandchildren in this way. After the first year a child is spoilt by over-protection, by never being allowed to do things for himself, by never being allowed out of his mother's sight. He is spoilt by lack of discipline because of fear of " repressing " him. He is spoilt by being allowed to wreck the furniture, walk on the table, draw on the wall and ride around the drawing-room on his tricycle. He is spoilt by deprivation of love and affection and security. He is spoilt by determined efforts to avoid spoiling him.

Over-protection and Over-anxiety

The term " over-protection " signifies a great deal more than excessive protection of a child against danger. It includes a failure to allow him to grow up and look after himself. The mother continues to feed him, dress him and attend to his eliminations long after a properly treated child has learnt to take full responsibility for these functions himself. It includes restriction of outdoor exercise in case he should catch cold or get his feet wet. It includes over-indulgence with his toys and play behaviour, with excessive domination in other ways. It includes yielding to wishes and actions which no normal parent would tolerate. It consists of preventing him playing with other children because they are " rough." It consists of what Kanner called "smother love " instead of " mother love." One of my patients had not been allowed to mix with other children for fear she should pick up the local accent. I saw two boys, whose father had died in their infancy, who had their temperature taken by their mother every day for 15 years.

Over-protection is due to a variety of factors. It may occur when the parents have had a long wait for the child, especially if on account of age or other reasons it is not possible to have another. It is apt to occur when there has been a succession of miscarriages, or a particularly difficult labour. It occurs when parents, determined to have a girl, eventually achieve their ambition after having a succession of boys. It may arise when a child arrives many years after the last one, or when a child returns home after a serious illness in hospital. It is likely to be a feature of institutional care or of care by a nanny. It occurs when a mother regards her child as delicate because of an illness, physical disability or premature delivery. It may occur when a child is adopted after a long period of sterility or when a previous child has died. A mother who has had an unhappy childhood, or who is unhappy in her married life, or who has been thwarted in her ambitions, may turn to her child to satisfy her own needs for affection. Psychologists say that over-protection may be a mask to compensate for hostility or a rejecting attitude of which, as a rule, they are unaware.

Over-anxiety is due to the same causes as over-protection. Both are related in part to the mother's personality. It may be engendered by doctors or nurses or by books on child care. It is often manifest as soon as the baby is born. The mother is then apt to be worried about her ability to feed the baby, and is nervous and anxious when the baby is put to the breast. If in addition the baby is irritable, lactation is liable to fail. When she gets the baby home she weighs him daily, and if the baby is breast fed she carries out test feeds every day. If he does not take as much as she thinks he ought to take, she tries to force him to take more, and food refusal occurs. She constantly goes in to see him in the evenings, in case he has suffocated, and keeps him in her bedroom long after he ought to have moved into his own room. She worries about his bowels and the amount of sleep he has, and so adopts forcing methods and meets with bowel and sleep refusal. She never leaves him alone for a minute in the daytime, however quiet and contented he is, always picking him up and playing with him. She grossly overclothes him and keeps him out of the sun. She keeps him indoors if it is at all cold outside. She prevents him from sitting, standing or walking as long as she can, in case his back will be weakened. In the weaning period she becomes very worried if he refuses a mouthful of food and tries to force him to take it, only to be met with further refusal. She may even regard him as delicate and make him too fat by overfeeding him. She constantly seeks advice from her mother, her neighbours and from various doctors. She reads one book after another about child management in an effort to find out how the child should be brought up. She fails to let him feed himself in case he will choke ; she will not allow him to go outside and play in case he hurts himself ; when he plays with other children she constantly interferes with the play in case he should be injured.

The result of over-protection is serious. The child's conduct is immature. He remains utterly dependent on his mother and so is late in learning various skills—in feeding himself, attending to the toilet and in dressing himself. He is insecure. He does not play well with other children. He is afraid of getting hurt and he wants to control the games himself. He runs to his mother for protection and he is accident-prone. Later on he fails to make friends. If the over-protection is associated with over-domination he is likely to be aggressive and boastful or submissive, timid and effeminate.[29, 32] In adolescent life and later he is unable to make any decision for himself without consulting his mother, for he fails to acquire normal independence. He does not take part in ordinary games with his fellows, preferring the shelter of home life. If the over-protection is associated with over-indulgence there are apt to be temper tantrums and other manifestations of aggressive behaviour. Obesity due to over-eating is sometimes a problem.

Over-anxiety in the mother is a very common picture familiar to all pædiatricians. In general, however, it is a diagnosis which is made far too frequently. It is very easy to criticize a mother for being over-anxious, but it is not so easy for a parent to avoid over-anxiety, particularly when there has been a long wait for the child, or when he has been born prematurely or had some serious illness. One should always be sympathetic and understanding with such mothers, particularly when the child is her first one, and constantly bear in mind the fact that over-anxiety springs from love.

Favouritism and Rejection

Of all parental attitudes favouritism and rejection are probably the most harmful. Both of these are always vigorously denied by the parents, largely because they spring from the subconscious mind and are in no way deliberate or voluntary. The favouritism is quite obvious, however, to everyone else but the parents.

Favouritism arises from a variety of causes. If there has been a sequence of four boys and finally a much-wanted girl comes, she is apt to be treated as a favourite. The more intelligent bright child, or the child with the more pleasing and affectionate personality, or the child who is blessed with good looks, is apt to be favoured at the cost of her siblings. To a certain extent the causes of favouritism are the same as those of over-protection. When a child comes, for instance, several years after the previous one—especially when he was much wanted—he is apt to be favoured. It often happens that the mother's favourite is the boy, the father's is the girl, and the third is no one's favourite.

Favouritism is shown in scores of little ways, all mounting up to a great deal in the child's mind. The favourite one is not reprimanded as much as the other ; he can do things which the unfavoured one is not allowed to do. He is given sweets, rides on the father's back and trips to the town, which are denied the unfavoured one. When the favoured one gets into trouble with one parent, the other parent defends him ; when the unfavoured one gets into trouble, both parents attack him. The favoured one is given just a little more of the pudding or cake than the other. Grandparents are frequently guilty of marked favouritism.

Parental rejection occurs for similar reasons. It may be due to the fact that the child was of the wrong sex. It may be due to his appearance or to the fact that he has a lower intelligence than that of his siblings. It is manifested by an excessively critical attitude to the child. The mother makes the most of his shortcomings, clearly exaggerating his bad behaviour and belittling his understanding and intelligence. She does not hesitate to make unfavourable comparisons between him and his siblings in his presence. She fails to give him the love which she gives to the others. At all times he is the unfavoured one. She is liable, if she can afford it, to hand the child over completely to a nanny to bring up. In the severest cases there is outright cruelty. The frequency with which a step-parent rejects a child is well-known.

When there is favouritism, the unfavoured child, in addition to the general signs of insecurity, may feel resentful against the parents. He shows little affection for them, and as a result a vicious circle is set up, the parents in turn responding by showing less affection for the child. He is secretive, and naturally will not confide in them. He is very likely to be jealous of the brother or sister who is favoured by the parents and is liable to dislike them. The favoured child also suffers by being spoilt, by having all his own way, and by lacking discipline.

The result of rejection or of insecurity is considerable. Some of the reactions are merely exaggerations of features of every normal child : excessive fears, shyness, timidity, lachrymation, aggressiveness, quarrelsomeness, destructiveness, disobedience, jealousy, attention-seeking devices, clinging to the mother, thumbsucking, masturbation, night terrors and attention-seeking devices. Other reactions include bedwetting, fæcal incontinence, temper tantrums, tics, cruelty to animals, stuttering and head banging. Nearly all these arise through the subconscious, so that the child cannot help them. It follows that it is useless to try to treat the symptom ; one has to treat the cause.

Misjudgment of the Child's Developmental Level

The variations in intelligence and personality in children are so great that the only rational way of training them is to adapt the methods to the level of development reached. It is wrong, for instance, to instruct the mother to give her child solids as soon as he is 6 months old. She should give him solids when he can chew, which an average baby can do at 6 months, while others begin later. It is obvious that a child with a very high intelligence quotient is ready to learn things long before an average child. In general the understanding of children tends to be under-estimated rather than over-estimated, partly because the mental processes are so far ahead of the powers of speech. If attempts are made to teach him before he is ready, he feels thwarted and insecure. One has seen children of 8 or 9 months smacked for taking an object to the mouth, a child of 15 months smacked for running alone across the road, and a child of the same age smacked for passing urine into his pants. One sees attempts being made to inculcate adult table manners in an 18-month-old child. Children of 2 are expected to be tidy. A child of nearly 3 can be taught the rudiments of tidiness by having to put toys away before a meal, but it should not be made an occasion for a fight and he should be helped in the task. A child of 2 is expected to have a conscience and to be unselfish, and he is scolded when he falls short of expectations. I saw a child of 3 being scolded for playing engines on a railway-station platform on the grounds that it was "silly."

Some parents cannot stop teaching their children. They are

perfectionists and demand far too much for their level of development. They are often the sort of parents who want to show off their child in order to compensate for their own feelings of inferiority.

If, on the other hand, a child is not taught when he is developmentally ready and enjoys practising his new skills, he may lose interest and not want to learn later. It is common enough to see a child of 5 or 6 years who is unable to dress or undress himself, because he was never given a chance to do so at a time when he would have enjoyed learning, between 2 and 3 years. At 5 or 6 he is quite content to let his mother do it for him. He should be allowed to feed himself as soon as he is ready, in spite of the mess ; he should be allowed to attend to his own eliminations as soon as he is developmentally ready, in spite of occasional accidents ; he should be allowed to help to put the china away, in spite of occasional mishaps ; he should be allowed to dress himself, in spite of the tremendous time it takes him to do it. He should be allowed at 2 years or so to have his own possessions, including books, and to assume responsibility for taking care of them.

Owing to the great differences in intelligence and personality in children there are wide variations in the ages at which children are ready to learn new skills. Rigid methods of training do not take these into account and so are apt to lead to unhappiness and insecurity.

Attitudes to Sex

The attitude to sex is of vital importance to the developing child. From the age of 15 months or so the child shows tremendous interest in the excreta. Parents must know that this is normal, and no notice should be taken of it. After the age of $2\frac{1}{2}$ children are likely to notice anatomical differences in the sexes. Their loud comments on such matters when in the grocer's shop may be embarrassing to the mother who has little sense of humour, but on no account should the child be reprimanded or laughed at for what he says. A simple question should be answered simply and truthfully in a way which he can understand. The parents may wrongly try to teach the child modesty at this age and by so doing suggest that nudity is evil and wrong. They do the child grievous harm. They should avoid being shocked when the first-born goes out of her way to peep at her young brother's genitals, and perhaps to handle them.

Sex play between small children is common and normal. They may handle each others genitals. Unfortunately many mothers are seriously disturbed when they see it happening. They should be reassured and advised not to show the least interest or anxiety in the matter. They should make no attempt to stop it. The most they can do is to distract the children, but that is not usually advisable. (See also Masturbation, p. 307.)

CHAPTER 22

DISCIPLINE AND PUNISHMENT

Discipline

DISCIPLINE is essential to every child. He has to learn the limits to his freedom, not only for his own physical safety, but in order that he may conform with social custom as far as is reasonable for one of his developmental level. Bakwin and Bakwin,[39] in an excellent discussion on the subject, said: "Training and discipline are implements to direct the child's energies into useful and socially acceptable channels, to assist him in outgrowing less mature modes of behaviour, and to curb excessive emotional demands." The child has to learn to accept needful restraint. He has to learn respect for and obedience to reasonable authority. He has to learn respect for the property of others. He has to learn that there are others who matter as well as he. As the Bakwins put it: "Proper child rearing requires a balance between encouragement for self-expression and freedom on the one hand and training for conformity on the other. He has his rights and privileges, but he has his duties and responsibilities as well." "He needs increasing freedom as his legitimate needs and capacities grow, but this freedom must be limited by his ability to take responsibility. As he matures he may be told the reasons for restrictions and the consequences which might result from transgression. He should be encouraged to use his own judgment where possible, but this cannot be done without direction and guidance. Too few restrictions, like too many, are undesirable." To use Stott's words, [405] "the best relationship between parent and child is one in which the child feels secure as long as he behaves himself, but knows that naughtiness will jeopardize that security." Authority which is firm, kind, reasonable and consistent gives the child that sense of security which is essential for his emotional development. He needs discipline so that he can learn self-discipline.

Lack of discipline is seriously harmful to the child and "spoils" him. It is practised largely by parents who have heard or read that firmness leads to repression, and by the ignorant, who as children themselves never learnt discipline. The result is the spoiled, insecure child, the child thought by all but the parents to be a horror, the child whom other parents do not want to mix with their own children because of the undesirable tricks which he teaches them.

He knows that he can get his own way by demanding it, if necessary with a temper tantrum. He is particularly difficult when taken out to friends, revealing his bad behaviour when faced with other children.

He is apt to wreck the furniture, throw hard objects about the room, and generally to set a bad example to other children. He is aggressive to other children and apt to injure them by kicking them. He grows up to be an unpopular spoiled school child who does not fit in well with his fellows. Food fads and accident proneness are common.

Stott wrote that lack of discipline in the first years is a major factor in juvenile delinquency. It is also an important factor in accident proneness [38] and in other undesirable traits in later life. To use the Bakwins' words : "The child reared without discipline has only a false freedom, for without the help of adult guidance and control he grows up uncontrolled and unsure of himself, uncertain of what to do and what not to do, slow in making decisions and angry when he has made the wrong one." It seems to be a common belief that, if there are children in a house, it is inevitable that the furniture and carpets will be ruined and that there will be pencil marks and scratches and stains on the walls. Accidents are always apt to occur, but with reasonable discipline damage should be rare.

Excessive discipline is hardly less harmful. Discipline is always excessive if it is not related to the level of development which the child has reached. It is always wrong if it is exerted not as a benefit to the child but as an outlet for the parents' offended sense of dignity. Some parents insist on obedience over a completely unimportant matter because they fear loss of face. A woman causes a scene in a tramcar over a trivial matter because she fears that others will be critical of her for not being able to command instant obedience from her offspring. She fails to realize that by her behaviour she merely reveals the short-comings of her own character. Some parents are far too sensitive about what people will think of their children ; they think that they will frown on what any well-informed adult will know is normal behaviour for the age.

Parents who are constantly saying "No, no, don't do this, don't do that," produce the child who rebels, has temper tantrums and other manifestations of insecurity. Obedience based on repression is never permanent. Parents who apply rigid forcing methods are the parents who have most trouble with their children. As Vining [430] says, "Most of us are well acquainted with the food-forcing, bowel-forcing, sleep-forcing and obedience-forcing parents, to whom belong all those children who refuse to eat, to sleep, to have their bowels moved and to obey." Some children brought up in this way are unduly submissive and timid. Most react by doing the opposite of what is expected of them. They respond by dawdling, by appearing not to hear commands, or by deliberate disobedience. Some children respond by aggressiveness, negativism, and temper tantrums ; some respond by excessive shyness and other signs of insecurity ; others respond by rebellion and bad behaviour at school. Accident proneness commonly results from excessive discipline, just as it does from over-indulgence.

Discipline must be accompanied by love or it fails. Excessive correction, excessive discipline which the child cannot understand, are apt to be indulged in when the parents are tired, harassed or in a hurry, so that they are irritated by trivial things. When irritated at work they take it out of their child at home. A sense of humour is essential; but unfortunately one loses one's sense of humour when tired and overworked. The mother with thyrotoxicosis or an anxiety state is apt to be excessively demanding for obedience.

It is undesirable for both parents to join in an attempt to discipline the child. There is often a tendency for both parents to pounce on the child for trivial misdemeanours. Frequently, owing to the housing shortage, the house has to be shared with relatives. I saw a disturbed child who was being constantly pounced upon and reprimanded by five adults who were living in the house.

Discipline should be consistent, though parents must learn to look the other way when there are trivial breaches. If a rule is made, however, it should be kept, but rules should be few, reasonable and necessary. A child will not learn to obey if obedience is insisted upon on some occasions and not on others. It is useless to try to teach discipline when a child is tired. It will not work. One must be sure, when one is insisting on obedience, that one is on safe grounds. All too often there is no real justification for one's stand. There is no doubt that the wiser the parent and the greater the patience, the less resistance there will be and the fewer will be the tears. The child does not learn because of scoldings, ridicule, admonitions and fear of punishment, but because of love, respect and the example set by his parents. The basis of good behaviour is praise and love, not blame and punishment. He will learn more from encouragement and judicious awards than he will from reprimands and smackings. He must never be bribed to do what he is asked to do, but an unexpected reward, such as a sweet, for obeying an unpalatable request is another matter. The aim is to teach discipline without tears.

Punishment

It is obvious that punishment is necessary, but when a possible occasion for it arises it is very much easier to mete out punishment than to say whether punishment is justified. The wiser the management the less is punishment needed. A good teacher in a nursery school practically never needs to administer physical punishment. She learns to avoid the need for punishment by avoiding the causes for the need. She removes the child from the source of danger instead of warning and threatening him of what will happen if he disobeys. The less frequent the punishment, and the better the relationship between child and parent, the more effective is the punishment and the less severe need it be to produce the desired effect. It is *never* necessary to inflict pain. The most trivial scolding, the mere tone of voice, can produce as great an effect in the wisely managed child who is rarely punished as a severe physical punishment in a child who is used to it. The more frequently punishment is given the less effect it has, except that it leads more and more to rebellion and insecurity. When punishment is frequent its severity has to be increased in order to produce an effect. It is common to be told that a child does not seem to care at all when he is beaten. The parent feels thwarted and angry if he does not show that he has been hurt, for he fails to obtain the emotional release which he needs.

All too often punishment is meted out purely because of parental loss of temper. It is hardly untrue to say that in the majority of cases physical punishment is merely due to loss of temper in the parent. Excessively frequent punishment is a sign that the parents have failed in their upbringing ; it is likely to be due to parental rejection or to unhappiness in their own lives. It may represent frustration in marital life, or a display of power in the home to compensate for failure and frustration at work. It may be because the father as a child was punished excessively and he was powerless to resist it. As a father he finds release from the repressions of his childhood. He excuses himself by Samuel Butler's dictum, " Spare the rod and spoil the child." He fails to realize that the whipping which he received has made him the sort of father he is and has led to rebellion in his children.

Of greater damage to the child than physical punishment is mental punishment. Some parents have gathered that physical punishment is harmful and replace it by something worse—chronic scoldings, disapproval, reasonings, threats, warnings of consequences and ridicule. I was told by a mother, who had brought her son to me because of fæcal incontinence, that she had tried to shame him out of it by showing his soiled trousers to his school friends and neighbours. A child with enuresis was ostracized by other members of his family and made to sit at a table alone for all meals because of the smell.

Repeated threats of punishment are useless and harmful. The child rapidly learns to take no notice of them, because the threats are never carried into effect. Repeated threats with occasional punishment are equally useless. They inevitably lead to disobedience. As said above, if a rule is made it should be kept. If it is broken, punishment should be inevitable, and that should be understood by the child. It is always absolutely wrong for a mother to threaten the child with such words as " I shan't love you if you do that." Bed or threats of bed should never be used, because they are apt to lead to sleep refusal, bed becoming associated with punishment.

Before punishment is decided upon it is essential to try to understand the child's motives. It is very easy to punish a child for doing wrong by adult standards when, with his limited experience and undeveloped conscience, he could see nothing wrong in what he was doing. Punishment in such circumstances is wrong. An explanation and warning should suffice. A child who is old enough to understand should be reminded of the behaviour which is expected of him. It must be remembered that screaming at night may be due to a nightmare. It would be very wrong to smack a child for this.

The reason for the wrongdoing may lie in boredom, jealousy or insecurity. Destructiveness and the throwing of objects about a room may be due to lack of sufficient freedom and outlet for his energies. It would clearly be wrong merely to punish him for his wrongdoing without trying to remove the underlying cause by trying to give him space to let off some energy without doing harm, removing breakable objects, and giving him a chance to play out of doors. A child may be punished for drawing on the wall, but he should also be given paper and pencil or a blackboard so that his desire to scribble and draw can be satisfied.

The parents must agree on punishment. The child does not take long to discover that what one parent disapproves the other condones. As Ogden Nash said :*

> " The wise child handles Father and Mother
> By playing one against the other.
> ' Don't,' cries this parent to the tot.
> The opposite parent cries, ' Why not ? '
> Let baby listen, nothing loth,
> And work impartially on both.
> In clash of wills do not give in.
> Good parents are made by discipline.
> Even a backward child can foil them,
> If ever careful not to spoil them."

Punishment must be consistent in another way. The punishment meted out is likely to depend more on the result than on the nature of the act. No punishment, for instance, is given when the child gently rocks a small table. He is merely told not to do it. But when in the process of rocking the table a little later an expensive piece of china is caused to crash to the floor, the child gets a severe beating. It is difficult for him to understand the reason for the different attitude now adopted and he feels confused.

* Ogden Nash (1943). " A Child's Guide to Parents," in " The Face is Familiar." London. J. M. Dent & Sons.

When a punishment is given it should be immediate, so that there is no doubt in the child's mind as to the reason for the punishment. It should never be given because of loss of temper. It should only be given to help the child. The severity of the punishment should be reduced to the minimum necessary to produce the desired effect. If the child has confessed to some heinous sin, punishment should not be very severe, for if it is severe confessions will not be likely in the future. Severe punishment is wrong for another reason. It is apt to cause repressions, insecurity and a feeling of hostility ; and other behaviour problems will then arise.

The punishment should be accompanied by as little fuss as possible, for if there is a great deal of fuss and anxiety the child may repeat the performance as an attention-seeking device. After the child has been punished it is unwise to insist on repentance, for he is in no mood to give it except from fear. There must be no prolonged disapproval, as so often happens. When he has been punished he should be treated as if nothing has happened. It should not be discussed with others in his presence.

The method of punishment must vary with the circumstances and the child's level of development. The unpleasantness of the consequences must be greater than the pleasure of the act. In the first year at least no punishment is ever justifiable. In the second year a mere firm expression of displeasure or deprivation of privileges is usually sufficient, as soon as he is old enough to understand. He may need a tap on the hand if doing something particularly dangerous and if it is thought that he will understand its significance. The odds are, however, that he will not understand, and the punishment is therefore useless. It is very easy in the latter part of the first year and first part of the second year to laugh at a child who takes no notice of "No, no," or does what he is forbidden to do with redoubled speed, laughing loudly as he does it. He will inevitably repeat the performance laughed at. This trait, together with the negativism and desire for attention so characteristic of this age, make discipline difficult.

In the third year mild physical punishment may be needed, but only rarely. Simple deprivation and expression of displeasure is usually enough. He may be deprived of his books or taken indoors when he wants to play outside. In general the form of punishment should as far as possible be the logical outcome of what he has done, so that the child cannot fail to connect his action with the result. If, for instance, he throws cutlery or food about the table during a meal, the food can be peremptorily removed or he may be caused to eat the next meal alone. If in spite of a warning he tears paper up into small pieces and scatters them over the floor, he should be made to pick them up and perhaps be prevented from going into the garden or having his dinner until he has done so, though he may be helped in the process. He may be isolated or caused to stand in the corner on account of a temper tantrum or wilful damage. If he throws his books about or damages them, they should be confiscated. If he kicks a sibling, his shoes may be removed. If the 4-year-old fails to come in from the garden to dinner when told to do so (after being given 10 minutes warning that dinner will be ready in a few minutes), he is not smacked for it, and dragged in screaming ; he is given one reminder, and if he fails to come in then, he just misses his dinner. He will soon learn.

The final test of any punishment is the effect it produces. If it makes him worse it has failed and a mistake has been made. Having punished the child, it is always a good thing to ask oneself whether it was justifiable. Usually it is not.

CHAPTER 23

ANOREXIA AND OTHER EATING PROBLEMS

Anorexia

OF all behaviour problems anorexia is the commonest, the most easily prevented, the most easily caused and the most easily cured. One pædiatrician saw so many cases in consultation that he claimed that he built his house on anorexia. McCloy [280] visited 100 " normal " children in their own homes and found that 40 had feeding problems. Brennemann said that the child who will not eat represents probably 10–20 per cent. of children in private practice between the second and fifth year inclusive. It is a commonplace to be told in the out-patient department that the healthy well-fed-looking child in front of one " does not eat enough to keep a sparrow alive," " never eats a thing " or " has been losing weight ever since the day he was born." The mother says that she has tried everything to make him eat. Therein lies the trouble, for if she had tried nothing there would have been no difficulty at all.

Methods commonly Employed

In the treatment of any behaviour problem it is essential to discuss the management of the child in detail. In order to do this one must be conversant with the methods commonly employed by parents to deal with the problem. Brennemann's description [60] of efforts to make children eat is worth giving verbatim : " In innumerable homes there is a daily battle. On the one side the army advances with coaxing, teasing, urging, cajoling, spoofing, wheedling, begging, shaming, scolding, nagging, threatening, bribing, punishing, pointing out and demonstrating the excellence of the food, again weeping or pretending to weep, playing the fool, singing a song, telling a story, or showing a picture book, turning on the radio, beating a drum just as the food enters the mouth with the hope that it will keep going in instead of returning, even having the grandmother dance a jig—all regularly recurrent actual procedures encountered daily. On the other side a little tyrant resolutely holds the fort, either refusing to surrender, or else capitulating on his own terms. Two of his most powerful weapons of defence are vomiting and dawdling."

An excellent description of a typical food-forcing scene was given by Benjamin.[43]

I have seen all the following methods used, many of them in scores of children.

Coaxing Methods. The mother tries to persuade the child to eat. She watches his plate and asks him to eat just a little more to please her. She asks him to take a bite for Santa Claus, for Auntie Lizzie or for Guy Fawkes. She tells the boy that the food is good for him—but he is not interested, neither does he understand what she means (nor does the mother). She asks him to eat just a little more so that she can tell Daddy when he returns from work.

Distraction Methods. The mother turns the wireless, gramophone or television set on, or sings to him. One mother said that for a while the boy ate well when she and her husband sang to him at mealtimes, but then the boy joined in the singing and they had to try something else. The mother tells stories or recites nursery rhymes. The father neighs like a horse, or moos, and pretends to be a dive-bomber. One child would eat only if the father crept about the room on all fours, pretending to be a dog. Another child would only eat if his brother set off an alarm clock at frequent intervals near him, so distracting him and enabling his mother to slip some food into his mouth. One mother spent 4*s.* a week on comic papers to make him eat. Others have tried putting a mirror in front of the child so that he can race the image in getting the food down. It is a common practice to allow the child to have his meal while walking or running round the house or garden, in order, presumably, that he will forget to refuse to eat.

Bribes. Most parents faced with food refusal have offered their child bribes to make him eat. In most cases the bribes consist of sweets, ice-creams and excursions to the cinema or park. Some parents offer to let the child stay up longer in the evening if he will eat the dinner. One intelligent girl of 6 years was making between 3*s.* and 4*s.* a week in pocket-money out of the bribes. A boy of 4 would only eat if he was given a toy motor car, and he had collected a garage of between 200 and 300 motor cars in this way.

Tonics. Most parents have tried various "tonics." One mother said that the only way which she found to make her 3-year-old eat was to give her a mixture of Ribena and brandy.

Threats. The commonest threat is the warning that the child will not grow up big and strong like Uncle Bob unless he eats his dinner. The child apparently could not care less. Some mothers are unwise enough to threaten to go and leave the child unless he eats his meal. One mother said, "Tom, I shan't love you any more if you don't eat that." The boy replied disarmingly, "Mummy, whatever happens I shall always love you." Another told her girl that she would die if she did not eat more. The prospect did not seem to disturb her. Some mothers threaten to bring the child from next door to eat the dinner, but as this threat is never carried out the child does not take any notice. Many mothers threaten to punish the child if the food is not eaten. Others threaten to take him to a doctor, as if this is a severe punishment.

Forcing Methods. Most parents have tried and discarded food-forcing methods. They hold the child's nose and push the food in with a spoon. Any intelligent child resists violently, sends the spoon flying with a well-aimed blow, spits the food out or vomits.

Punishment. One father regularly beat his boy with a leather strap for not eating what he was told to eat. Most mothers have tried smacking their children for not eating. As Anna Freud said, "The meal becomes forced labour rather than wish fulfilment."

Food between Meals. The mother is so afraid that the child will starve that she gives him food whenever he asks for it. The usual story is that he has constant snacks of milk, sandwiches, cake, fruit or sweets. When the regular mealtime is reached he refuses everything. One mother said that she always carried a packet of biscuits with her wherever she went, so that if ever the boy asked for something to eat she would be able to give it to him immediately.

Allowing the Child to choose the Menu. Astonishing food fads are allowed to develop. One mother really believed that her 4-year-old child could eat nothing but bacon and eggs. He would not touch anything else, and that was all he had. Nearly all food fads in children arise from food forcing or over-anxiety about food.

It need hardly be added that the mother is not the only one who employs these methods. The father joins in, tending to be firmer than his wife and to use more physical punishment and forcing methods. If the grandmother lives in the house, she too joins in the fray. To the child's delight, the whole house revolves round what he will eat. His morale is good, for he always wins.

The Basic Causes of the Problem

Relevant Developmental Trends in the Child

Negativism. The Development of the Ego. Some babies quite suddenly between 6 and 9 months refuse the breast or bottle, and will only take food if it is given by spoon or cup. Some babies will refuse to eat if they are not allowed to help to hold the spoon and feed themselves. It becomes increasingly difficult to change from breast or bottle to cup after 8 or 9 months, or to change from thickened feeds to solids. Food refusal in these babies is due to the increasing determination in the child and his developing ego.

Of all principles of infant and child feeding probably the most important is the avoidance of food forcing. Food forcing is by far the most important of all causes of feeding problems. Children cannot be forced to take food. There is an old saying that any man can lead a horse to water, but twenty men cannot make him drink. Children rapidly learn that they can prevent their parents from forcing them to take food. They can fight, knock the contents of the spoon on to the floor, spit food out, refuse to chew it or vomit it up when once it has been swallowed. They discover that in mealtimes there are most satisfactory opportunities for creating a fuss and for attracting attention. A child discovers that his mother is most anxious for him to take a particular foodstuff, such as milk or meat. He refuses to take it, or refuses to chew it, or else he retains the food in his mouth for an hour or two, revelling in the consternation which he causes. He particularly enjoys the scene when he spits food out or vomits it up. His parents are foolish enough to talk about his terrible appetite in front of him, and so suggest to him that he is expected not to eat. He soon has the whole house revolving about his appetite, and he certainly makes the most of the situation. It is quite an achievement for a 2-year-old to compel his parents to play games, read to him, dance jigs, creep about on all fours, pretend to be animals and dive-bombers, in order to get him to consent to eat, when in fact he is hungry, wants to eat and would on no account be prepared to do without.

Another most successful attention-seeking device is dawdling. In my opinion it is the commonest cause of food forcing and so of food refusal. Up to a point dawdling is normal between the ages of 9 months and 2½ years, and all children do it. The child plays about with his food, patting it with his spoon and putting his hands into it. He drops some on the floor, puts some into his hair and anywhere but into his mouth. He has no understanding of time and therefore sees not the slightest reason to hurry. He is particularly likely to dawdle with the first course, much preferring the pudding. It is not surprising that the mother, failing to realize that all children do the same, thinks that he has no appetite and is not eating enough, and so she tries to hurry him and to persuade him to eat. This makes him all the slower, and the mother then tries to force him to take food. The mother, in addition, is in a hurry, because she wants to get the washing-up done and to clear the table, and for this reason too she hurries him, threatens him and tries to force him to eat. The dawdling, which began as a perfectly normal stage in eating behaviour, becomes exaggerated and nothing more than an attention-seeking device. This dawdling may persist for years if the parents persist in their efforts to hurry him. It passes from the conscious to the subconscious and the child cannot help it. I have seen a child who at a boarding school was compelled to sit alone at a special table because of the time he took over his meals.

The Development of Likes and Dislikes. At 5 months a child may have firm likes and dislikes. It is amusing to watch a 6-month-old baby sampling a food which he has not tasted before and deciding whether he will eat more of it or not. He may flatly refuse a dish which he does not fancy. He becomes used to a particular dish and cup and refuses food from any other. This is harmless within reason, but I once saw a 9-month-old baby who refused all fluid unless it was given to him in a wine glass !

He may refuse food merely because he wants to have a drink first. After he has had a drink he will eat the rest of the dinner without difficulty.

He is much more affected by the appearance of food than is commonly realized. From the age of 6 months or so he is more likely to take a red brightly-coloured food than a colourless nondescript mush. He likes variety and may readily become tired of a food which he is offered over and over again. Some mothers show little ingenuity in supplying variety and in making the food look attractive. Whatever happens, there should be no attempt to force him to take disliked foods. This would cause not only food refusal, but often a permanent dislike of the food in question.

The Desire for Independence and the Practice of New Skills. Failure to allow the child to practise his new manipulative skill in holding the cup or spoon may cause him to refuse food.

Children are likely to want to hold the bottle or cup when they are able to grasp objects at 5 or 6 months, and at any time from 6 months to a year they may demand to hold the spoon and help to feed themselves. The sooner this is allowed the better, for it is most desirable that they should learn to be independent and look after themselves. An independent child may be extremely annoyed if not allowed to hold the cup or spoon himself. Some babies would rather starve than be fed by their mothers in this age period. The mother is apt to refuse to let the child feed himself because she is in a hurry to get the housework done, or because she is afraid of the mess he will make. She should spread a sheet or paper under the chair to catch the droppings and only help when it is absolutely necessary. She does nothing when the food gets into his ear or hair, but has to step in when an attempt is made to place the inverted food dish on the head as a hat. If she laughs at the mess which the child is making, he will repeat the performance and make a bigger mess. Some children of a placid disposition show no interest in this age period in feeding themselves. Others are extremely insistent. One 7-month child was referred to me on account of "acute indigestion." The story was that when the first mouthful of food was given she screamed and refused to take more. Further questioning showed that after the first mouthful the girl tried to get hold of the spoon, and the mother smacked her hand and would not let her help. The child thereupon refused to take any more.

Individual Variations in Appetite. There are big eaters and little eaters. Some children need to eat much more than others to achieve an average weight gain. The quantity of food which a child eats is in part related to his personality. The placid child tends to eat more than the highly active determined one. There is no doubt that a very occasional child does have a particularly bad appetite without any parental mismanagement and without any illness or disease. These cases are very rare. Thorough investigation fails to reveal any cause. In the vast majority of cases of so-called anorexia, however, the cause is simply the food-forcing methods of the parents. I have only seen 2 cases of severe chronic anorexia of the type mentioned above in otherwise well children.

The child's appetite varies, like that of an adult, from meal to meal and from day to day. The appetite is particularly liable to be poor at breakfast. Failure to recognize these variations causes mothers to worry about their child's appetite when they remember the appetite of a previous child or see the appetite of the child next door. Food forcing then results.

Unhappiness. It is natural to expect that a child who is unhappy, whether because of parental rejection or insecurity or for any other reason, will have a poor appetite. When mealtimes have been allowed to become a misery for a child, it is not surprising that when he approaches the dinner table his appetite disappears. I saw a child who began to cry every time the dinner gong sounded. He knew what was in store for him as soon as the meal started—a prolonged fight, threats and smackings.

Lack of Fresh Air and Exercise.

Association and Suggestion. Any painful experience, such as taking a food when it was too hot, is likely to be well remembered by a child as young as 6 months of age, and he may refuse food looking like it or the dish which contained it for several days after.

Likes and dislikes are readily suggested by the parents.

The Attitude of the Parents

The Mother's Love for her Child. Realization that this is the underlying cause of most cases of anorexia will prevent one from being critical of the mother's mistaken methods.

Undue Preoccupation with the Child's Weight. This is partly the fault of weight charts and articles in popular magazines. Mothers do not realize that there are great differences in the build of children owing to a variety of factors, such as size at birth and family history. They make the mistake of thinking that a child who is not up to the average weight is abnormal, and so they try to force him to take food. They do not know that normal children differ in the speed at which they gain weight. They do not realize that after the third month there is a rapid falling off of weight gain, and therefore of appetite. They think that at 12 months the child should be gaining about 7 oz. a week as in the first month or two. It is my practice to explain to them that, if a child had to continue to gain weight at the rate of 7 oz. a week, he would weigh 23 stones by the age of 14, which would be too much. I have seen two doctor's children who were given a test feed at every feed for 9 months.

When a child has been ill or was prematurely born, a mother is apt to consider him " delicate " and so try to force him to take more food than he wants.

A Little Knowledge of Nutrition. Many popular books teach rigidity in feeding methods, particularly in the feeding schedule and in the quantity of food to be given. Mothers acquire the idea that they must give an exact quantity of milk, and if the baby refuses it or goes to sleep before the feed is finished they try to compel him to take more. After the first year parents are apt to insist on children taking foods which they have been told are " good " for them—vegetables, meat and milk. A recent textbook gives diets for normal children of all ages, and the diet for a child of 2–7 years includes the following quantities for dinner : 2 tablespoonfuls of mince, 1–2 tablespoonfuls of potato and 1–2 tablespoonfuls of pudding. The exact quantity of each foodstuff is laid down for every meal. Some doctors give " diet sheets " to mothers. Mothers reading such instructions may unfortunately try to adhere to them, and apply compulsion if the child refuses to eat what the diet sheet recommends. They completely ignore the individual likes and dislikes, the variations in appetite from meal to meal, day to day and child to child. Some children show a great preference for the sweet course at dinner and dawdle with the first course or leave it altogether. Mothers imbued with the vital importance of the meat course may try to compel their children to eat it and so meet with food refusal.

Mothers over-estimate the quantity of food which a small child requires. Many fail to realize that the apparently small quantity which he takes is quite enough for an average weight gain. The inevitable result is that they try to force the child to take more food.

Constant Nagging. Undue insistence on good table manners is apt to make mealtimes a misery. Such insistence is due to the wrong idea of training and of the age at which good table manners can be expected. In the first 3 years all children make some mess. The amount of mess made rapidly decreases in the second and third years and patience is necessary.

Attempts at Discipline (see p. 243). Many parents are obsessed with the idea that the child must learn from an early age that their will is law, and that he must be taught to do what he is told, so that he will not be spoilt. If this is applied to mealtimes food forcing results, and therefore food refusal.

Other Factors in the Mother. Over-anxiety and over-protection lead to food-forcing methods. Psychologists say that the rejecting mother tends to concentrate on the mechanical sides of upbringing—the eating and elimination—and so to cause food refusal. Impatience in the mother as a result of pressure of work may cause the child to refuse food. When a mother has gone to a great deal of trouble to prepare a special dish to " tempt " the child and he refuses it, it is not surprising that she becomes annoyed and may smack the child or try to force him to take it.

To summarize, by far the most important single factor in the genesis of anorexia is food forcing. The most important cause of this is the dawdling which is characteristic in the early days of self-feeding. Children cannot be forced to take food. In a fight over food the child always wins.

The great majority of appetite problems commence between 6 and 18 months of age, at the time when the child is developing independence of character and so resists domination.

Prevention

This lies simply in the realization that the vast majority of children are born in working order, with an appetite which is sufficient for their needs. The child's likes and dislikes should be respected within reason and he should be allowed to help to feed himself and, as soon as he is ready, to feed himself completely. It should be fully understood that there is never any need to persuade or force a properly managed child to eat.

In the weaning period the addition of new foods should be a gradual process, one new food being added at a time, and that only in small quantities.

Treatment

The lines of treatment to be adopted are implicit in the remarks made above. It is futile merely to say that there is nothing wrong or that he will grow out of it. That is quite untrue. There is something wrong, and it is very likely that he will not grow out of it as long as the mismanagement persists. The worst possible advice to give is that more force should be used and that the child should be compelled to eat.

As with all behaviour problems, one must avoid appearing to criticize the parents for their management. The measures which so many of them adopt to make their children eat are so fantastic that it is often difficult not to criticize or ridicule them. On the other hand, they must be brought to understand that the trouble lies entirely in them and not in the child. If the child has ever been away from home, emphasis should be laid on the fact that he ate perfectly normally when away from parental influence. It should be made clear that, as this is purely a matter of management, all tonics and medicines are totally unnecessary. All attempts at forcing the child to eat must be stopped. When a child refuses food in the weaning period, it is a good plan to offer him the breast or bottle first and then to offer him the new food when he is in a better temper. If he still refuses it he should be tried again a few days later. At this age, as in older children, there must be no persuasion, no coaxing, no bribing, no threatening and no punishment. All tricks to make him eat must be stopped absolutely. There is no need to let him walk about the room or garden in order that he will eat what is set before him. He should sit up to the table and eat the food or leave it. The mother must avoid anxious looks at the plate. The child senses anxiety from the mother's tone of voice and facial expression. There is no need for praise when the child eats his dinner. The food should be put before the child and it should be taken as a matter of course that he will have what he wants. It is as silly to praise a child for eating his dinner as it is to praise him for playing games in the garden. There must be no punitive attitude if he does not eat and no suggestion that he is being naughty. He should not be prevented from doing what he wants to do because he has not eaten his dinner. This suggests to the child that eating is a duty. If he does not want it then it is given to the cat, and no interest should be shown in the fact. There should then be absolutely nothing between meals. When a child is eating normally it does no harm at all to allow him to have occasional foodstuffs such as fruit, milk or sweets between mealtimes, but if he is being difficult about eating he should have nothing and be brought to realize that he will have to wait till the next regular mealtime ; and mealtimes should be regular—at least after the first 6 months.

The parents inevitably ask what they should do when he will not touch a meal. The answer is that he is left without any food until the next meal. They then ask what they should do if he refuses that. It is extremely unusual for such a refusal to occur. I have never seen it happen. If it did happen the child should still be left without food. *No healthy child ever starves because he is not forced to eat.* He will soon capitulate when hunger overtakes him as long as no one makes a great deal of fuss about what he eats.

There should be no undue insistence on any particular food. It has been shown experimentally that animals show considerable wisdom in deciding what food they require. Young[464] and Richter[352] have written excellent reviews of this work. Richter showed that when rats were given complete freedom of choice between eleven pure food elements—three solid foods and eight liquid, in separate containers—they took constant daily proportions of the various food elements, all of which were necessary for life. When special circumstances were introduced, such as pregnancy, lactation or removal of a gland, the rats knew how to alter the proportion of foodstuffs taken. If, for example, the parathyroid gland was removed, the rats took additional calcium. The implication for human beings is that there need be no excessive insistence that the meat or greens be eaten before the sweet. It is no disaster if a small child eats some of the meat course, then eats the pudding and returns to the meat. It will not cause bad habits. He will grow out of it. Up to a point the child's strong likes and dislikes should be respected, but that is a different thing from allowing him to choose the menu. A child nearing his third birthday will readily, if permitted, say " I don't like this," " I don't like that," " I don't like currants," " I don't like fish." Such a child is merely asserting his ego and is displaying what is commonly termed bad manners. This should be stopped. The mother should make it quite plain that the food in front of him is all there is and that if he does not like it he can leave it, but there will be nothing else.

The food should be made to look attractive, bearing in mind the child's fondness of bright colours. No over-facing excess is put on his plate. It is always better to put a small amount on his plate and let him ask for more than to let him habitually leave his plate half emptied. There should be reasonable variety so that he does not get tired of any one foodstuff.

As long as the child's appetite is poor it is unwise to give more than about a pint of milk per day. Excess of milk may take the appetite away and prevent him from having other more important foods. I saw a child with anorexia who was drinking 5 pints of milk a day, and the cream off a further 3 pints. As long as the child's appetite is normal there is no need to restrict the quantity of milk which he takes.

He should be encouraged to practise his new skills and to help to feed himself as soon as he is interested in so doing. At the age when domestic mimicry is a characteristic feature of the developing child—from 15 to 18 months of age onwards—he should be allowed to help to prepare the meal himself, helping with the potatoes, fruit and pastry. The child's appetite for products of his own handiwork, however horrible they look to the adult, is tremendous. Milk refusal can often be managed by allowing him to pour the milk out of the jug himself. It is a good thing for him to have his meals with his parents or with other children.

Dawdling over the food is difficult to treat. The child should certainly not be rushed. He should not be allowed to create a fuss and anxiety, or else the dawdling will continue as an attention-seeking device. He should certainly not be forced to take food more quickly. The inevitable result would be food refusal. Part of the dawdling may be due to over-insistence on the meat course. The child is much less likely to dawdle with the pudding or sweet course. One has to decide exactly how long the meal will be allowed to take. If the child is still playing with his food when the rest of the table has been cleared, and certainly when the washing-up has been done, the food should be removed. There may be a wail of dismay. The only way to deal with the problem is to make no fuss, but simply to allow a reasonable time for the child to eat, and then, without further ado and without any threats or argument, remove the food.

The child should get as much outdoor exercise as possible, and over-fatigue should be avoided.

It is not always easy to persuade the parents to carry out this treatment. In my experience most parents do, and the response is extremely satisfactory. As soon as the child realizes that he cannot cause any more fuss and attract any more attention in this way the food refusal abruptly stops.

Other Eating Problems

Obesity

The word " obesity " is derived from the word " *obesus*," which is translated in Lewis and Short's Latin Dictionary as meaning " Fat, stout, plump, stupid, that has eaten itself fat." Obesity is not a common problem in the first five years, but it can be a serious problem as soon as the latter part of the first year. Obesity at this period usually rights itself, in that there is usually a notable loss of fat in the second year, but this excessive deposition of fat should act as a warning that the child is liable to respond in future to a positive food balance by laying down fat. It is difficult to define because it is not possible to draw a line between normal weight and the abnormal. It is not entirely a behaviour problem, but it is in part, and for that reason it is discussed here. I have reviewed the problem in detail elsewhere.*

Ætiology

The ætiology of obesity is obscure. Few will disagree with Newburgh's [309] finding that " obesity is invariably caused by an inflow of energy that exceeds the outflow. This disproportion is brought out by abnormality of appetite." He could find no evidence of an endocrine

* *J. Pediat.*, 1958, **53**, 117.

disturbance in an exhaustive study of the subject. Bruch,[71, 72, 73 74] in an investigation of 142 obese children, reported that the families of 80 per cent. of the children thought that the food intake was greater than the average, while the remaining 20 per cent. thought that it was normal or less than the average. Their idea of the average, however, was likely to correspond to their idea of what the child ought to take. The cause of the over-eating is not clear. Bruch thought that an increased desire for food and obesity frequently became manifest after an emotional disturbance. She thought that such emotional upsets might cause a functional disturbance of the hypothalamus. Kennedy[232a] found that if the tuberal part of the hypothalamus of rats is damaged by electrolysis the animals became very fat by over-eating. From the first day after the operation they ate two or three times more than they had been eating before. The increase in weight was entirely due to the deposition of fat.

The cause of the over-eating is often over-protection. According to Steiner,[400] " over-feeding and over-protection may become symbols of motherly care and substitutes for real affection." Over-feeding commonly results from over-protection as a result of an illness, which has led the mother to consider that the child is delicate. Premature delivery may also implant the same idea in the mother and cause over-feeding. Other behaviour problems and other signs of insecurity are common in obese children. I was asked to see a 6-year-old child on account of severe food refusal of four years' duration. The mother said that she was " hardly eating a thing." She weighed 73 lb. Investigation in hospital showed that in fact her appetite was very excessive.

Over-eating is clearly not the only factor, because many over-eat but do not become fat, and it is often quite impossible to demonstrate that the diet of a fat child is greater than that of an average child. Mossberg[303] and many others have discussed the strong hereditary tendency. Van Noorden[424] said that 70 per cent. of his obese patients came from families in which obesity prevailed. Danforth[102] described a strain of yellow mice in which there was a great tendency to obesity at maturity, particularly in females, so that they weighed three times more than the average. Sometimes what superficially appears to be a hereditary factor turns out on further investigation to be merely a familial liking for good food and for over-eating.

Another difficulty is the fact—pointed out by Bruch, Mossberg and others—that obese children tend to have large body proportions, to be taller than the average and to have advanced bone age. The reason for this is obscure, but the explanation may lie in an abnormal secretion of adrenal cortical hormones. Simpson[384] reviewed the role of these hormones in the production of obesity, including work which showed that they can cause obesity without an increase in diet. He wrote[385] :

"It is as inadequate to state that adiposity is due to overeating as it would be to state that diabetes insipidus were due to overdrinking." According to Mayer[274] there are two symmetrical centres in the lateral part of the hypothalamus, which are sensitive to variations in the blood sugar. Hunger is produced either by a decrease in the blood sugar or by an impairment of the phosphorylation or utilization of sugar. Pennington[331] thinks that one factor is a defective capacity of the tissues for oxidizing pyruvic acid.

There are still some who diagnose Frohlich's syndrome of adiposo-skeletogenitodystrophy in cases of obesity. The diagnosis is almost invariably wrong. I have never yet seen a case. Wilkins[458] wrote that in eighteen years of experience in endocrinology, he had only seen one or two cases of Frohlich's syndrome, which includes diabetes insipidus. Others make the mistake of diagnosing thyroid deficiency. That diagnosis, too, is almost invariably wrong. Wilkins only found two obese children in over 200 cases of hypothyroidism. The basal metabolic rate is normal in obese children.

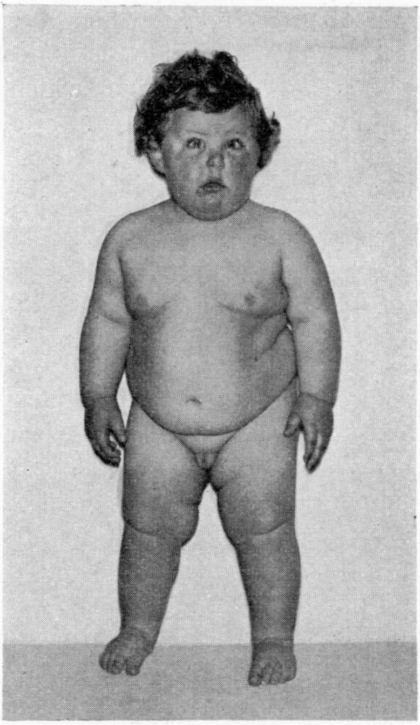

FIG. 69. Simple obesity, responding well to dietetic measures. Boy, $1\frac{10}{12}$, weight, 63 lb. Bone age, $3\frac{1}{2}$–4 years.

Mismanagement of feeding is undoubtedly a factor in many cases. It has been suggested that the common American practice of introducing cereals and soups (in the second to the fourth week of life) may lead to excessive weight gain. Excessive use of starch in later months (e.g. at the age of 4 to 6 months) may have the same effect. I have seen two fully breast-fed children who weighed 32 lb. at the age of 10 and 11 months respectively. It is probable that they each were taking 4 pints or more of milk from the mother. The children should have been weaned long before such obesity developed.

I have no doubt that much obesity is due to faulty eating habits in the home. Perhaps the major fault lies in the sweet-eating habit. Children are encouraged from an early age to eat large quantities of sweets.

Sometimes competition between siblings leads to excessive eating.

A certain amount of overeating is simply due to imitation. Many mothers unwisely press their children to have second helpings of food. In many families snacks are frequently eaten between meals.

In conclusion, one can say with certainty that though we do not understand the mechanism of obesity, children only become too fat if they eat more than they need.

Treatment

Prevention is better than cure. It is far easier to prevent obesity developing, when a child is beginning to show an excessive weight gain, than to treat it when obesity is fully developed. Although preoccupation with weight is undesirable, there is much to be said for a weight chart (see p. 84) on which a child's weight is plotted at intervals. I would only advise this in a child who showed any sign of excessive weight gain, especially if there was a family history of obesity. As Stuart [407] wrote, an excess weight gain of 2 lb. a year may easily pass unnoticed ; but it adds up to a considerable excess as the years go by. The earlier excessive weight gain is checked the better, and the easier is it achieved by a simple modification of food habits.

Early weaning is advisable in breast-fed babies who show a tendency to obesity. In bottle-fed babies a gradual change from an all-milk diet to mixed feeding should be made. In general it is wise to commence mixed feeds when a child reaches 16 lb. if he has not already started them on account of his age. He may otherwise take an excess of milk and continue to put on weight excessively. Care should then be taken to avoid giving excess of starchy food, such as cereals. The quantity of milk taken should be limited to 20–30 oz. per day. Purèed fruit and purèed vegetables are to be preferred to tinned soups, which have a high carbohydrate content. Jelly is useful for the second course at dinner, because it is liked by most babies and has little food value. Vitamin D may be given in concentrated form instead of cod-liver oil, because of its lower caloric value.

In the older child aged 1–3 care to avoid excess of starchy and fatty foods may be enough to correct the tendency to excessive weight. Fried foods should be avoided. Milk should be limited to 1 pint per day. Sweets should be eliminated and no food should be given between meals. It is not always possible to satisfy the child's large appetite without such foods, and in an occasional case amphetamine (beginning with 2·5 mg. per day, increasing to 10–15 mg. per day, before meals) may be given to reduce the appetite.

Attempts to make the child lose a great deal of weight are dangerous. The growth needs must be remembered, particularly when he is tall for his age, as most obese children are. It is safer to aim at keeping the weight fairly stationary while he is growing in height, at the same time giving him an adequate supply of vitamins (e.g. a mixed vitamin preparation).

Drugs are used only in the most extreme cases. Thyroid extract should not be used, as there is no thyroid deficiency, and there are possible undesirable side actions. Amphetamine may be used, but it may cause insomnia, and it is hardly ever necessary. A new sympathomimetic amine (" preludin ") is now being used to reduce appetite, but it may cause insomnia if used in the late afternoon. Methyl cellulose wafers (" Melozets "), which swell in the stomach in contact with fluid, are of some use in older children, but are unnecessary in younger ones.

It is much more important to discuss details of management with the parents, and to deal with their attitudes and habits. Care must be taken not to talk to the older pre-school child so much about his diet that anxiety is conveyed to him, with resulting insecurity. The parents should themselves set a good example, particularly in the avoidance of sweets.

Vomiting of Psychological Origin

Vomiting may occur from a variety of psychological causes. Excessive crying at almost any time in the first 3 years may make a child vomit. In the infant it is probably largely due to air swallowing which results from prolonged crying. The cause of the vomiting associated with crying in the 2–3-year-old child is not clear. The very difficult problem of the child with sleep refusal, who when left to cry makes himself vomit, is discussed elsewhere (p. 274). Food forcing is a common cause of vomiting in a child after the age of 5 or 6 months of age. It is commoner after the first birthday. It may occur when he is given food which he does not like, as an attention-seeking device. It inevitably causes considerable disturbance if it takes place at the tea-table, and other children may imitate it.

Any sort of excitement may make a child vomit. The excitement of an impending party may be enough to make him sick. In motion sickness there is a psychological element, the excitement of the prospect of a long trip in the car to the seaside or other desirable place being at least a contributory factor in causing the vomiting. If the vomiting is the subject of unwise conversation in front of the child, and if he realizes that there is a great deal of anxiety about it, it is likely to recur, partly as an attention-seeking device and partly as a result of suggestion.

CHAPTER 24

SLEEP PROBLEMS

The great majority of children sooner or later in the first 4 years develop sleep problems. These include crying when put to bed, refusal to go to bed for one parent and not for the other, refusal to lie down, awaking with or without crying in the night, prolonged failure to go to sleep, sleep rituals and early morning awakening. Often the "crying" begins as soon as the mother's back is turned. It starts as a mere shout without tears, the so-called "testing cry," but sometimes if she does not return promptly tears are shed and true crying begins.

The fussing and crying when the toddler is awakened from a nap are of no importance.

Methods commonly Employed

The usual story is that the parents coax the child and tell him to be a good boy and go to sleep. They play games with him, sit and read to him or tell him stories. They smack him for staying awake, lie at his side till he falls asleep, leave his light on or even bribe him to go to sleep. It is a very common practice for parents to take the child into their own bed. One 3-year-old child seen by me kept both parents occupied for 4 hours every night in trying to get him to sleep. Another bounced about the bed so much that the parents, aided by the grandparents, tried to get him to go to sleep by holding his four limbs down on the bed. Some doctors, and others, drug their child every night for months.

Relevant Developmental Trends

(i) THE DURATION OF SLEEP. The duration of sleep depends on a child's age, personality and intelligence and on the duration of his afternoon nap. The new-born baby sleeps most of the day. At 3 months the average baby has three or four sleep periods, at 1 year two or three, and at about 3 years of age he discards the afternoon nap. The more placid child sleeps a great deal more and may still sleep for most of the day at 4 or 5 months. He may continue to have an afternoon nap until he is 4 or 5 years old. The active child sleeps a great deal less. At 5 months he is awake for the greater part of the day and may refuse to have an afternoon nap by the age of 2. Various workers quoted by Despert [108] found that the more intelligent child tends to sleep less than the less intelligent.

The duration of the child's sleep at night is related to the duration of the nap during the day. Many parents make the mistake of allowing the 2- or 3-year-old to have a three-hour nap from 2–5 p.m. and then expecting him to be ready for the night's sleep at 6 p.m. It is very convenient to have a rest from the child in the afternoon and to get on with one's work, which is impossible when the child is around, but it does very often mean that the child will be wide awake and active for the rest of the evening. Chant and Blatz [87a] tried to correlate the duration of the daytime nap with that of the night's sleep. They concluded that before the age of 2 years children who have a long daytime sleep had a long sleep at night, and that from 3 years onwards those who had a long nap in the daytime slept less at night. This may be true for most children. I doubt it, and certainly in my limited domestic experience it is not true at all. When a child is 1 year old a long afternoon nap (of, say, an hour) is quite enough to reduce greatly the duration of the night's sleep, considerably postponing the time when he is ready to go to sleep in the evening. It must be admitted, however, that over-fatigue may delay sleep and shorten the duration of the night's sleep. Sometimes parents awaken their child from the mid-day nap too soon, and he is then very tired in the later afternoon and sleeps badly. Over-fatigue can shorten sleep in some children as much as the absence of fatigue does in others.

It is normal for any child from 18 months onwards to lie awake for a long time in the evening talking or playing, or to waken up in the early hours of the morning and sing. It is normal for a child to finish his sleep by 5 or 6 a.m. Some children are not tired at the time when one would expect them to be ready for bed. Gesell remarks that the bedtime of the $2\frac{1}{2}$-year-old is often 8–10 p.m. It is remarkable how a small child may go to bed tired out and awaken half an hour later, having apparently completely lost all fatigue, sleepiness and desire to sleep. He is then liable to cry for company. If taken downstairs he is then socially at his best.

Roberts and Schoellkopf [353] studied the sleep requirement of 783 children at Rochester (Minnesota) at the age of $2\frac{1}{2}$ years, and found that the duration of sleep varied between 8 and 17 hours, averaging 12·9 hours.

Because of these differences it is wrong to lay down rigid times for the amount of sleep required. The best guide to the adequacy of sleep is the absence of fatigue in the daytime. It must be admitted, however, that even if the child is unduly tired during the day it may be very difficult to increase the duration of his sleep. He is particularly liable to be tired in the afternoon when he is first doing without his afternoon nap. If he refuses this there is nothing that one can do about it. It rights itself in a very few weeks.

(ii) GOING OFF TO SLEEP AND FUSSING ON AWAKENING. Whereas the new-born baby cannot help going to sleep, after about 9 months it becomes a voluntary process which can be inhibited at will. A child can resist sleep for hours on end if he wishes, even though tired. Between 9 and 21 months going to sleep may be associated with rocking on the hands and knees, bed shaking, head banging, head rolling and finger sucking.

The child between 2 and 3 years often shows difficulty in awakening, crying and fussing for a while. Such difficulty is more likely to occur if there is also resistance to going to sleep. It is better not to hurry the awakening process.

(iii) THE SOUNDNESS OF SLEEP AND THE CAUSES OF AWAKENING. In general, the older the child the less sound the sleep. Practically nothing will awaken a young baby who is sleeping after a good feed, but from 4 months or so noises may readily awaken him. There is no doubt that some babies sleep much more soundly than others. Boys tend to be more restless in their sleep than girls. It is said that the more intelligent child tends to be more restless in sleep than the less intelligent. A late evening meal is associated with restlessness in sleep. Children, like adults, may sleep badly in unduly hot weather.

In the first 4 weeks most babies awaken twice for feeds in the night. Most of them drop the night feed by about 10 weeks. After that age babies only waken up for a feed under special circumstances, such as thirst on a very hot night or as a result of the compensatory increase of appetite after an illness such as gastro-enteritis. Discomfort of any sort may awaken a baby—colic, flatulence, excessive heat or cold, a rash, a wet napkin, teething or tight clothes around the limbs. I saw a child brought downstairs on a cold winter's night on account of crying. The overclothing was so excessive that clouds of steam were rising from the child. When the cause is merely a wet napkin the child goes to sleep when he has been changed. Teething is particularly liable to cause sleep disturbance. Some children have very little discomfort with teething. Others have severe pain, and consequently troublesome sleep disturbance, during the eruption of each new tooth. Most sleep disturbances, however, which are ascribed to teething, are in fact due to bad habit formation and therefore to mismanagement.

A common cause of sleep disturbance is the presence of parents in the same room. The child is disturbed by their coughing, snoring, arguing or by the squeaks of the springs. When a child awakens in his own room he is likely to go to sleep again without difficulty. When he awakens in his parents' room he soon realizes that his parents are there and he may cry for them. His mother, furthermore, would not know that her child had awakened if he were in another room, provided that he did not cry or talk, while if he is in her own room she is apt to get out of bed and look to see if he is safe. The child is then further disturbed.

It is an undesirable practice for the parents to have to creep about the house in the evenings for fear of wakening the child. Every effort should be made to get the child used to sleeping in spite of the ordinary household noises.

After the age of about 6 months children are apt to awaken with a sudden scream. It is not due to a wet napkin or other discoverable cause. It is probably a form of nightmare, and the child rapidly settles when the parent goes in to see him and gives him the desired security.

Between the age of 2 or 3 years children usually acquire sphincter control at night, and the full bladder may awaken the child and cause him to cry for help.

It must be admitted that often there is no discoverable cause for the child's awakening.

(iv) HABIT FORMATION AND ASSOCIATIONS. The child rapidly forms associations with sleep. The association of sleep release with head banging, head rolling and finger sucking has already been mentioned. It was also mentioned that a child with "three-months' colic" who was rightly picked up frequently in the evenings may continue to cry for the parents long after the colic has disappeared, until it is realized that the colic has been replaced by a habit. When a toddler is picked up at every whimper a bad habit is rapidly created, and the child then cries until picked up. If he can postpone bedtime by arguing or throwing temper tantrums, it becomes a habit and he causes trouble every night when bedtime comes.

The child becomes used to his surroundings, and even at 16 weeks a move from a bassinet to a crib may cause trouble. At 28 weeks a baby may refuse to sleep in a strange room. The whole rhythm of sleep may be upset as a result of taking the baby away on holiday. If he is allowed to sleep with his mother on account of an illness he may refuse to sleep alone for a time after recovery.

A child who is frequently rocked or sung to sleep soon becomes unable to sleep without it. Most children above the age of 18 months come to associate a particular rag, teddy or other object with sleep and will not go to sleep if deprived of it. Sometimes a double association can be seen. As soon as the child is given the special teddy he puts his fingers into the mouth and goes to sleep. After about 21 months the great majority of children develop some sort of sleep ritual, demanding this, that and the other before going to sleep. The child demands a drink, asks to be placed on the chamber and then asks for a doll. He commonly asks for the door to be left open for a specific width. If the parent is not careful he will keep adding to the ritual and successfully delay the departure of the mother from the bedroom.

Roberts and Schoellkopf described a girl whose ritual required at least half an hour. She always lay on her mother's bed after her shower with a towel around her, said her prayers, looked at three pictures on the wall, insisted that her three dolls be in their special places, and finally got into her own bed alone and asked for her wash-cloth, which she then sucked. Despert [108] described a 4-year-old girl who every night stroked a pair of clean pants, took an aspirin and asked her father to blow her feet. She then sucked her thumb and turned over to go to sleep. Most children discard these rituals shortly after the third birthday.

(v) THE EGO AND NEGATIVISM. These are major factors in sleep disorders. If the child discovers that he can cause a great deal of fuss and anxiety and can attract a great deal of attention to himself, causing the whole house to revolve round his sleeping, he will certainly continue to be difficult. Many parents are unwise enough to discuss the child's sleeping problem in front of him. Attempts to force him to lie down or to go to sleep will almost inevitably cause sleep resistance. In a fight the child almost always wins.

(vi) DESIRE FOR LOVE AND SECURITY. Most of the crying in bed is due to the desire for the parents' company. The phase of increased dependence on the parents between 18 months and $2\frac{1}{2}$ years makes the child's separation from the mother a matter of difficulty. This separation is all the more difficult if he has been deprived of her company all day because she has been at work or for other reasons. If the mother works all day in industry or leaves the child for long periods during the day so that she can " get away from him," playing Bridge and so forth, it is quite likely that he will cling to her in the evening and be particularly reluctant to leave her. It is always wrong to go out in the evening and leave the child without telling him, as soon as he is old enough to understand. He must never feel that he is being put to bed so that he can be out of the parents' way ; he will feel considerable resentment at being excluded from the family circle.

The happier the child is during the day, the greater his feeling of security, the fewer the scoldings which he receives, the more likely it is that there will be little trouble at night. The more tense he is during the day, the more tired and impatient the mother, the greater is likely to be the difficulty at night. As a result of his bad behaviour at night the mother has insufficient sleep and so is impatient and irritable with him during the day, and a very troublesome vicious circle is set up.

A child's sense of security may be broken by admission to a hospital, particularly if he undergoes a painful experience there, such as an operation.

(vii) FEARS AND NIGHT TERRORS. Fear of the dark is extremely common in children, especially after the age of 2. Not only is there fear of the dark but there may be fear of strange shadows or moving curtains. The fears may be suggested by alarming stories about ghosts and giants before bedtime.

Sleep walking is not usually a problem in the pre-school child. There are no known causes of the condition. It has been suggested that it is related to insecurity, but I very much doubt this. It may follow a late meal just before going to bed, and this can readily be avoided. Otherwise no specific treatment can be recommended, nor is it necessary.

(viii) THE USE OF BED FOR THREATS AND PUNISHMENT. It is very common to threaten to put a child to bed if he is naughty. This is always wrong, for it inevitably causes the child to associate bed with punishment.

(ix) OTHER PSYCHOLOGICAL CAUSES. Psycho-analysts offer various theories about the causation of sleep disturbances. Sperling [394] says : "According to psycho-analytic theory and practice, repressed infantile sexuality, particularly the œdipal conflict, is the principal cause of neurotic sleep disturbances in children. Sibling rivalry, with the repressed hostility and resentment toward the mother and death wishes directed toward the sibling, I would place second highest in the ætiology of such disturbance." She thinks that sleep rituals are aimed at counteracting such repressed feelings. Night terrors she regards as "the repression of intense sexual and aggressive impulses stemming from the œdipal complex."

(x) UNEXPLAINED PHASES. When children misbehave parents can always take refuge in the excuse that they are teething, or that they are merely "going through a difficult phase." There are often good grounds for such excuses. There is no doubt that children do go through such phases, for which no adequate reason can be found. Properly managed they rapidly pass ; badly managed they become perpetuated and fixed.

Parental Attitudes to Sleep

(i) A WRONG IDEA OF THE AMOUNT OF SLEEP NEEDED. Parents are often ignorant of the normal variations in sleep requirements and are seriously disturbed when the child lies awake, happily playing or talking with her dolls, or awakens at 1 a.m. and sings a few songs. Instead of leaving her alone they go in and try to persuade her to go to sleep. Rigid ideas of sleep requirements are liable to lead to sleep-forcing methods and so inevitably to sleep refusal.

(ii) OVER-ANXIETY AND EXCESSIVE DOMINATION. Over-anxiety, over-protection and excessive domination are important factors in the genesis of sleep problems. Many mothers frequently visit their children in the evening to see if they are safe and are apt to disturb them. Children often stay awake expecting such visits. The mother's anxiety is soon sensed by the child. Others go in to see the child and pick him up when there is the smallest whimper. Impatience in the parents to go out for the evening often causes trouble. A child is apt to be put to bed before he is ready for it or deliberate efforts are made to force him to go to sleep, with the opposite of the effect desired. The child may sense the fact that the parents want to get rid of him, as in fact they do. They want to eat their meal in peace and be on their own, but the child reacts accordingly and cries. Attempts to discipline the child and to make him obey cause sleep refusal just as much as food refusal.

(iii) RIGID METHODS OF MANAGEMENT. *It is thoroughly desirable to create good habits in the child, and as far as possible a fixed bedtime is eminently desirable. The child becomes used to a regular routine and accepts bedtime as a matter of course.* One cannot, however, agree with Blatz,[49] who wrote : "The most common error of training is to permit the child to put off the sleeping time even for five minutes." Such rigidity of management, though working well in many children, leads to a great deal of trouble in others, for it completely fails to take into account the different sleep requirements of children. It is not reasonable to expect small determined children to go to sleep smoothly when they are in no way fatigued.

(iv) SOCIAL FACTORS. A major cause of trouble after 4 or 5 months of age is allowing the baby to share the room with the parents. It is almost inevitable that he will be awakened. Overcrowding frequently makes the provision of a separate room impossible, but it can often be arranged that the baby's cot is carried out of the bedroom and put into the kitchen when the parents go to bed.

Of equally great importance is the proximity of neighbours or the presence in the same house of complaining relatives. The mother who has a small child in part of the house, particularly in part of one floor of a house, is in a very difficult position. If the child cries, immediate complaints come from the neighbours. As a result she is almost compelled to keep picking the child up and trying to force him to go to sleep. The inevitable result is the opposite of the effect desired.

Prevention of Sleep Problems

There should be some elasticity with regards bedtime, for reasons stated. If the toddler is not ready to go to bed at the usual time in the evening, one should try the effect of cutting down the afternoon nap.

Open-air exercise is a good source of healthy fatigue. Fatigue must not be excessive, for an over-tired child is apt to be difficult about going to sleep.

A wise pre-bed routine is essential. It is a good practice to read a story before the child goes to bed. There must be no argument about whether it is time to go to bed or not. Once the child sees that the mother is undecided, or changes her mind when pressed by him, he will certainly take advantage of it and try it again another night. Tears at this or any subsequent stage should be avoided. It is easy to become impatient when the child dawdles in putting his toys away or in putting his toys down to come up to bed. He should be allowed to help to prepare the bath—to turn the tap on, to throw the sponge in and to undress himself, even though it takes a lot longer than doing it all oneself. Children from earliest infancy enjoy the bath, and this should be encouraged. Much as one would like to complete the job as quickly as possible, the child should be allowed some time to have fun in the bath and help to wash himself. He should then be allowed to help to dry himself if he is old enough ($2\frac{1}{2}$–3 years) and put his nightie on. The bed in winter should be warmed by a bottle, which is taken out when he gets in. From the age of about 5 months, when he learns to grasp objects, he should be allowed to have toys in bed with him. It is no use expecting the toddler's bed to be tidy. The wise mother does not mind if he lies asleep in strange positions in bed, with his feet on the pillow (as long as he can be covered up), with a mass of toys all around him—his bits of rag, bobbins, bricks, old tins and toy dogs—for she knows that he is very much more likely to be quiet in the morning after early awakening if he has some toys than if he has none. He should not be tucked in excessively if he does not wish. The room should be well ventilated. The effect of a dark blind may be tried if there is difficulty in the summer. It is exasperating after fitting a dark blind, however, to be compelled to supply a nightlight because of the development of a fear of the dark. Overclothing must be avoided. The child should be put to bed with an air of certainty, for the child recognizes uncertainty and anxiety with astonishing rapidity. It is wise for the parents to take turns, because if no one else but the mother puts him to bed, difficulty might arise in the event of the mother's illness. It is wrong to tell him to be a good boy and go to sleep. This is asking for trouble in the shape of negativism. No one can go to sleep on request.

The rapidity with which children form habits must be remembered. There is no need to fear, however, that bad habits will be started if a child is given night feeds in the first 10 weeks if he demands them. It is wrong to refuse to pick up a child with colic, pain from teething or other discomfort because of the fear of habit formation and of spoiling the baby. A child should be given all the love and security which he needs when he is suffering discomfort. Habit formation may arise as a result, but once diagnosed it can readily be treated. It it not always easy, however, to draw a distinction between crying from discomfort and crying from habit. When one is really satisfied that the child is no longer having colic or other discomfort and that a habit has developed, the habit must be broken.

It is harmless to rock a child or sing him to sleep occasionally, but it readily leads to habit formation, so that he cannot go to sleep without such rocking or singing. He must get used to going to sleep without such devices. They may be used on odd occasions, as when, for instance, a child who normally sleeps without trouble awakens without apparent reason and seems to be unable to go to sleep again. In the same way it is harmless on occasion to take the crying child downstairs, but such a procedure readily becomes a habit and it must not therefore be frequently repeated.

No hard and fast rules can be laid down about the advisability of lifting a child out in the late evening to pass urine. It is futile before about 18 months of age, because he has not sufficient retention span to make it profitable. It should only be practised after that age, when the retention span is such that if lifted out he is likely to be dry in the morning, and if not lifted out he is liable to be wet. The practice should in any event be dropped as soon as possible in order to allow him to take responsibility for being dry in the night. Such lifting out does not usually disturb him. In my opinion there is no need to awaken him when lifting him out. He should otherwise only be visited when necessary, in order to see if he is adequately covered up. Children are likely to learn soon after the second birthday to cover themselves up if cold. Before that much anxiety can be avoided by the use of a sleeping bag in winter, and by clips which hold the blanket in place. Care must be taken, however, when a sleeping bag is used, or when bedclothes are tightly tucked in or held in place by clips, to see that there is no chance that the baby can wriggle down and suffocate himself. Many children kick all the bedclothes off in the process of finding a comfortable position in which to go to sleep, and the bed is in such a state of confusion that they can hardly be covered up without being disturbed. The mother should in these circumstances keep a blanket on a chair at the side of the bed so that this can be put over the child after he has gone to sleep. She may keep his hands warm by sewing mittens to his bed jacket so that they cannot be pulled off.

The Treatment of Sleep Problems

The treatment can be very difficult, and it is wrong merely to tell the mother to leave the child to cry it out, to smack him or to put him to sleep every night with drugs. The treatment is not nearly so simple. It has already been explained that the whole daytime management of the child has to be reviewed. It is necessary to explain the relevant features of normal child psychology in order that she can understand the reason for the approach suggested and the reason for the necessity of avoiding forcing methods, loss of temper and anxiety. The mother needs to lose any sense of guilt she may feel for failing to manage the child better. She needs to understand that the child's behaviour is in no sense naughtiness, a sign of nervousness or other abnormality. She needs to understand habit formation and, for that reason, the importance of being consistent. It is clearly wrong, if a child cries when put to bed, on one day to take him downstairs, on the next to sit and play games with him and on the third to leave him to cry. He can never learn that way. She must realize the importance of breaking a bad habit which has already formed. The mother herself may have to be given a sedative drug so that she is calmer in her management of the child in the daytime as well as at night.

The treatment of specific problems can be summarized as follows :

Crying. It is normal for the 6–12-month infant to cry for a minute or two when put to bed (the " testing cry "). No treatment is necessary. The child is put to bed and the mother leaves the room.

It is another matter if there is prolonged crying every night when he is put to bed. This is a habit, and it has to be broken. In the first place, he should be left to cry. If there is a danger that he will fall out of his cot he should graduate to a bed. If there is a danger that he can open the bedroom door (as many children can at about 2 years of age) and fall downstairs, then a catch may have to be put on the door. It must be emphasized, however, that it is thoroughly undesirable to lock a child in the bedroom, and it must only be done as a very temporary expedient.

It is difficult to say how long a child should be left to cry. A good mother finds it difficult to leave him crying at all, but it must be done to break the habit, which otherwise may continue for years. Some children show an astonishing capacity for crying for hours on end even though extremely tired. It is incorrect to say that if a child is left to cry it out for 3 or 4 days the habit will be broken. It is broken in most children but not in all. Spock [399] said that 9 out of 10 children so left cry for less than an hour. Most cry for less than half an hour on the first night, 15 minutes on the second, and not at all after that. He agrees that an exceptional baby may cry for hours, becoming more hysterical as time goes by, and so suggests that the mother should not allow him to cry for more than an hour or two. In any case it is absolutely essential for the mother to glance into the room at intervals to see if he is safe. A mother would never forgive herself or the doctor if, acting on his advice, she left a child to cry and he met with a serious accident as a result. The greatest difficulty of all is the fact that many children make themselves vomit by crying. In infants the vomiting is probably due to air swallowing. The increasing distension of the abdomen in a screaming baby is easy to observe. When a child can make himself sick by crying he cannot be left to cry for long. As has already been said, social factors, particularly the proximity of complaining neighbours, make it impossible to leave a child crying for long. In such cases there is only one way of breaking the habit, and that is the use of a drug.

Drugs should be used as a preventive rather than as a therapeutic measure. They should be used not after the child has begun to cry, but rather to prevent him crying. The drug is used not merely to break a bad habit, but to start a good one. It should be given before the child goes to bed, so that when he gets to bed he is very sleepy. It may have to be used to break a habit such as taking the child into the parents' bed. It should certainly be used to ease the pain of teething. It would be cruel to withhold the drug if the child is having considerable discomfort from an erupting tooth. One of the safest drugs to use is chloral. The dose has to be adequate and can only be determined by trial and error. In a child of 1 year of age one could begin with 3 gr., and increase each day if necessary by 2 gr. till the desired effect is achieved. As much as 10 gr. may be required even at that age. It should only be necessary to use the drug for 5 or 6 days. The prolonged daily use of the drug is quite unnecessary and merely a sign of defeat. Drugs are no substitute for careful history taking and a frank detailed discussion of the child's needs and management.

It is impossible to say with certainty in an individual child whether shortening or lengthening the afternoon nap will help. It is a matter for trial and error. It is certainly unreasonable on the one hand to expect a child to go to sleep when he is not in the least fatigued. On the other hand, excessive fatigue often postpones sleep. However tired a child is, he possesses the power of screaming and resisting for prolonged periods if he so wishes.

When a child of any age wakens up in the night and cries, the line of action depends on the nature of the cry and on the frequency with which it occurs. When there is a sudden half-hearted cry, gradually decreasing in intensity, it is usually better not to go in to see the child. It is another matter if he emits a full-throated shriek. It is then essential to go in to see him immediately. He does not make such a noise without reason. The causes of night awakening have already been mentioned. He may have vomited, had a nightmare or be strangling himself. He may want to empty the bladder. Whatever the cause, his needs should be attended to without delay. The longer he is left to cry the longer it takes to pacify him. Crying, if allowed to continue, becomes hysterical, the child becomes greatly distressed and continues to show the sudden jerky respirations known as sobbing long after he has been picked up. A stay of a minute or two is usually enough to give the 2-year-old awakened by some fear the security which he needs. When the younger child has been awakened by a wet napkin, the napkin is changed and the room is then immediately left. As has already been said, if he is occasionally rocked or sung to sleep no harm is done.

It is another matter when the child wakens up every night and screams. One mother complained that her child awakened twelve or fifteen times every night and screamed, and she went in to see her every time. Such crying is a habit, and the habit must be broken. It is always wrong for the parents to take the child into their own bed. This inevitably creates a habit very rapidly, and sooner or later the habit has to be stopped. It is always wrong for the same reason to sit and play games with him or to make a practice of taking a hot drink to him whenever he awakens and cries. The necessity of avoiding a scene, of not having a fight with the child or smacking him has already been described. It is stupid to smack a child for wanting the company of the mother whom he loves, for that is the cause of the crying. Only occasionally is smacking justified in the older child, when there is deliberate screaming in the night unrelated to night terrors.

Refusal to go to Bed for one Parent and not the other. As has already been said, this may be due to the child's greater dependence on the mother, especially between 2 and 3 years. The father should, if possible, put the child to bed every day for a week or so, and then the mother should take over, being careful to avoid any show of anxiety or doubt about what the child will do. The habit may have to be broken with the aid of a drug.

Refusal to Lie Down when put to Bed. He should be left sitting or standing up. The child of 2 is usually able to cover himself up in bed. The use of a sleeping bag in the winter is a help to keep the child warm. The mother may have to look in on him as soon as he has gone to sleep in order to cover him up.

Sleep Rituals. These have to be broken, especially when the child is adding to them.

Failure to Sleep or Awaking without Crying. It is normal for children, especially after 1 year, to lie awake in the evening and talk and play. It is normal for a child of $2\frac{1}{2}$ to waken up at 1 a.m. and sing. On no account should the mother go in to see him or do anything about it. He will go to sleep when he is ready to do so.

Early-morning Wakening. I do not know any answer to this problem. The child has no sense of time. He cannot be blamed for thinking it is time to get up at 5 a.m. The problem is almost confined to the child of 18 months onwards. There is not likely to be much difficulty if there are two children who are old enough to play with each other. If he merely awakens and plays with his toys and sings, there is no need to do anything about it. When he cries or insists on going into his parents' room, it is not so easy. It is quite futile to leave him to cry it out, hoping to break the habit that way. Not being tired, he will continue to cry incessantly until the parents are worn out. He should, of course, be given a plentiful supply of toys to have in his room. One can try the effect of changing the napkin or giving him a drink or placing him on the chamber, but it usually does not help. He is wide awake and full of energy, and he sees no reason why his exhausted parents are not as pleased to see him as he is to see them. One may try changing the child's napkin or lifting him out at 10 or 11 p.m., in the hope that he will at least not be awakened early by a wet napkin or a full bladder. One might think that if the child were put to bed later that he would awaken later, but the reverse may occur. One can only console oneself with the thought that this is usually a temporary phase. When the child is old enough to sit on the chamber without help (from 2½ onwards) and when the bladder capacity increases, as it does with age, there is likely to be less early-morning disturbance. The greater the child's intelligence at this age the greater the likelihood that one can persuade him the previous evening not to cry for his parents when he awakens in the morning. An average 3-year-old child is certainly old enough to understand that he should not disturb his parents when he awakens. Often no measures succeed, but he grows out of it.

Conclusions

Enough has been said to indicate the difficulties which may arise with sleeping problems. Every sympathy should be shown with the mother, who feels at her wit's end. She feels quite powerless with the child. She has discovered that smacking is useless. She cannot reason with him, because he does not understand. She cannot explain to him that she is tired out and longing for sleep. She cannot leave him to cry, because the neighbours complain or he makes himself sick. A full, careful history is essential in order that the mother can be helped to deal with the problem. It is wrong to think that the problems are easy to solve. They can be very difficult and there is no answer to early-morning awakening. One cannot agree with Blatz [49] when he says : "There are no problems of training so easily dealt with and which respond so readily to adequate treatment as those connected with sleeping. A reasonable routine rigidly but patiently enforced is always successful." Would that it were always so easy.

CHAPTER 25

PROBLEMS OF SPHINCTER CONTROL

Most children develop minor problems of sphincter control. Most of them have phases of refusing to sit on the chamber. Other problems include delay in the acquisition of control of bowel or bladder, or loss of control when once it has been acquired ; deliberate withholding of urine or stools, either at all times or merely when placed on the chamber ; constipation, sometimes causing diarrhœa and incontinence ; frequency of micturition and stool smearing.

The Normal Development of Sphincter Control

The very infrequent bowel action in many breast-fed babies is discussed elsewhere (p. 69). In any child there may normally be 2 days between motions.

The frequency of urination in babies varies from child to child. According to Gesell,[147] there is often a temporary phase of increased frequency at the age of about 21 months. At 2½ years there is often a retention span of about 5 hours. The retention span then rapidly increases with age.

Babies commonly empty the bowel and bladder immediately after a meal, especially in the first 8 months, and they can very often be "conditioned" to use the chamber any time after 2 or 3 months of age. This conditioning frequently breaks down as a result of teething or some disturbance of routine, particularly between 12 and 18 months. It is important to realize that there is no voluntary control at this time, for voluntary control does not begin till about 15–18 months of age.

The first indication of voluntary control is awareness at about 15 months of having passed urine, the child pointing it out to the mother. By about 16–18 months the child is able to say "No" with reasonable correctness when asked if he wants to urinate. He now begins to tell the mother just before he passes urine, but he does not give her time to "catch" him. The urgency decreases as he grows older, and by 18–24 months he tells the mother in sufficient time for her to place him on the chamber. By 2–2½ years he is able to pull his pants down and go to the lavatory and may climb on to the lavatory seat unaided. He takes pride in so doing and may refuse to pass a stool if his mother tries to attend to him. In a study of 783 children at Rochester (Minnesota) Roberts and Schoellkopf[353] found that 92·2 per cent. of girls and 77·5 per cent. of boys were taking responsibility for going to the toilet for a motion at the age of $2\frac{1}{2}$. Bowel control is usually acquired before bladder control. Children at a similar age also take responsibility for not wetting their pants, and as a result the napkin is discarded during the day. The child is still wet at night. By $2\frac{1}{2}$ the retention span is longer, and between $2\frac{1}{2}$ and 3, if he is lifted out at 10 or 11 p.m., he is dry in the morning and the night-time napkin is discarded. The chamber is placed at his bedside and he gets out of bed and attends to his own needs. Roberts and Schoellkopf found that 58·8 per cent. of 783 children were wet at some time of the day or night at $2\frac{1}{2}$. At about $3–3\frac{1}{2}$ he is dry by night, though occasional accidents may occur till he is 4 or older. He rarely soils his pants after the age of 2 years, though an accident may occur if the stools are temporarily loose. Girls tend to acquire sphincter control earlier than boys.

Temporary relapses of control occur as a result of teething, an infection, a change of surroundings or some other change in routine. Short phases of refusal to sit on the chamber occur from time to time without apparent reason. In some instances such refusal occurs with the eruption of each new tooth, the child's behaviour returning to normal in 2–3 days.

The extreme urgency in the early days of voluntary control is worthy of emphasis. Once the child feels the urge to pass urine or a stool he cannot wait a minute without doing it. He soon develops a genuine desire to be clean and the desire to pass urine is often shown by a shriek, as if some dreadful accident has occurred. The urgency rapidly disappears. There is a gradual transition from the entirely unconscious voiding of the baby through the stage when the child is fully conscious of the act (15 months), past the stage when he becomes conscious of the desire immediately before emptying occurs, to the stage when he can wait as long as circumstances make it necessary.

Shortly after control has been acquired children commonly go through a phase of deliberately withholding the urine or stool. The child knows that he wants to empty the bowel or bladder but does not want to drop his toys or stop his game. He " holds " himself below, characteristically jerking himself up and down, and has to sit down as if he dare not stand up. Accidents commonly do happen at this stage. He emits a shriek and is unable to move from the spot. Even though the child is old enough to look after himself, the wise mother sees that accidents are avoided when he is concentrating on some exciting game, and reminds him to go to the lavatory. Some children find it difficult to pass urine after a long span and have to be placed in a warm bath before they can empty the bladder.

Children often pass through a stage of stool smearing between the age of 1 and $2\frac{1}{2}$, especially at 18 months. They have a tremendous interest in the eliminations at this age.

There are considerable variations in the age at which sphincter control is acquired. In some conditioning is acquired early and there is no breakdown. Voluntary control is acquired without difficulty and the child is completely dry by day from 9 months or so. This is exceptional but not rare. In others there is little sign of voluntary control until after the second birthday.

Methods commonly Employed

I have frequently seen all the methods described below.

Mothers try to insist on the child passing an " adequate " and regular stool, and compel him to sit on the chamber for long periods (e.g. 20 minutes three times a day) in order to " train " him. They coax him, offer bribes (trips to the town, sweets), threaten punishment if a stool is not passed and smack him for " failure." He screams and kicks to get off the chamber, but he is held down by force. He learns to withhold the urine or stool until he is off the chamber and then passes it in his pants or on to the floor. I have seen several cases in which paper was regularly spread out on the floor for the child to pass a stool on, as he would never pass it into the chamber. Such children usually pass the stool away from the paper. One child who was accustomed to receiving bribes for passing a stool would daily say, " What will you give me if I use the pottie ? " Trouble begins even before the child is placed on the chamber. I was impressed by the screaming and kicking of a boy who was being undressed so that he could be examined. The mother said : " He is always like that. He thinks that he is going to be put on the pot." Mothers sit with their children when they are on the chamber and play games with them. They may sit on the lavatory themselves in order to set the example. They place hot water in the chamber, thinking that the steam will enable the child to pass a stool. Even when the child is 8 or 9 years old the mother insists on staying with him and inspecting the product to see if it is adequate. Some go to the trouble of building a special seat for the child, as he refuses the ordinary seat. One child of 9, with fæcal incontinence as a result of constipation, was every morning placed in charge of his elder sister, whose duty it was to see that he passed a stool.

Mothers say that they have " tried everything " to get the bowels moving. They have " really persevered." They have tried numerous patent medicines, inserted soap sticks into the rectum and given enemas, and still the child is no better. The mother says that his bowels are the despair of her life. One despairing father said that his daughter regarded " all time spent on the pot as so much time wasted."

The Basis of Disturbances of Sphincter Control

The basic causes of problems of sphincter control can be summarized as follows :

The Wrong Idea that Children need to be Trained to be Clean. They are not trained. They can only be helped when they are developmentally ready to learn. Numerous books advocate strict " training " methods. As Halliday [179] put it, " When the clock strikes certain hours little pots are punctually applied to little botts." Such methods frequently cause the mother to keep the child on the chamber against his will, and rebellion then results. Bostock and Shackleton,[53a] in discussing the frequent delay in the acquisition of control in children who are rigidly trained, and the frequent breakdown of control in children so managed, considered that unwanted children are particularly liable to be trained by strict rigid methods.

Ignorance of the Normal Variations. Variations which occur in the age of acquisition of control are very great. If the first child acquires control early the mother is apt to expect the second one to acquire control at the same age, and she punishes the child for his " failure."

Ignorance of the Normal Bowel Action. Mothers have a greatly exaggerated idea of the importance of a daily action. When a child misses a day they try to force him to have a motion or give purgatives. Many cases of chronic constipation have started with the mother's anxiety about the infrequent motions of a breast-fed baby. The child who normally has motions at irregular times is the one who is apt to be forced to sit on the chamber for long periods against his will. Parental over-anxiety is a major factor in the genesis of the problem. The mother who carefully inspects every stool which the child passes in order to decide whether it is adequate or not is the sort of mother who owns the child who refuses to empty his bowels.

Ignorance about the Development of Sphincter Control. Mothers think that the " conditioning " of a child to pass a stool or urine is synonymous with voluntary control. When conditioning breaks down, as it does in the majority of babies, they interpret it as a refusal by the child or naughtiness and punish him. The child then rebels.

Mothers fail to understand the normal sequence of events in the development of control and think that a child is naughty for telling them about his need too late. The boy is then smacked. Later, when accidents occur, he is punished and a display of fuss and anxiety is shown. He then deliberately does the opposite of what is wanted.

Development of the Ego and Negativism. Nothing pleases the child more than to have the whole house revolving round his bowels. He discovers that not only can he refuse to take food in without his parents being able to do anything about it, but he can refuse to let anything out. Both achievements cause untold anxiety, fuss and attention, and he delights in it. As with food refusal, his morale in fights is good, for he always wins. He delights in the fuss which occurs when there is an accident or when he deliberately passes the stool into his pants as soon as he has been allowed off the chamber. He finds that there is no more successful way of annoying his parents. He likes to have his mother sitting with him in the bathroom, playing games with him, coaxing and trying to persuade him to have a motion, and he delights in refusing to oblige. He uses the chamber for anything but what it is intended for. He roams the room on it, plays games when sitting on it or wears it as a hat.

A baby may withhold stools deliberately because he has passed a hard one which hurt him or because he has a painful fissure *in ano*. More often he withholds it because he finds that by so doing he can draw attention to himself and cause a great deal of fuss and anxiety. It should be understood, however, that when this voluntary inhibition of defæcation continues for some weeks stools become hard, considerable dilatation of the colon (megacolon) occurs and dyschezia develops, so that the rectum becomes insensitive to distension. The final result is that the child cannot have a motion if he tries. The hard scybala irritate the mucosa and cause diarrhœa, and there is frequently associated fæcal incontinence. The picture is then a strange one of diarrhœa with masses of hard fæces to be felt in the rectum, and often in the abdomen. The abdomen may become severely distended and the diagnosis of tuberculous peritonitis or even of malignant disease is not uncommonly made. Hirschsprung's disease is closely simulated, but fæcal incontinence and a full rectum make it very unlikely. The hard scybala may themselves cause anal fissures, so that further retention occurs as a result of painful defæcation.

A child can satisfy his ego, his craving for attention, by means other than the mere retention of stools or of urine. He enjoys the fuss which is made when he has an accident and is very apt deliberately to repeat the performance. It is unfortunate that the period of the early acquisition of sphincter control coincides exactly with the phase of resistance or negativism. The majority of functional disturbances of sphincter control are due to efforts to force the child and the child's refusal to be forced.

Another attention-seeking device is excessive frequency of micturition. The child discovers that when he asks to use the chamber the mother immediately drops everything, and probably carries him upstairs. He is then apt to demand to use the chamber every few minutes. It is difficult for the mother to refuse to answer his call, because she assumes that the request is genuine and that he will not learn to be dry unless he is given immediate attention. It is true that there is genuine urgency at this age and that children genuinely desire to be clean and dry if properly managed. It is not easy, therefore, to decide just how much is natural urgency and how much is a deliberate attention-seeking device. If it is decided that it is the latter, it has to be treated in the usual way by ignoring the call except at what are considered suitable intervals. The urine should always be examined in these cases so that a urinary tract infection or polyuria can be eliminated.

Laziness. On a cold night, particularly if the lavatory is at the other side of a yard, a child may prefer to wet himself rather than to go to the lavatory.

Unhappiness in the Child and other Psychological Causes. Unhappiness or insecurity for any cause may lead to a reversion to infantile habits, including the loss of sphincter control. The insecurity may be the result of jealousy, a spell in hospital, domestic friction and over-strictness on the part of the mother. Agatha Bowley [56] wrote : " Soiling and wetting are the natural symptoms of the deprived child. They arise from libidinal satisfactions being withheld and represent the child's attempt to obtain substitute gratifications."

Whatever the cause of the reaction, most would agree that unhappiness is a common cause of sphincter disturbances.

Freud [137] explained the deliberate withholding of stools as follows: " Children utilizing the erogenous sensitiveness of the anal zone can be recognized by their holding back of fæcal masses until through accumulation there result violent muscular contractions." " One of the surest premonitions of later eccentricity or nervousness is when an infant obstinately refuses to empty his bowel when placed on the chamber." " The retention of fæcal masses, which is at first intentional in order to utilize them as it were for masturbatic excitation of the anal zone, is at least one of the roots of constipation so frequent in neuropaths." I personally feel that the problems mentioned are due simply to the developmental trends and parental attitudes described above.

Neglect and Failure to Help the Child. The acquisition of sphincter control is later in children brought up in an institution than in children at home. Unhappiness together with a failure to help them in the learning stage is primarily the cause of this.

Mothers who have themselves had enuresis may regard it as an act of God and fail to help their children to acquire control. They regard them as having " weak kidneys " or " a weak bladder " and do nothing to help them when they show a desire to pass urine. One mother told me that she had never placed her 4-year-old daughter on the chamber because " she did not mind washing nappies."

There is often a strong history of nervous instability in the parents of enuretic children.

Organic Causes. Tilney and Casamajor,[415] Hardcastle [182] and others have shown the intimate relationship between myelination of the nervous system and its function. It seems likely that the development of sphincter control is related, like other skills, to the myelination of the appropriate part of the nervous system. There seems to be a familial rate of myelination. This theory would explain the finding that in about half of all cases of enuresis there is a history of similar trouble in other members of the family, particularly the mother or the father.

Bakwin [33] considered that enuresis (defined as incontinence of urine after the third birthday) consists of " a hereditary abnormality of bladder function, the chief characteristic of which is the urgent need to empty the bladder. Cerebral control is normal, but the urgency of the call is so intense that voluntary inhibition may be overcome." There is a persistence, in other words, of the state at 18 months, when the child, once he feels the urge to void, cannot wait.

Meredith Campbell [80] described the frequency of structural abnormalities in the urethra in cases of delayed acquisition of control of the bladder. The abnormalities consist of anomalies of the bladder neck, valves in the urethra, enlargement of the verumontanum in the male and urethro-trigonitis in the female.

It is always essential in cases of severe constipation to examine for organic causes. The simplest is a painful fissure *in ano*, which causes the child to withhold the stool because of painful defæcation. A prolonged period of constipation may readily result from the passage of a single hard stool with pain for any reason. Other organic causes of constipation are rare, but they include congenital stricture in the anorectal region and Hirschsprung's disease.

It must be admitted that in many cases of severe constipation in young children, no cause can be found, and there is no history of mismanagement. Further research into this problem is required.

It need hardly be added that a mentally defective child is likely to be late in acquiring sphincter control, as he is in all other skills.

There is no relationship between these problems and spina bifida, except in the very rare case where the spina bifida is associated with a paralysis of the legs.

Prevention

The management of the child must be adapted to the level of his development. He will not learn voluntary sphincter control until he is developmentally ready for it, and all attempts to " train " him before he has shown himself ready are likely to lead to the opposite of the result desired.

There is a difference of opinion as to when " conditioning " should be attempted. I do not think that it matters as long as the difference between conditioning and voluntary control is fully understood, so that there is no anxiety when breakdown occurs. Provided that there is never a fight to keep the child on the chamber and the child does not resist, "potting" is a harmless procedure, and it does undoubtedly save dirty napkins. When there is a phase of resistance to the chamber there must on no account be anxiety and attempts to compel the child to sit on it. Most children sooner or later develop such phases. The motto should always be "Placid painless potting." The child is placed on the chamber when he awakens from a nap, immediately after a meal and when he comes in from outside. If he does not void in a minute or two he should be taken off it. I disagree entirely with opinions on bowel training expressed in various books. Wright [463] advocated the use of an enema at the age of 3 months in order to "train" the child in regular bowel action. Blatz [49] advocates the use of a soap stick or glycerine suppository at a similar age. It is extremely doubtful whether any device like this alters the rhythm in a child whose rhythm is naturally irregular. Enemas and suppositories should never be given unless absolutely necessary.

The mother should know the normal development of control and realize the great individual variation in the age at which it is achieved. She should get out of the idea that she is training the child. All she can do is to help him when he is ready by enabling him to reach the chamber in time. She can also help him by allowing him to take responsibility for looking after himself as soon as he is ready—thus satisfying his ego, his pride in new skills.

It is futile to allow him to do without a napkin too soon, before he has shown himself able to tell the mother when he wants to void. When he is able to manage without a napkin during the day, he should be tried without one in his daytime nap. At night it is wrong to let him do without a napkin until, having been picked up at 10 p.m., he is usually dry in the morning, unless he can be persuaded to get out of bed and use the chamber unaided. This is not likely to happen till after the age of $2\frac{1}{2}$. If the napkin is discarded too soon frequent accidents are inevitable, and they upset both mother and child. If the child is allowed to wear a napkin after the time that he is ready to do without, the mother merely retains all responsibility for his dryness and the child is late in learning control.

The age at which a child should be picked up at 10 p.m. is a matter of trial and error. It is a mistake to think that one is "training" a child by picking him up. Usually the child is not even awakened. I cannot agree with those who feel that it is essential that the child so picked up should be thoroughly wakened so that he knows what he is doing. Parents are rightly reluctant to waken children at this time.

They may be slow to go to sleep again and be fatigued next day as a result. If a child is disturbed by being picked up it should as a rule be avoided. It is useless to pick a child up if he is found to be wet at that time. This would mean that his retention span is not long enough. On the other hand, it is sometimes found that picking a child up delays his early-morning awakening. Sooner or later it will be found that if a child is not picked up he is wet in the morning, while if he is picked up he is dry. Picking him up will now enable him to do without a napkin and so take responsibility himself.

Some children are not dry at night unless they are given a chance (without a napkin) to get out of bed to use the chamber when they want. This is impossible if the child is in a cot, but most children after the second birthday are quite ready for a bed. Naturally, he cannot get out of bed in winter if he is in a sleeping bag.

Every effort should be made to prevent the stools being hard and so causing painful defæcation. Any tendency to this should be treated by attention to the diet (increasing roughage and fruit) and, if necessary, by giving a mild aperient such as milk of magnesia.

The child should become accustomed to using a toilet outside home ; otherwise he may refuse to void when visiting friends.

The most important single point in the normal establishment of sphincter control is the absolute necessity of avoiding a fight with the child, of trying to force him to sit on the chamber or to void when he does not wish to do. At all costs there must be no fuss when a lapse occurs, when he refuses to sit on his chamber or when accidents happen. The placid, understanding mother who takes everything in her stride has little trouble with her child in the difficult days when sphincter control is being acquired. A few extra weeks of napkin washing when the child is 1 or 2 may save months of pants and sheet washing when he is 3 or 4.

Treatment

The treatment is implicit in the remarks made above. A careful detailed history of the whole management of the child has to be taken before the treatment can be discussed with the mother. It is essential to know how the mother tried to " train " the child and how she deals with " accidents." One has to understand her attitude to the problem, and that of her husband and relatives in the house. The mother must know a little about the normal development of sphincter control and the relevant features of the psychological development of children, in particular the negativism and desire for fuss and attention in the age group in question. She must learn that no harm will befall the child who fails to have a motion every day as long as the stool is not very hard. Every effort, in other words, has to be made to remove her anxiety, which is usually the basic cause of the whole trouble.

All forcing methods must stop. She must stop showing anxiety or making a fuss when accidents occur or when the child refuses to sit on the chamber. She must on no account punish the child for an accident, scold him, try to shame or ridicule him or show anger. She must not discuss the problem with anyone in front of him or do anything else which encourages him to use the difficulties as an attention-seeking device. She should, in fact, show no interest in accidents apart from clearing up the mess. There is no place for bribes or rewards in treatment. She must be told about the wide normal variations in the age at which control is acquired, and she must be brought to understand that forcing methods and anxiety will do nothing more than postpone the age at which control is established.

Even without any mismanagement most children have temporary phases of refusal to sit on the chamber. The refusal should be respected and no attempt should be made to persuade the child to change his mind. An effort may, of course, be made to distract him by giving him a toy, but if he still refuses nothing further should be done about it. Provided that no forcing methods are applied the phase will be a temporary one only.

When serious harm has already been done the problem is indeed a difficult one. When a child has for some weeks displayed complete rebellion against the chamber, there are only two alternatives which are likely to work. One is for the mother to stop "potting" him at all for a sufficiently long period for him to forget all about it—and this depends on the child's memory. The period may be one of, say, 3 months. The mother then starts again after the doctor has given the necessary advice about management. The other alternative—in many ways undesirable but sometimes necessary—is to take the child into hospital, where a tactful nurse will soon cope successfully with the problem. The disadvantage of this method is that the child is likely to relapse as soon as he returns home. It is better for the mother herself to correct the mischief that has been done.

When a child, aged about 18 months, who is in the process of acquiring voluntary control of the bladder, demands the chamber every few minutes, one has to decide whether this is purely an attention-seeking mechanism or a genuine fear of an accident. It is usually the former. It is difficult for the mother to decide on the correct course. She will have to try to ignore the very frequent demands and only place the child on the chamber at reasonably frequent intervals—say, after a meal and halfway between mealtimes. If the diagnosis of an attention-seeking mechanism is correct the problem will then resolve. It is important that frequency of this nature should be distinguished from the constant dribbling of urine which is sometimes found in boys in association with urethral valves.

When a serious relapse occurs in a child who has acquired full control of the sphincters there is usually an underlying emotional disturbance, which must be sought and treated. An organic cause should be eliminated by examination of the urine for an infection or for polyuria, but it is very unlikely that any abnormality will be found. Much the most likely causes are rigid training methods, with an excessive display of anxiety when accidents occur, or some cause of insecurity, such as jealousy. As with the other problems mentioned, the less anxiety which is shown about it and the less the scolding which the child receives, the more rapidly is it likely to clear, particularly when the underlying emotional disturbance is properly managed.

When the child is nearing his third birthday and is not showing any sign of acquiring control of the bladder, in spite of reasonable management on the part of the parents, the problem is a very difficult one. One often sees children like this, who show no resistance to the chamber, who have been given every chance to urinate into the chamber or in the lavatory without any undue fuss or anxiety having been shown, and yet they constantly wet their pants. In the majority of these there is a family history of similar lateness in the acquisition of control, and the age at which control was established in other members of the family may provide a useful indication of when control can be expected in the child in question. It is worth while performing a routine examination of the urine to exclude a renal lesion, such as a chronic pyelonephritis or chronic renal insufficiency, but the chance of finding any abnormality is a remote one. Apart from this one would hardly advise a full urological examination until after the third birthday, when a thorough search for an organic basis should be made. Medicines will not help and there is nothing to be done except to continue with the ordinary management of the child as outlined above. Vigorous efforts to train the child will do nothing but harm.

In the case of gross constipation, especially if there is diarrhœa and incontinence, it is advisable to admit the child to hospital in order to ensure that the bowel is completely cleared out. This is achieved by olive oil enemas and colonic wash-outs. Manual removal of hard scybala is sometimes necessary, an anæsthetic being used for the purpose. Tremendous dilatation of the colon occurs, and the rectum is apparently quite insensitive to the loading and distension. The bowel, therefore, has to be re-educated. After it has been cleared out normal bowel actions are maintained with the aid of non-irritating aperients. A combination of syrup of figs and magnesium sulphate is satisfactory, the dose given being adjusted to give the desired action without causing diarrhœa. Preparations which act entirely by increasing the bulk of the motions, such as agaragar, are ineffective.

A wetting agent, dioctyl sodium sulphosuccinate, has been recommended[461] the idea being that it would promote penetration of water or mineral oil into the hard fæces. A controlled study at Sheffield [346] indicated that the drug was not of value. In my experience prostigmine does not help. It is doubtful whether rectal suppositories are of much value. The objection to them is that they involve further interference with the anal region. Every effort should be made for psychological reasons to discard the use of enemas and suppositories as soon as possible. It is obvious, however, that unless sufficient doses of the drugs (syrup of figs, salts) are given by mouth the motions become hard and are either not passed for a long time or cause pain when they are passed.

An essential part of the cure consists of encouraging the child to pass a stool in the usual way without forcing or fussing. As soon as he is passing a normal daily stool without the help of enemas or suppositories he is returned home, the necessary advice being given to the mother. For a time a mild aperient is needed every day, but this is reduced and stopped as soon as possible. It should not be thought that cure of this condition is easy. It is very difficult.

With the exception of the treatment of gross constipation there is no place for drugs in the treatment of the problems of sphincter control.

The problem of stool smearing is discussed in the section on Attention-seeking Devices (p. 318).

CHAPTER 26

CRYING—TEMPER TANTRUMS—BREATH-HOLDING ATTACKS

Crying

Crying may begin *in utero*. It is termed vagitus uterinus. King and Bourgeois [234] collected 127 cases from the literature after 1800. St. Bartholomew and Mahomet are said to have cried *in utero*. Mclane [279] described a case in an operating theatre. The cry was heard by all present, and a superstitious nurse spent the rest of the time on her knees in prayer. It can only occur when the membranes are ruptured and air has entered the uterine cavity. It is of no significance.

According to Adler * the first cry represents an "overwhelming sense of inferiority at thus suddenly being confronted by reality without ever having had to deal with its problems." This feeling of inferiority at least serves a useful function in ventilating the lungs. Another psychologist [342] wrote that birth represents "a loss of paradise," but it is not clear how he knew this. After birth crying is largely a signal for need. Babies can demonstrate their displeasure long before they can show pleasure, yet there are not many stimuli for displeasure in the new-born period. I have reviewed the subject fully elsewhere.[214]

By far the commonest causes of crying in the new-born period are discomfort and loneliness. The chief cause of discomfort is hunger. On a self-demand schedule crying is quickly checked by a feed, provided that the quantity of food is adequate. Even in the new-born period personality differences manifest themselves. Some cry a great deal more readily than others. Some will not brook a moment's delay when they are hungry and scream so vigorously that the mother is compelled to take action. Others are much more tolerant of hunger. Some babies are well suited by a rigid feeding schedule because the times laid down for their feeds happen to coincide with their needs. Others find themselves hungry long before the clock says that they ought to feel hungry, and cry a great deal as a result. There are still many who say that a child should never be fed in the night in the first few weeks because it may lead to bad habits. Instructions to this effect inevitably cause a great deal of totally unnecessary crying at night.

Crying from hunger may also be due to fixed ideas of the duration

* Quoted by Valentine.[423]

of feeds or of the quantity which a child should take. Babies are individuals and some suck better and more quickly than others. The milk flows from some breasts more slowly than from others. The crying may be due to nothing more than not allowing the baby sufficient time on the breast (p. 20). Some babies require much more than the average amount of milk for an average weight gain and for satiation of their hunger and thirst. Wallgren [435a] investigated the amount of milk taken by normal healthy breast-fed babies and found that the variations were very considerable. If " heavy eaters " were compelled to take a quantity of milk which was an average one and sufficient for most babies, a great deal of crying resulted. Rigid rules for the duration and quantity of feeds should not be laid down. They are apt to cause unnecessary crying (pp. 20, 74).

Some babies are of the irritable type and scream when they approach the breast,[293] or suck for a minute and then withdraw and scream. Some scream vigorously when taken off the first breast prior to being given the second. Others do not fuss in this way.

Another cause of discomfort in the new-born period is flatulence, the causes of which are discussed on pp. 58, 75. Colic is a common cause of crying in the first 3 months (p. 60). It occurs mostly, but not entirely, in the evenings. Colic may also be due to substances in the milk if the mother is taking senna, excess of fruit or pickles.

Other causes of crying are overclothing, excessive heat or cold, a wet or soiled napkin, an itching rash or an unpleasant smell or taste, such as that of vomit. A baby cries when there is a sudden noise or when a light shines in his face. Sometimes the new-born baby cries when the light is put out and he finds himself in the dark.

Another common cause of crying in the new-born period and onwards is loneliness. It is surprising how many mothers fail to realize that even the very young baby cries for company. The crying stops as soon as he is picked up, whereas the crying of hunger does not stop, or else there is a minute's quiet and then he cries again even though he is in his mother's arms. I saw a mother who was completely worn out as a result of following the instructions given to her by a nursing home. She had been told never to pick her baby up when he cried, never to feed him at night and always to feed him strictly by the clock. The baby did not approve of this. He settled immediately when managed with common sense. The usual cause of excessive crying due to loneliness is the fear of spoiling. It does not spoil a baby to pick him up when he wants it.

Failure to realize that loneliness causes crying leads many mothers who are using the self-demand method to give unnecessary feeds. It is surprising that Aldrich and his co-workers,[8, 9, 10] in their studies of crying in the new-born, failed to mention this in their list of causes of crying. They drew attention to the frequency of crying "without known reason" and remarked that such crying is far commoner in hospital than in the home. They also found that the average number of prolonged crying spells in the home was 4 per 24 hours as compared with 11·9 in the new-born nursery. They found that in the nursery the average time spent in crying was 113·2 minutes per day. When more nurses were added and the care of the babies was individualized the time spent in crying was 55 minutes per day. It is probable that these differences lie chiefly in the extent to which the babies are picked up when they cry for company. A baby will be picked up at home a great deal more than in the nursery. For the same reason there is much less crying when the baby in hospital is kept constantly at the mother's side, as in many British hospitals and some American ones, rather than in the nursery.

Crying commonly occurs when the position of the baby is suddenly changed, particularly if he is allowed suddenly to fall back from the sitting position. He is likely to cry when his clothes are being changed or when his cot is being made, but this may be partly a cry to be picked up and loved. Some babies cry when placed in the bath, but most enjoy this. An almost certain way of making a baby cry is to hold his limbs or head so that movement is impossible. For the same reason clothing which prevents movement should be avoided. Aldrich and his co-workers [8, 9] showed that crying in a new-born nursery is not contagious.

As the baby grows older crying decreases, though the number of different stimuli which cause crying increases. At 6 months a child endures hunger, thirst or a wet napkin longer than a month-old baby does. Any sort of discomfort still causes crying, though some cry much more readily than others. The commonest causes of discomfort are a wet or soiled napkin, hunger, fatigue or teething. A baby may emit a scream when he passes urine, as if it causes discomfort. He cries if he feels tired or poorly. He objects to having his nose or ears cleaned. The breast-fed baby may cry at the time of the mother's menstrual period (p. 25).

After 5 or 6 months fears may cause crying. The baby may cry when he sees a strange face, particularly when a stranger speaks to him. He cries when he gets into difficulties in his cot. Any time after 5 months he may cry when put to bed in a room to which he is not accustomed. He may awaken with a sudden shriek which is not due to a wet napkin or to other discoverable cause. It may well be a nightmare. From 9 months onwards the baby may show signs of jealousy and cry when he sees his mother pick up another baby. A 6-month-old baby may cry when he sees his brother fall and hurt himself or when he sees him smacked.

Loneliness comes into greater prominence as a cause of crying after the new-born period. The importance of loneliness as a cause of crying depends on the child's personality. Some babies are quite content to be left out in the pram all day. Others at 3 or 4 months cry incessantly if left outside. They are perfectly content when lying in the pram in the kitchen where they can see what the mother is doing. At 4 months the baby may cry when approaching the cot. He is very reluctant to see his mother leave the room.

Any thwarting of the baby's developing powers is apt to cause crying. Reluctance to be left outside in the pram is partly due to the child's developing interest in the activities of the kitchen. Many mothers fail to realize this and think that the child is crying to be picked up. Fearing that they will spoil him, they leave him to cry. It is surprising how many mothers are apparently deaf to the crying of their babies, leaving them to cry for hours on end. When a child is ready to be propped up in the pram he is reluctant to be left lying down. When he can sit he may well cry if not given the opportunity to do so. When he can grasp objects he may cry if not given a chance to play. It is common to see a baby over the age of 5 or 6 months left for hours without any toys ; he cries from sheer boredom. A baby cries when a pleasurable experience is stopped, as when he is removed from his bath or when the mother stops playing with him, or when, having held him in her arms, she puts him into the cot. He cries when he is unable to reach for an object which he wants or when a wanted object is removed from him.

The development of the ego and personality leads to crying from 6 months or so onwards. Even at 5 months the baby may show striking likes and dislikes and cry when given food which he does not like, or when fed from a cup or dish which is not the usual one. A determined independent child at 6 or 7 months may refuse to take food unless he is allowed to help to hold the spoon. Efforts to make the child take food which he does not want or to sit on the chamber against his will, lead to crying.

Excessive crying in this period is almost always due to failure to answer the child's basic needs for comfort, love and security, and for opportunities to practise his new-found skills.

After the first birthday there is a further reduction in the frequency of crying. Crying is particularly liable to be the result of conflict with the developing ego and with his newly-found interests. Many tears are the result of wounding of the child's pride. When he has learnt to do things for himself—to help to set the table, to dress himself, to attend to his eliminations—he is very likely, if of an independent character, to respond to interference by tears. He becomes more and more determined to have his own way. He wants to play without interference. Adults often interfere unnecessarily in children's play and thereby cause tears. The father, for instance, steps in when he sees his boy pushing his engine about on the floor instead of winding it up and letting it run on its own. The child does not want to stop doing what he is so much enjoying, and has no sense of time. He wants to do something which for reasons of safety his parents forbid. He wants a toy which another child has. Crying as a result of the most trivial knocks or falls is often purely an attention-seeking device. He may find wailing during play an effective way of getting an older sibling into trouble. It is stopped by ignoring it, or punishment.

His great need is for love and security, and any apparent deprivation of this causes tears. His fear of the dark may be largely fear of separation from his mother. He cries when he feels lonely or when he is left behind because he walks so slowly. If given a chance he will cry every night for company. After the age of 1½ he develops a variety of fears and cries for the security of his mother's company. He may cry outside because of the discomfort of wind and rain. He cries because of the pain of teething, because he is tired or because he feels unwell.

As in the younger child, the frequency of crying depends in part on his personality. Excessive crying is almost always due to mismanagement, in the form of failure to give the child the love and security which he needs and failure to allow him to learn independence and practise his newly-found skills. It is greatly increased by constant interference—by perfectionism, domination and attempts to " train " him before he is developmentally ready. It is increased by insecurity, whatever the cause. It is greatly increased by irritability and fatigue in the parents. It is similarly increased in the child as a result of insufficient sleep.

When there is excessive crying, whatever the cause, there is always something wrong in the child's management. A child does not cry without reason.

There are many who feel that a child is spoilt by picking him up when he cries. I do not agree. No child is spoilt by being picked up when he cries for love and security, or when he has fallen and hurt himself or has pain or discomfort. It is never right to leave a child to cry for prolonged periods. The less he is allowed to cry in the first 2 or 3 years the happier he is likely to be in later childhood. This does not mean that he should always have his own way. It does mean that the wiser parental management, the greater the parents' tact, patience, common sense and sense of humour, the fewer tears will be shed by their children.

There is no place for drugs in treatment, except only in certain sleep problems (p. 272). Neither do I think that there is any place for the dirty unhygienic " dummy " or pacifier.

Temper Tantrums

The usual age for temper tantrums is 15 months to 3 years or more. A determined child may give displays of temper long before that age, from 6 months onwards, but typical tantrums hardly occur before the first birthday. Their appearance corresponds with the period of resistance, of the development of the ego and negativism, and of the normal aggressiveness in the transition stage from infancy to the independence of the mature child. The frequency and character of temper tantrums are familiar to all. In the worst forms the child may do considerable damage by throwing china on to the floor, valued objects into the fire and in kicking the furniture. Breath-holding attacks are intimately related to temper tantrums, but owing to their distinctive nature they are discussed in a separate section.

The methods used to deal with tantrums are also well known. The child is likely to be soundly smacked and he very often succeeds in getting his own way after them.

The Basic Causes

(i) The Personality of the Child. Tantrums are not a problem in the placid, easy-going child. They occur in the active, determined child with abundant energy.

(ii) The Period of Resistance and the Development of the Ego. In essence tantrums represent the clash of the child's developing personality with the will of his parents. His increasing desire to show his powers, to gain attention and to have his own way gets him into trouble, particularly when his parents are perfectionists and of the domineering type. If he finds that by screaming and a display of temper he can attract attention, secure bribes or sweets to pacify him, or get his own way and do something which he wanted to do or avoid doing something which he did not want to do, he will certainly repeat the performance. His tantrums give him control over his environment. He finds a tantrum a successful device for avoiding punishment. When parents have been foolish enough to talk to friends in his presence about his dreadful tantrums, he realizes immediately the anxiety and interest which they have aroused and repeats the performance. A single tantrum badly managed is very liable to develop into a habit. The child soon realizes that he has discovered a most satisfactory way of annoying his parents. This reaction is not one of naughtiness. It is merely a normal sign of the development of the ego.

It is an obvious fact that the child's negativism is greatly increased by fatigue and boredom, and to a certain extent by hunger.

(iii) The Desire to practise New Skills. Bound up with the above is the child's desire to practise new skills and to take responsibility for doing things which he has recently learnt. There is little doubt that many tears are due to the thwarting of this pride because the parents, perhaps in order to save time or to prevent possible accidents (e.g. with china), have not allowed him to help or do things for himself which he is able to do.

(iv) Imitativeness. The child who sees his parents display bad temper, throwing things on to the floor and banging the doors in rage, is very likely to copy them. He is also likely to imitate tantrums thrown by his friends.

(v) Insecurity. Insecurity for any reason is a potent cause of temper tantrums.

(vi) The Level of Intelligence. Though temper tantrums are common in children of any level of intelligence, including those of mental superiority, they are especially liable to occur in children with some degree of mental retardation. Such children are apt to be thwarted because too much is expected of them or because they are unable to understand the limits of their freedom.

(vii) Ignorance of the Normal Personality Differences in Children. An attempt to bring children up by rigid rules instead of by elastic methods adjusted to the needs of the individual is apt to lead to various difficulties, including tantrums. When a first child has been of a placid easy-going disposition and the second one has an active determined character, methods applied to the first often cause considerable trouble in the second.

(viii) Over-indulgence, Over-protection and Domination. One of these is almost always present. The temper tantrum is one of the commonest manifestations in the child who has suffered from over-indulgence or over-protection. The child who has never been taught discipline, when eventually he goes too far even for his over-indulgent mother and is rebuked, throws a tantrum in order that he can still have his own way. If ever he has difficulty in getting his own way he knows that he will get what he wants if he has a tantrum.

Excessive strictness with the child is equally liable to cause temper tantrums. Insistence on unreasonable demands which are unsuitable for his level of development and on immediate obedience inevitably causes trouble. Excessive interference with the child's normal pursuits by the mother or grandmother because of perfectionism, an excessive desire for tidiness or a determination to make the boy "good," is apt to be met by rebellion. The mother who is saying "No, no" to the child all through the day, when in reality his pursuits are harmless, must expect to meet resistance if the child has any character at all. The temper tantrum is the child's best defence reaction against such repression. A vicious circle is apt to be set up, the resistance being met with more repression, and the repression by more resistance.

Sometimes the excessive repression is due to a social problem, the mother being compelled to prevent the child making a noise because of unpleasant critical neighbours or relatives in the house.

(ix) Parental Inconsistency. If the parents vacillate, sometimes insisting on a particular line of behaviour and sometimes not taking any notice, or if they constantly threaten and never carry out the threats, the child becomes confused or reacts by a tantrum when eventually the parents take action. More often the parents disagree with each other. If one parent forbids a child to do a particular thing and the other permits it, the child is apt to throw temper tantrums in order to get what he wants.

(x) Parental Fatigue, Impatience or Unhappiness. The irritating characteristics of the small child have been mentioned elsewhere (p. 233). They are particularly relevant here. The mother has to put up with her very exasperating offspring morning, noon and night. One can hardly blame the mother who complains that the child is getting on her nerves and is driving her to distraction. The more tired she gets, the more irritable she becomes, and the more her fatigue and irritability is reflected in the child's behaviour. He is worse when she snaps at him or tries to hurry him. Domestic unhappiness has a similar effect. When the mother is badly treated by her husband and is not happy in her relationship with him the child almost invariably suffers from her irritability, over-protection or fatigue.

Prevention and Treatment

It is essential to look behind the temper tantrums for the underlying cause. In the first place, organic disease must be eliminated. A chronic infection such as tuberculosis may cause undue fatigue in the child and so lead to bad temper. Bad behaviour with screaming attacks may be due to deafness, the child being unable to make his wants known. When in addition to the bad temper there are personality changes, one must not forget the possibility of a cerebral tumour or of a degenerative disease of the nervous system. Miller and Lennox [295] drew attention to the occurrence of electro-encephalographic abnormalities in some children who had been thought to have simple behaviour problems.

In the vast majority of cases, however, no sign of organic disease will be found. One then has to review the whole management of the child in order that the parental attitudes can be understood and corrected. Any underlying insecurity in the child, over-protection, over-indulgence and over-strictness in the parents, has to be remedied. No excessive demands must be made on him. The opportunities for resistance must be cut down to a minimum, for the essence of treatment lies in prevention. He should be kept occupied (see p. 326). He should have playmates of his own age. He should frequently have them in his own house and go out to visit them in their homes. He should be encouraged to practise skills and to take pride in what he can do. As far as possible sources of danger must be removed, and he should be removed bodily when he is approaching them or when it is seen that a storm is brewing. Most children at this age are very distractable, and this trait should be utilized. It is far better to remove him and distract him than to sit and say "No, no," thus inviting defiance. The mother must be reasonable in her requests and not rush him, but she must be consistent and there must be no disagreement between the parents. Once she has given the child an instruction she must see that it is carried out.

If the request involves tidying up after games, she should help him rather than risk meeting with resistance. She may reduce opportunities for resistance by deciding on a course of action for the child rather than asking him if he would like to do it. For example, when she wants to take the child out for a walk, instead of saying "Shall we go out for a walk now ?" her attitude will be "We are going to go out for a walk now." She must on no account try to break the child's will. He will need his determination and force of character in later years. As Arlitt [22] wrote, anger must be trained to such a degree that it functions only when it is socially desirable. Excessive inhibition of a child's normal aggressiveness is apt to lead to timidity, morose withdrawn behaviour, an inferiority complex or, later, to rebellion and excessive aggressiveness.

When a temper tantrum occurs there must on no account be a fight, a fuss, anger, anxiety or argument. There must be no reasonings and no attempt to force him to stop his behaviour. Reasonings and repression are useless. Scolding a rebellious child is as much use as pouring petrol on a fire to extinguish it. It is essential that the mother should herself not lose her temper. Smacking is likely to be merely the result of loss of temper and should usually be avoided. Sometimes smacking may help in the early stage of a tantrum, but it is not likely to be useful if the child has become hysterical. The best way to treat a tantrum is to ignore it. A display of indifference is a much more severe and effective punishment than any disciplinary method. On no account must the child be given the centre of the stage for his effort. He should certainly not be given what he wanted after the tantrum. As soon as he finds that he is achieving nothing by tantrums he will stop having them. He can be picked up and given a feeling of love and security after one, but he should not be given sweets or other awards.

After the tantrum the mother should ask herself exactly why the tantrum occurred. Was it really necessary to stop him doing what he wanted to do or to try to force him to do what he did not want to do ? Was she too hasty in scolding him ? Could she have achieved her ends by a loving request rather than by a hasty rebuke ? Was it because he was tired ? Did she insist on obedience or on a particular line of action to satisfy her own pride ? Was her request really reasonable for a child of his age who was engaged in a fascinating game which he did not want to stop ? Very many tantrums arise as a result of a totally unreasonable insistence on something which does not matter. Discipline and obedience are essential, but they must be reasonable. There is no doubt that the greater the parental wisdom, patience, common sense, tact and sense of humour, the rarer will be the temper tantrums.

Finally, when a vicious circle has developed as a result of maternal fatigue and loss of patience, the best immediate solution to the problem may be a short holiday for the mother away from the child, if that can be arranged. She will come back rejuvenated and rested and better able to deal with her exuberant children. Far too many mothers never have a chance to get away from their offspring and a stage comes when each gets on the nerves of the other.

Breath-holding Attacks

Breath-holding attacks are closely related to temper tantrums. They occur any time from 1 year to 3 years of age, but the great majority begin in the first 18 months. They are almost unknown after 4 years. In a minor form they are fairly common ; in the severest form, which is associated with major convulsions, they are rare. An excellent review of the subject was written by Bridge, Livingston and Tietze.[63]

Hippocrates * described an attack as follows : " The onset may be from some mysterious terror or a fright from somebody shouting, or in the midst of crying the child is not able quickly to recover his breath, as often happens to children ; but when any of these things happens to him, at once the body is chilled, he becomes speechless, does not draw his breath, the breathing fails, the brain stiffens, the blood is at a standstill. The French [105] term the attacks " spasme du sanglot "—sob spasms.

The usual cause of attacks is anger, thwarting, punishment or an effort by the child to get his own way. It may be due to a toy being snatched from him by another child or to an unsuccessful attempt to get a toy from him. It may be due to insistence of the parents that he should put his toys away, or to their refusal to allow him to do something which he has set his heart on.

* Quoted by Still.[403]

It is important to note that attacks may be due to pain from a fall or knock, or to fear. Repeated attacks are more common in mismanaged children, but I would not go as far as Hinman and Dickey [194] who consider that the attacks are " primarily an emotional disorder symptomatic of profound insecurity." I believe that the child's personality is important, some being much more likely to have them than others when faced with even mild thwarting or conflict with the parent.

In an attack the child utters two or three loud cries and then holds the breath in expiration. In the most trivial cases the apnœa lasts 5 or 10 seconds, he becomes blue and then promptly recovers. In slightly more severe cases the breath is held for an additional 5–10 seconds, he becomes severely cyanosed and loses consciousness, becoming pale and limp. He may fall. There is then a feeble cry followed by more vigorous crying, and after a few moments of confusion he is his normal self again. If the apnœa is prolonged for more than 30 seconds or so the child develops generalized rigidity and has a major convulsion indistinguishable from epilepsy. There is a marked bradycardia in the attacks. There may be only one attack in his life or they may frequently recur. I have seen children have several attacks in a day. If no treatment is given they tend to occur at less and less frequent intervals and disappear by about the fourth birthday. If they are due to pain they are less likely to be repeated than if they are due to a behaviour problem, unless undue fuss is made of them, when they will continue as an attention-seeking device. Livingston [257] studied 242 cases ; eighty-seven had one or more a day, thirty-three had less than one a month. In all but three the attacks disappeared by 5, and in the remaining three at 6. Electroencephalograms are normal.[257, 260]

The mechanism of the attacks was discussed by Bridge [63] and by Scharpey Schafer and his co-workers.[377] The latter workers, describing similar attacks in schoolboys and adults brought about voluntarily as a trick, concluded that the unconsciousness is due to the drop of blood pressure caused by the increased intrathoracic pressure due to breath-holding in expiration. Sharpey Schafer pointed out that, amongst other actions, over-ventilation increases muscle blood flow and increases cerebral vascular resistance. Breath-holding in expiration then causes a greater than normal drop in effective cerebral blood pressure and, since the cerebral vascular resistance is simultaneously increased, a very considerable drop in cerebral blood flow results. The cerebral anoxæmia then causes unconsciousness and possibly convulsions.

It is thought that the apnœa is due to spasm of the glottis, for contractions of the diaphragm have been noted in attacks, without any effect on the colour or ventilation. The attacks probably begin as a voluntary act, but the results are obviously involuntary.

The differential diagnosis is important. As the attacks are rarely seen by the doctor, the diagnosis rests essentially on a careful history. The orderly and rather slow sequence of events in the breath-holding attack, a few cries after a known precipitating factor, followed by breath-holding in expiration, the rapid onset of cyanosis, followed by limpness and convulsion in that order, differ from epilepsy, in which fits rarely follow a precipitating factor, except occasionally over-ventilation. In epilepsy, the so-called epileptic cry before a convulsion is unusual in children, and when it does occur it is usually different in nature from the child's ordinary cry. In epilepsy the clonic phase is preceded not by limpness but a tonic phase, and cyanosis, instead of preceding the onset of the fit, follows the beginning of the tonic spasm. The whole sequence of events in an epileptic fit is much quicker. After an epileptic fit the child, instead of being just momentarily confused, is likely to fall asleep. Though many epileptic fits are short lasting, some may last for many minutes or even for hours, while breath-holding attacks never last longer than 2 or 3 minutes. It is by no means always easy to distinguish the two conditions.

If the attack was due to pain nothing can be done to prevent the attack, which anyway is unlikely to recur. Otherwise the methods of prevention and treatment are the same as those for temper tantrums. Drugs are of no value. When an attack occurs every effort must be made to prevent injury. There must be a minimum of fuss and interest in the event. A colleague found that attacks in his own child were effectively stopped by holding him upside down. On no account must the child have his own way as a result of the attack. Some adopt the method of giving the child a sound slap as soon as breath-holding is observed, and there is much to be said for this. It must be admitted that, whatever the line of treatment, the attacks may persist for a time, gradually becoming less frequent and finally ceasing. They are not easy to stop.

CHAPTER 27

BODY MANIPULATIONS

Finger and Thumb Sucking

ALL children suck their fingers or thumbs at one time or another. A few suck their toes. Some suck part of the wrist or forearm. The sucking may be so frequent that soreness or callus formation occurs. The act is often associated with ear pulling, hair pulling or twisting, handling of the genitals, or with rubbing the nose or chin on some soft fabric or doll, or with sucking of the blanket.

There is a surprisingly extensive literature on the subject. Views expressed as to its ætiology differ considerably. Gesell [144, 147] considered that it is a developmental phenomenon. It may begin *in utero*. Most babies suck their fingers in the new-born period. There is then a lull in the activity until the child can voluntarily take his fingers to his mouth at about 3 months of age. When he can grasp objects voluntarily, at about 5 months of age, he takes everything to his mouth, for the mouth becomes the exploratory organ and it is natural that his fingers should go to it.

Finger sucking is apt to be associated with hunger, shyness, teething, fatigue and sleep. It may disappear at 5 months, only to reappear when each new tooth comes. The child is then seen to rub the affected part of the gum with his fingers and then to suck them. About half of all babies suck their fingers at 1 year of age—some much more than others. Finger sucking is apt to reach its peak between 18 and 21 months. It is apt to become associated with sleep, and the insertion of fingers into the mouth may actually induce sleep. The child who is wearing gloves out of doors may, when tired, removed his gloves so that he can suck his fingers and then fall asleep. The association with sleep becomes less marked by about 3. Whereas previously he had sucked his fingers throughout the night, by 3 or so he may merely suck his fingers when about to go to sleep.

Freud [137] wrote : " Thumb sucking is a model of the infantile sexual manifestations." "No investigator has yet doubted the sexual nature of this action." "The child does not make use of a strange object for sucking, but prefers its own skin, because it is more convenient, because it thus makes itself independent of the outer world which it cannot yet control, and because in this way it creates for itself, as it were, a second even if an inferior erogenous zone. The inferiority of this second region urges it later to seek the same parts, the lips of another woman. ('It is a pity that I cannot kiss myself' might be attributed to it.)" Melanie Klein [237] explained thumb sucking in a 6-year-old child who was being psycho-analysed as being due to "phantasies of sucking, biting and devouring her father's penis and her mother's breasts. The penis represented the whole father, and the breasts the whole mother." According to English and Pearson [122] the cause of much of the unnecessary alarm in parents is that they unconsciously realize the connection with masturbation, and their own early conflict with masturbation is brought to the surface.

Levy [248] thought that the most important ætiological factor is insufficiency of sucking experience in feeding. He found that there was more often a history of spontaneous withdrawal from a too rapidly flowing breast or bottle, or forced withdrawal from sucking at the end of a set period of time, in thumb suckers than in controls. They had a longer interval between feeds and a shorter feeding time than controls. In the controls there were more unscheduled untimed feeds, more frequent feeds and more frequent night feeds, and there was a greater use of dummies. He could find no relation between the type of feeding—breast or bottle. He showed [249, 250] that when the feeding of animals was interfered with before satiety was reached, corresponding sucking habits developed. Dogs would lick the paw or body of another dog and suck various inanimate objects. Calves licked the ears of other calves, painted boards, clothes or other objects. Chicks pecked excessively. Puppies fed from nipples with large holes, so that the sucking time was short, acquired vicarious sucking habits to a greater extent than puppies fed from nipples with small holes. Margaret Mead [281] wrote: "In most primitive societies of which we have any knowledge children are suckled whenever they cry; as a result infants seldom cry for more than a few minutes, unless they are sick. This suckling at any time seems to have one important result—no primitive child whom I have ever seen or heard of sucks its thumb or fingers." Freeden,[133] on the other hand, after 10 years' experience of feeding babies by cup from the new-born period onwards, found that there was no greater incidence of thumb sucking than in those fed on the breast or bottle.

Spock,[396] probably rightly, thought that no one explanation is sufficient for all cases, and suggests that the ætiology may vary with the age. In the younger age group the satisfaction of the sucking instinct may be of importance, whereas after the first birthday insecurity and boredom may be important factors, though he agreed with Gesell that the finger sucking in connection with sleep is probably related to neither, but is merely a developmental phenomenon. It seems to me that not all finger sucking is related to insufficient sucking experience. Two children in a family fed in precisely the same way on the breast may differ considerably in the extent of their finger sucking. There are probably, in fact, constitutional factors which govern the amount of finger sucking in which children indulge. It might be supposed that Nature made sucking a pleasant occupation so that babies would suck to keep themselves alive. It would then be expected that babies would enjoy sucking the nipple, bottle or thumb, and that they would suck the thumb or other object when tired, bored or unhappy.

Prognosis

Bragman [59] and Mazzini [275] found thumb sucking in various paintings and sculptures of Italian masters of the early Renaissance. As Kanner [226] wrote, the notion that it is bad and harmful did not arise till the end of the nineteenth century. Alarmists then stated that thumb sucking causes scoliosis, enlargement of the tonsils and adenoids, flatulence and colic, dental caries, digestive disorders in adult life and changes in facial expression. It was commonly believed that the habit was the cause of severe malocclusion.

Sillman [381] took serial casts from impressions of upper and lower jaws from birth to 14 years in 60 children, 20 of whom were thumb suckers. The habit did cause some deformity of the jaws, but by the age of 4 it had corrected itself. He thought that hereditary factors were much more important in governing the development of oral structures. Lewis,[253] in a study of 170 children over a 5-year period, found that in 24 of 30 thumb suckers there was some malocclusion of the deciduous teeth, but that if the habit was stopped before the age of 6 the deformity corrected itself spontaneously. Massler and Wood [273] agreed with this. They found that persistence of the habit beyond the age of 6 caused severe deformity. Lewis [254] described a similar defect from lip sucking. Bakwin [28] wrote that there is no evidence that the habit causes any deformity of the palate, air swallowing, oral infection or gastro-intestinal upsets. He thought that dental malocclusion is much more likely to be hereditary in origin. Freud, however,[137] claimed that " children in whom this (thumb sucking) is retained are habitual kissers as adults and show a tendency to perverse kissing, or as men they have a marked desire for drinking and sucking."

Treatment

In the past a wide variety of ingenious mechanical devices was used to stop thumb sucking. It is unanimously agreed now that no devices should be used, at least until the age of 5 or 6. They cause considerable psychological disturbance in the child and do nothing but harm.

In the new-born baby no treatment should be given, because it is normal. It is very doubtful whether anything should be done in the first year to check the habit. In view of Levy's work some recommend that the duration of breast feeds should be lengthened, or that the hole in the teat should be made smaller so that sucking is prolonged. This would seem unwise, as such a measure might well cause flatulence and colic. After the age of a year thumb sucking associated with sleep or indulged in occasionally during the day is a harmless procedure, and the child will almost certainly grow out of it. No treatment should be given. Dental or other appliances should not be used. Bitter substances should not be painted on the fingers. A direct attack on the problem is useless.

When in a 2- or 3-year-old child the thumb sucking is excessive and occurs in the daytime as well as at night, or when thumb sucking starts again after a long period without it, every effort should be made to determine the cause. If it is boredom the child should be kept occupied. If it is insecurity, repression or jealousy, the cause should be treated. On no account should threats or punishment be used. If a lot of fuss is made the child may deliberately continue to suck the thumb as an attention-seeking device. By about 3 years of age a direct appeal can be made to him to stop it on the grounds that it is an infantile habit and that he is too old for it.

Over-enthusiastic efforts to stop thumb sucking do a great deal of harm. There is apt to be constant nagging and reprimands, which cause unhappiness, resentfulness and insecurity. Ridicule is always undesirable as a means of dealing with such problems. All ridicule, teasing, shaming and threats should be avoided. The danger of thumb sucking lies not in the thumb sucking but in what the parents do about it.

The vast majority of thumb suckers grow out of the habit by the age of 5 or 6 if nothing is done about it.

Nail Biting

According to Massler and Malone [271] nail biting does not occur before the age of 3. This is not true, but it is not a common habit in the first 3 years. I have seen it in a 15-month-old child. Billig,[45] in a 90-page review, wrote that it usually begins between the ages of 8 and 10. Of 346 boys in Chicago aged 8 to 11,[268] two out of three were nail biters. In another study [442] 44 per cent. of boys and girls aged 12 to 14 were biting their nails at the time of examination. Similar figures were given by Birch.[46] He found that 51 per cent. of 4,000 school children in South Yorkshire were biting their nails at the time of examination.

Although these figures apply to the older child, they are quoted here because they suggest that the popular idea that nail biting is always a manifestation of insecurity seems hardly tenable. It is true that children (and adults) often begin to bite their nails when nervous, tense, or in deep thought. It may be learned from another child. According to Billig nail biters are nonconformists. " The nail biting is a form of revolt at having to comply." Wechsler [442] wrote that " it is nothing but a particular form of unconscious masturbating activity, a symptom of an incompletely resolved œdipus situation." Others regard it as a tic, a compulsive act, or as a sign of psychopathic personality.

I feel that insecurity may cause or increase nail biting, but in many children the cause is not clear.

Punishment and restraining devices will do nothing but harm. It must be treated by distracting the child when he is biting the nails, attending to any cause of insecurity, and seeing that the child is fully occupied. In the older pre-school child, an appeal to his pride may help. Ridicule and teasing never works.

Rocking

Rocking in the bed begins especially at the age of 40 weeks. It usually stops after one or two months,[203] but may last for many months. Some children cause their cots to disintegrate by the constant rocking. It pleases them to find that they can rock the cot from one side of the room to the other.

It is a difficult habit to stop. If a soft rug is placed under the cot, it may help by reducing the pleasing vibrations. It is useful to move an older child with this complaint from a cot into a bed. In an intractable case the child may be put into a hammock.

Head Rolling

Head rolling is practically confined to the first three years. It may cause the hair of the back of the head to be worn off. It is of no importance and no particular treatment helps.

Spasmus Nutans

This condition occurs in normal children, and is not associated with any known disease, or with malnutrition. It has been reviewed by Norton and Cogan.[316] It is characterized by head nodding, anomalous head positions and nystagmus. The head nodding is usually an irregular horizontal movement, but the movement may consist of turning or tilting. The frequency is about 1 to 2 per second. The movements increase with efforts to fix the eyes on an object, and disappear in sleep, or if the eyes are bandaged.

The nystagmus is always asymmetrical in the two eyes, and varies with different positions of gaze. It is lateral, vertical or rotatory in type. It is a fine rapid nystagmus, and it is increased by forced fixation of the head. It may be associated with a convergent strabismus. There is a tendency to look at objects out of the corner of the eyes, with the head partly flexed. The nystagmus is more constant than the head nodding, and is usually the last sign to subside.

The onset is usually between the fourth and twelfth month. It is rarely seen after the second year, but may last up to 8 years. There is no particular sex or familial incidence, and there is no relationship to mental deficiency or rickets. It is usually said that it is due to poor lighting conditions, but this is thought now to be untrue. The cause of the condition is unknown. No treatment is of value.

Head Banging

This occurs particularly in the child aged 7–12 months when put to bed. The head is banged against the mattress, top of the bed or other hard object. It occurs in perfectly normal children as well as in mentally retarded ones. It may be a manifestation of insecurity or an attention-seeking mechanism, particularly if the parents show great anxiety about it and try forcible means of stopping it. It is a relatively harmless pursuit which usually stops spontaneously between the age of 2 and 3 years, and no treatment is either advisable or necessary. In severe cases head banging in bed can be cured by putting the child into a hammock, but head banging involving furniture can be very difficult to stop.

Hair Plucking

This is sometimes called trichotillomania. It is apt to occur when the child feels frustrated or angry. It may be associated with finger sucking. When the cause has been removed and the act is ignored the habit stops.

Hair plucking is sometimes a feature of Pink disease (erythrœdema).

Ear Pulling, Lip Biting and Tongue Sucking

These are similar habits. The tongue sucker twists the tongue round the mouth with a loud sucking noise. The practices are harmless and disappear spontaneously.

Tooth Grinding

Though more frequent in mentally defective children or in children seriously ill with a disease such as tuberculous meningitis, it may occur in normal children. In such a case it is likely to be an attention-seeking device, perpetuated by the anxiety which parents show about it. It also occurs in sleep. No treatment can or should be given. If it is ignored it will stop.

Masturbation

Masturbation is practised at all ages, but it is rare before the age of 6 months. It must be distinguished from simple non-rhythmic manipulation of the genitals which is not accompanied by any excitement or evidence of particular satisfaction. It is natural that when a child learns to grasp objects, at about 5 months, he should grasp the penis. Mothers are apt to be very shocked by this and to try to stop it. They think that it is dreadful for the child to touch his genitals, although they themselves try to retract his foreskin in bathing him, and in the girl they clean the vulva. The less attention which is paid to such manipulations the sooner they will stop.

True masturbation is another matter. In the infant it is usually practised by rubbing the thighs together. This is often achieved by a variety of rocking movements—rhythmic elevation of the pelvis in the supine position, or rocking back and forth on hands and knees in the prone. This begins any time after the age of 5 or 6 months. It may be associated with head banging and is often particularly noticed at bedtime. A little later the child may learn to rub the genital area against the arm of a chair or against part of the play pen. Rhythmic manipulation of the genitals by the hand rarely occurs before the age of $2\frac{1}{2}$.

In all these rhythmic activities the child's face may become flushed while doing it, and the sweating of the face, fixed eyes, and sometimes pallor, with the bodily contortion, may well lead to a diagnosis of epilepsy. It frequently arises as a result of some local irritation, such as vulvovaginitis, pruritis from threadworm infection, balanitis, napkin rash or eczema. It could arise from excessive handling of the genitals by the mother when washing the child. It is also learnt by imitation of others. Bergman [43a] offered various other explanations. He wrote: "He may masturbate because he wants to call another person's attention to the excellent little organ he owns. He may do it because he wants to shock or irritate or shame the other person. Or he may want to convince himself that he can still produce pleasure in himself in spite of some frightening experience he may have undergone. He may wish to reassure himself that his organ is all right in spite of the fact that it is different from the organ he has noticed in the other sex. He may try to transform his organ into that of the other sex. He may have nothing else to do and resort to masturbation because of boredom. He may feel unhappy in his interpersonal relationship and console himself with masturbation. Masturbation may give a child the feeling of strength he needs to be stubborn and hostile towards his parents."

The practice is carried out quite openly unless the mother has scolded the child for it, when it is practised in secret. Mothers are apt to be very shocked by seeing their child masturbate and smack him hard, threaten that his penis will fall off or that something dreadful will happen to him. On no account should he be scolded, frightened or threatened. It is a mistake to " catch him " in the act and then try to shame him. He should simply be distracted as soon as it is seen and nothing should be said to him about it, the actual act being ignored. Any local cause of itching must be removed. There should on no account be any fuss about it. If there is it will be prolonged as an attention-seeking device.

In severe cases it is important to try to find the cause of the problem. It is likely to be due to worry or insecurity, and it has almost certainly been exaggerated and perpetuated by parental efforts to stop it. In severe resistant cases a local anæsthetic ointment applied to the genitals is a useful adjuvant to treatment. In general, however, the less attention is paid to the genitals the better.

It is essential to treat the parental attitudes, for it is those attitudes and the resultant actions which do the harm, rather than the actual masturbation. The parents must be made to understand that all children do it at one time or another and that their child is not therefore a sexual pervert. They must have their fears allayed that he will develop insanity, epilepsy or other disease.

CHAPTER 28

JEALOUSY, FEARS, SHYNESS AND OTHER PROBLEMS

Jealousy

JEALOUSY is a normal reaction which most normal children feel at one time or another. As Ziman [467] wrote in his excellent book on the subject, " Children are jealous as a matter of course. It is normal and proper and to be expected." Some of the manifestations of jealousy are obscure, and parents, not realizing this, are apt wrongly to think that their children have never shown jealousy. Jealousy is not a problem unless it is mismanaged.

Ætiology

The child fears that he is losing something which he had before—love, a feeling that he is important and that he is wanted. It is greatly exaggerated by anything which causes a feeling of insecurity—a feeling that he might lose his mother's love, that he might be deserted. Such feelings arise from any of the causes of insecurity—over-protection, excessive domination, parental impatience and irritability, domestic friction or indiscipline. They are especially liable to occur if the mother has ever been foolish enough to threaten to leave the child if he will not do what she wants him to do, or if she has been in the habit of leaving him a great deal. In a child rendered insecure in this way problems of jealousy are precipitated by the arrival of a new baby, and more still by what he rightly or wrongly interprets as loss of love and interest in him. He has already had a foretaste of what is to come when he was moved out of the bedroom which he loved so much to make way for the baby, and when later he was sent away from home to some people he did not know while his mother was in hospital. The mother on arrival home has little time for her first-born. She is tired, and therefore irritable, when the latter, feeling the first pangs of jealousy, is more than usually demanding of her love. Tactless friends come and admire the baby and bring him presents, not saying a word to the 2- or 3-year-old, who till then has held the centre of the stage. The more stupid ones make jokes to the older child about his feeling put out by the new baby. It so happens that the second baby is apt to come just at the very time that the first one is passing through a phase of increased dependence on the mother. According to Levy, the larger the age difference between one child and the next the less likely is jealousy to occur.

When the child is a little older there are new ways in which the older child is made to feel that he has lost his parents' love. The father, when he comes home from work, may make the mistake of always picking up the younger one. He is apt to be constantly warned not to touch the baby or to be careful not to hurt him. The baby snatches toys from the first-born's hands, and when the latter protests there is a chorus of reprimands from the parents. It is difficult for the parents to do anything else but come to the defence of the little one and to punish the older child for acts which are ignored in his young brother, for the simple reason that the brother is not old enough to understand that they are wrong. It is difficult for the older child to understand this difference in treatment, and he is apt to feel hurt and upset as a result. There is no doubt that the first-born's discovery that he is not the only one is painful and does cause a considerable emotional disturbance. The disturbance is all the greater if he has not been accustomed to mixing with other children and if he has been given all his own way.

Comparisons with siblings are a potent cause of ill-feeling in the home. The mother says, " John does not cry when he falls " ; " John would never do a thing like that " ; " Watch John and see how he eats." Not only does this sort of remark produce enmity between the children, but it leads to a feeling of insecurity, inferiority or rebellion. The little girl who is compelled to wear the clothes of her elder sister is apt to feel jealous when her sister has new clothes in place of the discarded ones. When the 3-year-old is taken with his baby brother into a restaurant or other public place, people admire and talk to the baby and never speak a word to him. The child may be jealous of his parents if they constantly caress each other in his presence and leave him out. The boy is apt to rush up and demand to be cuddled too.

The younger child may feel jealous when his older sibling first goes to school (and the older child may feel jealous when his younger sibling starts at school—the older one realizing that he is no longer quite so important as he was).

The importance of favouritism has already been discussed (p. 239).

According to Arlitt [22] there is no correlation between jealousy and the intelligence or personality characteristics. I doubt this. I feel that some children, however careful and wise the management, show jealousy more than others.

The ætiology has been discussed at some length, because a knowledge of the common causes of jealousy is essential to prevention and treatment.

Manifestations

The manifestations of jealousy may be obvious, but there are frequently occult signs and symptoms of emotional disturbance which only the most discerning can ascribe with confidence to underlying jealousy. When a child hits the new baby on the head or fusses when the baby or another child is picked up, it is not difficult to see that he is jealous. But when, shortly after the baby's arrival, he reverts to infantile behaviour, sucking his thumb again, wetting the bed, demanding to be fed, talking baby talk and constantly asks to be carried, or when he becomes quarrelsome and aggressive with his friends, becoming destructive and negative again, the cause of the behaviour may not be obvious. Observation of a girl's play with her dolls and of her conversation with them may give the mother a clue to the real nature of the disorders. The child cannot express his feelings in words, but his feelings are there and various behaviour disorders result. He may react, in fact, by any of the manifestations of insecurity (p. 240).

When jealousy becomes a serious problem and is allowed to continue, it may well have a permanent effect on the child's character, leading to aggressiveness, selfishness or an inferiority complex, which he will carry with him for the rest of his life and which will in time affect the character of his children.

Prevention

The most important preventive for jealousy is love, understanding and security with judicious discipline. When a new baby is expected, plans calculated to prevent undue jealousy should be made early in the pregnancy. The child should not start at a nursery school at the time of the baby's arrival, move from one bedroom to another to make way for the baby, or move from the cot to a bed. These changes should be made long before the birth of the baby. He should be allowed to help in shopping for the baby and be given money with which to buy necessary objects for it. When the mother goes to hospital it is better in general for the child to stay at home as long as there is someone whom he likes to look after him. Otherwise he should go to a relative whom he loves. It would certainly be a mistake to leave him in the hands of strangers, if this could be avoided. When the baby is brought home, the importance of the child's first impressions should be remembered. The whole house is apt to revolve around the new arrival. Though inevitable, it should be minimized, and on no account should the older child feel that no one has any time for him. He should be encouraged to help in bathing the baby and changing the napkin and in fetching things for him. It is easy to overdo this, however, and so let the " helping " become an unpleasant duty. When he wants to play with the baby the playing has to be supervised until he can be trusted not to hurt the baby, but parents are apt to issue so many admonitions and reprimands that he is reduced to tears or plays on his own. It is most desirable that the child should play with and get to love the baby. Jealousy then is much less likely to be a problem. When the mother picks the baby up the father or other person should go out of his way to pick the older child up. Every possible effort should be made to ensure that the elder child is just as sure as he ever was that he is loved and wanted.

Treatment

Half the battle is won when the parents understand the nature of the problem. They must on no account have a feeling of guilt that they have let the child down. They should realize that jealousy is not a crime, but that it is normal, and as long as it is managed with common sense and understanding it will not be a problem which will last. The whole management of the child has to be reviewed in order that the various manifestations of jealousy can be properly treated. All possible causes of jealousy have to be avoided. When an overt act of jealousy occurs it has to be treated wisely, or great harm can be done. When the child hits the baby he should not be unduly scolded or smacked, for punishment will merely make him worse and increase his feeling that he has lost his parents' love. The cause of the incident should be treated, not the symptom, and the cause is the child's fear that his mother no longer loves him. This fear must be attended to so that he is given that love and security which he needs. Smacking for bed wetting or other manifestation of jealousy would be equally harmful, for it would lead to greater insecurity. It is far better to try to prevent a child injuring the baby than to warn him or smack him after the act. He should be prevented from the act by distraction—by lifting him bodily away from temptation and giving him something interesting to do. Anything which contributes to the insecurity—anger, irritability, constant warnings and reprimands—must be avoided. Above all, there must be no favouritism and no comparisons with other children.

Fears

Probably all normal children have fears. Up to a point they are desirable, for a completely fearless child is particularly liable to become involved in accidents. Severely mentally defective children have practically no fear. Fears constitute a natural normal defence mechanism. It is only when they are exaggerated and anxiety develops that they are harmful.

It is very difficult to draw a line between normal and excessive fears. The infant in his first year is likely to show fear when there is a sudden noise, a sudden falling movement or when there is some sudden unexpected event which he cannot understand. At about 6 months he may show fear of strangers. Children between the ages of 2 and 3 characteristically develop fears of everyday objects—dogs, motor cars, the hole in the bath, the water-closet, noisy machines and darkness. During the phase of increased dependence on the parents, at about the same age, they may fear being deserted by their mother.

Ordinarily fears are not a problem in the first 3 years. They may become a problem if they are exaggerated by an underlying insecurity or by mismanagement by their parents.

The number and extent of fear reactions shown by children is governed in part by the sex and the personality of the child. Girls tend to show fear more than boys. Some show fear a great deal more than others. One factor is the child's imagination, the imaginative child being more apt to develop fear.

Ætiology

According to Watson and Morgan [441] all fears are the result of suggestion. There is no doubt that many fears are suggested by adults. Caution has to be taught and used by parents and it is almost inevitable that some fear is engendered in a susceptible child as a result. This particularly applies to fear of motor cars, animals, fires and other hot objects. The parents may very well show fear of thunder or of the dark, and the child by suggestion and imitation shows the same fear. Dislike of certain foodstuffs can readily be suggested by the parents if they express their own dislikes in front of a child. Fears may be caused by foolish threats made in an attempt to force him to eat, sleep or have the bowels moved. Fear of desertion is commonly suggested by stupid threats by the mother that if he does not do what she wants him to do she will go and leave him or send him away. Fears may be suggested by fairy stories which are unsuitable for his age or by other gruesome tales or pictures, particularly if he has a vivid imagination. Excessive shyness may almost amount to fear. It may result from his having been prevented from mixing with people outside his own home. He may show fear of objects and of noises when he is alone but not when he is in the presence of his mother. He feels unable to cope with the situation on his own. Fear may develop as a result of transference. Arlitt [22] described how in a party a paper napkin caught fire as a boy blew out the candles on his birthday cake. Thereafter the boy cried with fear whenever birthdays were mentioned. Fear may arise in the same way as a result of a fall from a tricycle. The child after such a fall may be afraid of all tricycles.

Gesell [141] thought that the role of suggestion is overdone. He emphasized the developmental aspect of fear, pointing out that the nature of fear stimuli is related to the child's developmental level and to the level of his experience. The child is afraid of those objects which his experience has not equipped him to cope with, so that objects, for instance, of which some immature 3-year-olds are afraid, have stopped frightening the more mature $2\frac{1}{2}$-year-old child, who has learned to cope with the situation in question.

There is no evidence that fears are inherited, but the personality which renders a child particularly likely to show fear because of his timidity or imaginativeness is largely a hereditary characteristic.

Prevention and Treatment

Fears cannot be entirely prevented, and in any case they may serve a useful purpose. Some excessive or undesirable fears can be prevented by care to avoid suggesting them. Still more important is the prevention of a feeling of insecurity by over-protection, domination and the other faults of management discussed elsewhere.

Fears cannot be stopped by teasing, ridicule, force or distraction. They are not stopped by reassuring the child (that a dog, for instance, will not hurt him), or by ignoring his fear. Children are not likely to forget their fears or to lose them by getting used to the feared objects. It is wrong to be impatient or unsympathetic with a child who is afraid. Such an attitude increases rather than decreases his fear, because he feels that he cannot rely on his parents for protection as much as he had hoped. It is wrong when a child is afraid of the dark to deprive him of a light in the hopes that he will get out of the fear. He should be given security, protection and reassurance. His fear is a real one to him and it should be respected. It is a good thing to try to let him become more familiar with the feared object. If he is afraid of the vacuum cleaner, he may be willing to play with some of the components and then with the machine as a whole. If he is afraid of water he should be encouraged to play with water with a bucket and ladle. If he is afraid of the dark he may play at putting the lights on and off. His natural imitativeness should be remembered. He should be enabled to see other children playing with the feared objects, such as a dog.

In every case the whole child must be treated. Children with excessive fears are often insecure, and as a result they show other behaviour problems. It is essential to review the whole of the management and to correct unwise parental attitudes. Most fears will be outgrown.

Shyness

Though all will agree that shyness is a common and important problem, there is a remarkable dearth of literature on the subject. It is not mentioned in the index of any of the books by Arnold Gesell referred to in the reference list in this book.

Perhaps the first sign of shyness is at about 4 months of age, when the baby shows some coyness when spoken to by strangers. After his first birthday he tends to cover his eyes up with his forearm when spoken to, he becomes notably quiet, pulls faces and hides behind his mother. The child of 2 or 3 cries if his mother leaves him with other children. He fails to play either alongside or with other children, merely standing immobile, quiet and unhappy. He will not say a word when he is spoken to.

Shyness is partly an inherited characteristic, but it is also partly developmental and partly environmental in origin. Any parent of two or more children knows how one child is more shy than his brother, although there has been no known difference in the management of the two children. This difference is probably due to inherited character traits. It is also developmental in origin, for almost all children go through stages of shyness. Environment is obviously a factor. The child who is never given a chance to mix with others, adults and children, is very likely to be shy.

Shyness can be partly prevented by allowing the child from earliest infancy constantly to mix with others. It can partly be prevented by wise upbringing in other directions—by giving him love, security and self-confidence and giving him a sense of pride in the skills which he has learnt.

Treatment is not easy. The causes must be treated. He must certainly not be ridiculed or scolded for his shyness. It is wrong to say anything at all about his shyness in front of him. It is stupid to tell him not to be shy. He cannot help it and ridicule can do nothing but harm. He should be allowed to have friends into his home at frequent intervals and he should go out to visit his friends, at first with his mother. He should be encouraged to play alongside friends in the first place and not be pushed into playing with them. Above all, his shyness must be respected.

Stuttering

Johnson [221] made the remark that stuttering develops after the diagnosis has been made rather than before it. He considered it a consequence of the diagnosis. Some lay person—the parent, grandparent or neighbour—suggests that the child is beginning to stutter. The parents become seriously concerned and do their utmost to check it. They tell the child to take a deep breath before he speaks, to repeat himself and to speak more slowly and distinctly. He becomes self-conscious about his speech and it becomes forced and artificial instead of natural. One is reminded of the story of the centipede :

"The centipede was contented quite,
Until the toad one day in spite
Said, 'Say! which foot comes after which?'
This so wrought upon her mind,
She lay distracted in the ditch,
Considering which came after which."

Johnson, at the Iowa Child Welfare Research Station, became interested in the normal repetitions made by children in learning speech. He found in a large group of normal children that 15–25 per cent. of their words figure in some sort of repetition. The initial sound or syllable of the word is repeated, or the whole word is repeated, or the word is part of a repeated phrase. Johnson considered that a great deal of stuttering is caused by the diagnosis being made as a result of failure to realise that such repetitions are normal. Children from $2\frac{1}{2}$ years onwards become so excited in recounting what they have seen that they stumble over themselves in a torrent of words and stuttering is suspected by the mother.

Perhaps half the children in nursery schools pass through a stuttering stage [223] which lasts a few days. The more sensitive and timid the child, the more likely he is to have spells of stuttering. Stutterers can usually talk normally when alone, or when speaking to animals, or to people whom they know well. Stuttering is precipitated by insecurity and anxiety.

There is a voluminous literature about stuttering, and there is little doubt that the problem is a highly complex one. A study of the previous development of stutterers shows that they have tended to be later in learning to walk than controls, and later in beginning to speak.

There is often a family history of speech disorder, and apart from the hereditary factor a child may readily stutter in imitation of another member of the family.

It is probably not related to handedness. It is more a behaviour problem than a speech defect. Eisenson,[120] in an excellent review of speech difficulties, quoted various studies to the effect that stutterers tend to come from a home in which there is excessive domination and discipline, overprotection and perfectionism.

The essential part of treatment is the relief of parental anxiety. The parents must be reassured about their child's speech. They must stop trying to make him speak distinctly. His diction should be ignored.

If he is still stuttering when he reaches his fourth birthday, he should have speech therapy, because it is important that his speech should be normal by the time he reaches school. Some recommend earlier treatment. I would certainly not advise any treatment before three years.

Tics

The term habit-spasm instead of tics, is not a good one, as tics are neither habits nor spasms. The common tics consist of blinking the eyes, wrinkling the forehead, rotating the head, or shrugging the shoulder, but a wide variety of other movements, some of them quite complex, may be seen. They are uncommon in the pre-school child. They disappear during sleep, and are increased by anxiety or tension. They are usually manifestations of insecurity.

Tics may lead to unpleasantness in the home. Mothers complain that they get on their nerves. Determined efforts by scolding and punishment are made to stop them, but they only aggravate matters and make them worse. They should be ignored completely. Any cause of insecurity should be removed.

It is wrong to say that all tics will disappear if ignored. They often do, but many tics last for years.[465] Sometimes one tic disappears, only to be replaced by another.

Hyperkinesis

This is an exaggeration of the constant activity manifested by all young children. The degree of activity shown by children depends very largely on their character, some being very much more active than others. Extreme activity, restlessness and fidgetiness is important because it is very exhausting for the mother. It may occur in normal children as a result of insecurity. It is particularly common in mentally retarded children.

Treatment is aimed at the cause. Any cause of insecurity must be removed. The child should be kept fully occupied and be given ample opportunity to play with his friends. Several workers have described the value of amphetamine when all underlying causes have been treated. Bradley [58] described a dramatic decrease of restlessness, noisiness and hyperactivity. The most frequent optimal daily dose was 20 mg., given in the morning on rising. It is usual to begin with a smaller dose (2·5–5 mg.) and increase every other day until there is a toxic or therapeutic effect. The drug may cause dizziness, nausea, vomiting, anorexia and insomnia.

The cure may lie in sending him to a nursery school.

Quarrelsomeness and Aggressiveness

All young children are aggressive, and no parent need be disturbed or surprised at games of killing and shooting. All young children are quarrelsome, though some are much more so, because of inherent personality, than others. Some bickering is inevitable in a family, however well the children are managed. Teasing and quarrelling are precipitated by fatigue, hunger (hypoglycæmia), and boredom.

The difficulty in management lies in deciding when to intervene in quarrels. On the one hand children have to learn to settle their own disputes. On the other hand good relationships with others are largely learnt in the home, and children have to learn in the home what is right and wrong. In general it is better to step in before quarrels develop rather than to wait till a quarrel occurs and try to stop it. One should anticipate by separating children when they are showing signs of having reached their limits of tolerance of each other, particularly if they are tired. The aim is to strike a happy mean between excessive interference and not interfering enough.

Excessive aggressiveness or quarrelsomeness is usually a sign of insecurity, and the cause must be looked for. It may, for instance, be due to overstrictness in the home, or to overindulgence. Determined efforts to stop a child hitting others are likely to lead to aggravation of the problem, for it will be continued as an attention-seeking device. A father told me that he had "tried everything" to stop his child hitting others. Although one cannot allow a child to injure others, the less that is done the better, because once the child recognizes the parental anxiety, he will enjoy the fuss and hit children all the more. It is better to treat the cause rather than the symptom, and the cause lies usually in one of the causes of insecurity (p. 223).

It is worth remembering that undue fatigue, which leads, amongst other things, to excessive teasing and quarrelsomeness, may be due to a slight degree of anæmia. It may, of course, be due to inadequate sleep.

Attention-seeking Devices

A very wide range of attention-seeking devices are adopted by children. Below is a collection of familiar ones. Most parents could add others. They are much more likely to be found in the insecure child than in the secure one, but it would be a mistake to think that they only occur in the absence of security. Any child likes power and attention, especially between the age of 1 and 3 years.

In connection with eating, the chief devices are food refusal, sometimes refusal of a particular food which the mother has shown a special desire for the child to eat, particularly meat, milk, eggs and vegetables. The child may drop it on the floor or take it into the mouth, then spit it out or refuse to swallow it. Many mothers have thought that their child had some mechanical difficulty with swallowing, such as a disease of the œsophagus. Children may carry the meat around in the mouth for 2 or 3 hours. Others discover the trick of vomiting the food out. Some discover the particularly impressive trick of bringing it up over the tea-table.

Dirt eating (pica) is only a problem when the child discovers that it is a good way of drawing attention to himself, though psychologists have other explanations. A question on paper-eating was asked in the Question and Answer Section of the *British Medical Journal.*[66] The reply ran as follows : " The eating of paper, which symbolizes cleanliness through its toilet use, is likely in the logic of infancy to represent inner cleanliness. Practical measures would include the avoidance in the diet of food which may arouse disgust, such as sausages or anything brown or of messy consistency."

In connection with sleeping, screaming when put to bed and refusal to lie down are the chief devices used. One 18-month child was brought to me because it was feared that he had "gone wrong in the head." Every night when the mother put him to bed and left him he screamed, and as soon as she returned she found him standing on his head.

In connection with sphincter control refusal to sit on the chamber, withholding of urine or fæces, and the deliberate passage of a stool or urine on the carpet are the chief attention-seeking devices. Some discover that when they ask to be placed on the chamber the mother immediately jumps up and attends to them, and so they demand it every few minutes, having great fun as long as it lasts. Some boys refuse to pass urine standing up, simply because of the pressure which is brought on them by adults to do so. Stool smearing becomes an attention-seeking device if mismanaged.

Body manipulations—masturbation, sex play, head banging, head rolling, nose picking, teeth grinding, hair plucking, lip pulling and other manifestations are similar devices, or at least they become so if the initial manifestation is treated with anxiety and fuss.

Children may discover that they attract attention by abnormalities of speech, by facial distortion, by making certain noises, by coughing or gagging. One child achieves it by pulling up the best flowers in the garden ; another by turning the gas tap on ; another by banging the table ; another by breath-holding attacks and tantrums ; another by dawdling in dressing, tidying up or in other tasks ; another by deliberate disobedience. One boy aged 3 greatly alarmed his mother, who feared that he was a sexual pervert, by frequently dashing up to ladies and lifting their skirts up. Another caused consternation in his mother's bridge parties by suddenly asking the ladies if they wanted to have a " we-we." Some children achieve their ends by feigning a pain or limp. A child may complain of pains in the legs when he does not want to go out for a walk, or abdominal pains at mealtimes when efforts are being made to compel him to take food. This is partly an attention-seeking device and partly a defence mechanism.

A successful device adopted by many children is frequently to ask the mother, " Do you love me ? " This is highly successful when asked at the right time, just when the mother is showing signs of becoming angry. Another, when reprimanded, says " I'm sorry " with such feeling that the mother's heart melts and he gets his own way. The ingenuity of small children is remarkable and their powers of annoying considerable.

Any prank is likely to be repeated if the child discovers that it has attracted attention and put him in the centre of the picture. All too often parents describe his wrongdoing in his presence, for his pranks do supply a good topic of tea-time conversation. The inevitable result is that they are repeated. It is disastrous ever to let one's child know how much one secretly enjoys his wickedness. A child very readily becomes conscious of his parents' admiration of his tricks even though it has never been expressed in words.

The treatment of these problems is usually easy, but some of them tax the ingenuity to the utmost. Half the battle is won when the cause — the desire for attention, the development of the ego — is recognized. Not all of these tricks can be simply ignored. One cannot ignore the turning on of the gas taps or other dangerous tricks. Clearly the least possible anxiety should be shown. He should be distracted as soon as it is seen that he is about to repeat the trick. Distraction is much better than warnings or threats before the act or punishment after the act. Punishment may help towards the latter end of the third year, but it may make the behaviour worse. It is a matter of trial and error. It is preferable at this age to explain to the child that he is too old for that sort of behaviour. If such an appeal fails, stronger measures may have to be tried. For anything but dangerous tricks much the most effective method of dealing with them is to ignore them. That is the worst punishment that the child can have. When, in spite of the above treatment a child persists in turning the gas tap on, other measures must be tried. One would consist of fixing a toy tap for the child to operate, at a safe distance but near the gas stove, making it quite clear that that is his tap while the other one (the real one) is " Mummy's." This sort of method is more likely to succeed than punishment.

In all cases it is important to look behind the attention-seeking devices to the underlying cause. In simple cases the cause lies simply in the normal desire for attention which any child has and shows. In severe cases these tricks suggest that the child's basic needs are not being met, that in the normal course of events he is not being recognized sufficiently as a person, not being praised and loved sufficiently and not being given the responsibility which he wants. He then finds that the only way he has of attracting attention is being " naughty " and doing one of the tricks mentioned above.

CHAPTER 29

THE PREVENTION OF ACCIDENTS

In Canada,[97] the United States,[339] Holland and other countries accidents are the chief cause of death in children of 1 year of age and over. In Canada they cause more deaths in children than the ten common acute infectious diseases combined. Dietrich[111] showed that accidents account for more deaths in children than the next six most common causes of death combined, and more permanent crippling. They kill 12,000 children each year in the United States and cause permanent injury every year to 30,000–50,000 children. Rowntree[363] found that in a National Sample of young children in England and Wales studied in 1946–48 the rate of injuries requiring professional treatment in the first 2 years of life was 79·6 per 1,000. In one year doctors and hospital departments treated about 15,000 severe burns or scalds, 16,000 bad cuts or bruises and 4,000 fractures among an estimated total of 1,740,000 children under 2 years of age in Britain in 1947.

The accidents consisted chiefly of burns and scalds from radiators or fires or from boiling liquids ; road accidents ; falls from prams, chairs and stairs ; suffocation ; poisons ; and electric shocks. Colebrook and Colebrook[94] analysed the causes of 1,000 examples of burns and scalds. One of the chief ones was the unguarded gas, electric or coal fire. Children either fell into the fire or their clothes became ignited by contact. They drew attention to the highly inflammable nature of many clothes now in use and to methods which should be employed in their manufacture to make them non-inflammable. Castle[84] gave a useful analysis of the causes of other types of accidents, such as falls. Old-fashioned houses, in a poor state of repair, and the absence of play space are responsible for many accidents. Other factors are absence of domestic help and the employment of women in industry.

Another important factor is accident proneness. It has been shown that some children and adults are more prone to accidents than others. Fabian and Bender[124] found that of 86 children with severe head injuries at the Bellevue Hospital, New York, 33 (38 per cent.) had been involved in two or more major accidents; 83 per cent. of the parents of children with the accident habit had psychopathological disorders. In half one or both were alcoholic. In many instances the fathers were domineering, abusive or rejecting. The mothers were submissive or over-protecting. Violent displays of temper and marital disharmony were common. Accidental self-injury, including bruises and bumps on the head resulting from deliberate injury in anger or otherwise, was discussed by Ackerman and Chidester.[4] It is a personality disturbance usually resulting from insecurity, over-protection or excessive domination by the parents.

The question of the prevention of accidents will be discussed under two headings : (i) Physical Steps to Prevent Accidents, and (ii) The Management of the Child.

Physical Steps to Prevent Accidents

All fires and stoves should be properly protected by guards which are secure. They should be held in place by expanding curtain wire attached to eyelets in the fire surround. All electric points must be of the safety variety so that pencils and other objects cannot be pushed into them. Gas taps must be safety ones. Portable stoves are dangerous. Flex must be kept in good condition. Electric apparatus is not permitted in the bathroom. There should be no gas fire or gas water-heating apparatus in a child's bedroom. The child should on no account be left alone in the house even for five minutes. The highly inflammable nature of most clothes must be remembered. Nighties are particularly dangerous in this respect, and pyjamas are preferable. Fireworks should not be allowed to go off in a room. The high chair and clothes horse should be well away from the fire. No child should ever be allowed to play with fire. He should never be allowed to climb over the fender to recover a lost toy. A hot water bottle should not be left in the baby's bed.

Pan handles on stoves should be turned in so that the child is less likely to reach them. The kettle, teapot and basins of hot fat should be out of reach. The teapot should not be on the edge of the table, where it will fall off if the table cover is pulled. The tablecloth should not hang over the edge of the table. Hot liquids such as tea should never be passed in front of a child, and no baby should be on his mother's knee when she is drinking hot liquids. Buckets of water should never be left about. Lily ponds in the garden have caused many deaths. The child should never be left unattended in the bath. The cold water should be run in before the hot.

Dangerous toys must not be allowed. Bows and arrows and airguns cause blindness. Eyes of cuddly toys should not come out. Metal toys should not have sharp corners. Colours should be fast.

Falls from the high chair are prevented by safe strapping. A bar between the legs prevents the baby sliding down. A gate at the top of the stairs may cause danger, for the child may climb over the top or push against it when it is not properly closed. The stairs should be properly lighted. Toddlers should not be asked to carry objects up and down the stairs. The window in the child's bedroom should be rendered safe so that he cannot climb out of it, but if all the windows upstairs are barred there will be difficulty in the case of fire. The floor on which rugs are placed should not be polished. If they are polished, non-skid devices should be fastened to the rugs.

When a child shows signs of being able to climb over the edge of a cot it is time he were given a bed. This is usually about the second birthday. Harnesses and straps to keep him lying down are dangerous. No baby should be taken into his parents' bed because of the danger of suffocation. The bars of the cot should not be more than $2\frac{3}{4}$ to 3 in. apart if they are flexible tubular rods, or 3 in. apart if the rods are of solid wood.[121]

Electric washing machines are a danger. One paper [263] described 295 cases of washing machine accidents, causing mangling of arms.

All poisons, including matches, camphor balls, cleaning materials, tablets and medicines should be placed right out of reach of the small child. In the garden there should be no poisonous berries. As soon as he is old enough it should be explained to him that they are only for birds to eat. Sharp objects, such as razor blades, scissors, pins, opened tins, and fragile ornaments should be out of reach.

Street doors should be securely closed. Car door handles should be safe. Parents should develop the habit, and teach others the habit, of opening and closing doors gently. Door banging games should not be allowed. The danger of swings in the garden, and particularly swings of the rotating type, should be remembered. When an older child is swinging, a younger one may run up behind him and have his skull fractured.

Many accidents arise in connection with prams. The chief accidents are due to the child climbing over the edge or tipping the pram over. Davies [104] discussed some of the reasons for pram accidents. He says that the pram may tip forwards through overloading at the handle end and by excessive weight in the shopping basket. Tipping may also be due to the wrong use of a single pram for two children. The pram may tip backwards through wrong use of the safety strap. This is often placed too near the hood of the pram. The correct position for the strap is 9–11 in. from the interior back of the pram, according to its size. This should bring the strap fastening to a position from which a vertical line will come within the wheelbase. It is essential to see that there is not too much play in the straps, for otherwise the baby may climb over the edge.

Mothers should be discouraged from working in industry at least until the child is about 3 years old. They should look after their children unless the strongest financial reasons make it essential for them to leave their children in charge of others.

The Management of the Child

The proper management of the child is an essential step towards accident prevention. The child who has never had any sort of discipline, who is permitted by his parents to climb on to window sills, tables and other dangerous places and who is allowed to do exactly as he wants is particularly apt to become involved in accidents. Occasional climbing in certain active children cannot be avoided. It can be minimized by proper discipline when it is seen. The over-protected child is equally liable to become involved in accidents.[38] The child who is constantly thwarted and prevented from any sort of ordinary activity because of some conceivable danger is very apt to rebel and so get into difficulties.

An excellent discussion of the problem of accident prevention was given by Dietrich.[110, 111] He wrote that safe behaviour, like any other form of behaviour, grows out of early parent-child relations. Accident prevention needs forethought, time and discipline : forethought—to think of and become sensitive to possible dangers to children ; time—to watch them ; and discipline—so that they learn how far they can go. " Mild, consistent, logical discipline is as necessary to a child's sense of security as it is to his life. It may be administered by a glance, a word, an act of deprivation, a tone of voice or the proper anatomic application of a dispassionate hand." In the first year there must be 100 per cent. protection, and any accident is entirely the fault of the custodians. If such absolute protection is maintained for a relatively few years the child becomes unusually vulnerable to accidents. Dietrich suggests, therefore, that after 1 year, while maintaining protection against serious accidents, the child should be exposed to minor painful experiences for their educational value. He should at all times be protected from severe burns or scalds and from catching his clothes in an electric radiator, but he should be allowed to feel the heat of a coffee pot. " Instead of forbidding him to touch commonplace objects one should simply and objectively state : 'That is hot ; if you touch it, it will burn you.' He does, it does, and a valuable lesson is learned." He must be prevented from reaching poisons, but a good lesson is learnt when a jar of vinegar or mustard is left in a place where the child cannot fail but discover it. He must not be allowed to fall from any dangerous height or on to a dangerous surface, but he may fall out of a chair as long as he has not a dangerous implement in his hand. In other words, there must be a constant balance between protection and education, beginning with absolute protection at birth and finishing with almost complete independence by about 10 years of age. In these short intervening years the completely protected, totally dependent 1-year-old infant must be transposed into a secure, self-confident school child armed with safe behaviour.

Certain dangerous practices should always be prevented or stopped if seen. Children should not be allowed to throw hard objects about the room, to play with fire, to recover a lost toy from the fireplace, to play on the stairs, to play with cord round the neck, to run about with food in the mouth, or run about with a sharp or breakable toy (e.g. a plastic trumpet) in the mouth, to remove a chair when someone is about to sit on it, to climb down from a stool with a fork in the hand, or to climb on the window-sill.

It is very difficult in teaching caution to avoid implanting fear. The average child of 20 months can be taught some degree of caution. He can usually be trained to keep away from the kitchen stove or electrical connections. The ease with which forbidden acts are repeated as attention-seeking devices must also be remembered. The greatest ingenuity has to be used to stop such dangerous habits as turning the gas taps on and other acts which cannot be dealt with simply by ignoring them.

CHAPTER 30

TOYS AND PLAY—NURSERY SCHOOL

It is very difficult, especially in wet weather or in winter, to keep a small child occupied. The problem is just as important in institutions for well children as it is in the home. The importance of keeping him occupied is very great, for boredom rapidly leads to bad temper, irritability, naughtiness and destructive behaviour. A vicious circle is set up, for the child's bad behaviour annoys and tires the mother, and her irritability and loss of patience makes the child worse.

In any discussion of ways and means of keeping children occupied the normal variations in the personality, interests, aptitudes and intelligence of children must always be borne in mind. Toys which will interest one child will not interest another. Some are better with their hands than others. Some by the age of 3 can draw as well as the average 5-year old. Others, though of equal intelligence, cannot draw any recognizable object at that age. Even when a child's interests and capabilities are known it is not usually possible to predict which toy will give the most lasting pleasure.

In all cases solitary play, though necessary part of the time, should be avoided in excess. The child must learn to play without constant help from his mother. Many mothers make the mistake of constantly interfering in play, so that he becomes utterly dependent on her and cannot entertain himself without her help. On the other hand, he should at frequent intervals visit the homes of others to play and to learn to give and take, and he should have friends into his house. All too often small children are denied the opportunity of mixing with others.

Children learn by their play. To a certain extent all toys have educational value, but some have more value than others. Some toys, particularly certain expensive mechanical ones, do not maintain interest for long. All children like to practise their new skills, and toys which enable them to do this, toys which make them think and experiment or which make them use their developing powers of imagination, are more likely to retain interest for weeks and months. Mechanical out-of-door toys, such as tricycles, are of value in giving exercise in the fresh air and in keeping the child out of doors. Most of the toys described below have some educational value. Many of these are not very easy to find in ordinary shops and are not readily thought of. It is assumed that the child has a supply of the usual cheap mechanical toys which are on display in every toy-shop.

Apart from the out-of-door mechanical toys there is no need to think that toys will cost a great deal of money. It is by no means the most expensive ones which give the greatest pleasure. The highly costly hand-made doll will not necessarily please the child any more than a cheap doll with some hand-made rapidly-knitted garments which the girl can put on and take off herself.

When in doubt about the suitability of a toy for a particular age, it is always wise to give one which is a little too difficult for him than one which is too simple. He will soon discard the one which is too easy for him. Fortunately, however, wisely chosen toys are popular for many months. A good miscellaneous assortment of wood blocks, for instance, is enjoyed just as much by the 5-year-old as it is by the 1-year-old. The use to which the blocks are put is different, but in each case they teach the child to use his hands and brain. When a child gets bored with a toy and loses interest in it, it should be put away for a few weeks. It is likely to be thoroughly enjoyed as if it were a new toy when it reappears one wet afternoon a few months later. Children who are given an excess of toys are apt to become bored and destroy or waste them.

In the choice of toys it is always important to see that the toys themselves, or parts which can be detached, are not sharp enough to hurt the child ; that the toys or detachable parts of the toys are not so small that they can be inhaled or swallowed, and that the paint does not come off when they are taken to the mouth.

A child should have a toy cupboard or a large box in which he keeps his assortment of odds and ends. A playroom is a luxury. It is of uncertain value in the first 3 years unless there are older children as well, for the child is likely to want to play near his mother, but it is of great value later, helping not only the mother, by allowing her to get on with her work away from the children, but helping the children by giving them a place of their own in which to play.

Between 3 and 6 months a wide-awake baby wants to see what is going on. He very readily becomes bored if left in the pram all day with nothing but a view of a brick wall in front of him. Even when taken out for a walk he is apt to be kept lying down with the hood up and other obstacles to his vision, so that he cannot see anything. He should be propped up so that he can see what is happening. He may refuse to lie outside in a pram. In that case he should be wheeled into the kitchen, where he can watch his mother doing her household duties. At about 3 or 4 months he can hold objects if they are placed in his hand, though he cannot reach out for objects and get them. He should be given objects, therefore, such as plastic rattles or large curtain rings, which he can hold and play with. Highly-coloured objects will be more popular than dull colours. A toy may be tied on his pram so that it dangles in front of him. As long as this is a reasonable distance from his eyes it will not do them any harm.

He should begin to get used to seeing other children. It is a mistake to isolate a baby from other children. When eventually he sees them he is apt to be frightened and shy.

At 5 months the average baby can reach for an object and grasp it. From this time onwards he should be given an abundance of toys which will help him to learn to use his hands. A discarded tin with something inside, such as small pebbles or lentils, will be enjoyed. Bobbins, cubes, large beads on string, bricks (not paper covered), spoons and other large objects are suitable for him. He should be propped up in his high chair so that he can play with the toys on the tray in front of him.

From the age of 6 months onwards an ever-increasing range of objects interests the child. He is rapidly learning to use his hands, and he should be given a variety of toys to help him. Cubes, plastic rings on chains, bobbins and rattles continue to be favourites. Between 9 months and a year or so babies take a delight in placing objects in and out of containers, and baskets, boxes, tins and bricks of various shapes and sizes are particularly popular. Nesting boxes and barrels, nesting pyramids and interlocking building bricks will be enjoyed. Stiff books are likely to be enjoyed at about this age. They should be made of stout card, which is virtually untearable. Linen books are useful but not so satisfactory. The pages rapidly curl up. It is surprising how few mothers think of giving their children books at this age.

In the second year books become of increasing value. They should now be of two types, hard card books which the child can look at himself without risk of damage being done, and ordinary books which the mother will show him and read to him and then put away out of reach. The latter type includes nursery rhymes. Even before a year of age babies often show great pleasure in the rhythm of nursery rhymes and anticipate with appropriate bodily movement when a particular line is being approached. Picture books should preferably be simple, showing one object on a page. Many of the available books show pictures which are too complex and confusing to the child. When objects are pointed out to children in this way they learn a great deal and they can then themselves point out numerous objects long before they can say the appropriate word. This helps in the development of speech. Towards the latter part of the second year story books become popular. The Beatrix Potter books may become great favourites. Other books show coloured pictures of common objects. Scrapbooks composed of coloured pictures cut out of magazines and stuck into Press cutting books or albums will be enjoyed and instructive.

Boxes, tins and cubes continue to be useful. Sets of wood blocks of different shapes and sizes will occupy many hours. Toys which can be pushed and pulled, particularly if objects can be put into them, will be enjoyed. Children should be given opportunities to hear music on the wireless or gramophone. They enjoy drums, whistles and trumpets. Pile driving with wooden pegs which have to be hammered through holes is a satisfying pursuit.

Domestic mimicry is a characteristic feature of the $1\frac{1}{2}$–3-year-old child. Cookery sets, tea sets, doll's furniture, sweeping brushes and toy carpet sweepers will enable him to spend hours in this way. A doll and teddy bear enable him to use his imagination and he is likely to become very attached to them.

Towards the latter half of the second year children are likely to be able to thread large beads (or cubes with holes through them). They often play with pencil and paper. At first it is a mere scribble, which the child may call a man or dog, but with practice the drawing rapidly improves. Lacing cards are useful. They consist of celluloid or similar material with holes punched through. Coloured laces are threaded through and through. Plasticine and modelling material will be used in this period. At about 2 children can pronate and supinate the wrists well enough to screw and unscrew jars. A sand-pit with simple wooden implements (rake, shovel, etc.) and tins will keep a child busy for hours. A bowl of water in the garden, with jugs and other containers, is always popular. Spinning tops, balls and trains have their uses. In my experience sets of farmyard animals have only temporary interest, in that they do not enable the child to think or use his imagination. There is nothing much to do with them.

In the third year books, building blocks, Plasticine, clay and other modelling materials find increasing use. Drawing books, paints, stencils, coloured shapes which can be stuck on to paper, bead threading, coloured pencils (with a pencil sharpener) all help to keep the child occupied. A blackboard and chalk can be provided. Domestic mimicry is now much more advanced. Children delight in "helping" the mother to cook, and like to make pastries, shell peas, pick the tops off fruit and to set the table. "Cakes" made by the child have a specially delightful flavour for him. Home-made clothes or discarded baby clothes for the doll, with suitably large buttons, enable him to dress and undress the doll. A doll's cot and pram, with bits of rag to act as sheets, and doll's furniture, give him full scope for his imagination. A "Wendy" house can be constructed from clothes-horses if it cannot be made by the handyman; it, too, helps in developing the imagination. Remnants from dressmaking find various uses if given to the child. There may be enough to enable her to dress up as a "nurse." The child should "wash up" his own cooking utensils. An hour or two may be spent in washing-up two or three cups. The doll's clothes may be washed and pegged out. He may play shops with the aid of his junk box.

Out of doors a small tricycle or pedal car will give great pleasure and provide him with exercise in the fresh air. A swing, rocking boat, wheelbarrow, balance bar, balls, sand-pit and bowls of water will keep him occupied for prolonged periods.

In the latter part of the third year simple jigsaws—beginning with those made of two or three pieces—may be given. Appreciation of size and shape is also learnt by peg boards and by a posting box with holes of various shapes carved in the side through which blocks of the appropriate size are "posted." There are simple form boards—pieces of wood with carved holes into which blocks of the right shape have to be fitted. Plastic mosaics serve the same purpose. Tracing books help in teaching finer manipulation.

Colour and picture matching is enjoyed. Sets of pictures of common objects have to be matched with corresponding pictures on a board ; sets of five of each of a dozen or more pictures have to be put together in their proper pile. Assorted wools of various colours may be matched in the same way. Cut-out numerals which have to fit into a board, cardboard counters and cardboard coins and cut-out letters of the alphabet have a similar use.

Tile pictures can be made by shaped pieces of wood with holes in the middle which are hammered by means of nails on to a piece of beaverboard.

In the latter part of the third year the child is old enough to use blunt-ended scissors. Plastic scissors are available, but it is very difficult to cut anything with them and they are of little use.

Gramophone records of children's stories, songs and other music may be purchased. On the wireless there are programmes of music which help to teach rhythm.

When the child is 3 or 4, many of the toys, such as building bricks, continue to be popular. Dinky cars and similar vehicles please the boy. Dolls, whose clothes can be put on and taken off, please the girl. Sets of paper dresses for dolls are very useful. A shoe box can be made into a house or garage, doors and windows being made by scissors, the child being left to arrange the colour scheme. A child may be given a discarded pattern book, from which he can cut out the figures and dresses. He may be allowed to colour pictures in old newspapers. Tracing and stencil books are popular. A dressing-up box, containing discarded clothes and pieces of material, provides endless pleasure.

The plastic building toy "Bildit" is a very good toy for this and subsequent ages. The Raphael Tuck "Panorama Books" and the various Golden Play Books, published by Adprint, London, are very much liked by boys.

Firms which specialize in educational toys include :

E. J. Arnold & Son, Butterly Street, Leeds, 10.
Wilkane Ltd., Eastbourne, Sussex.
Educational Supply Association Ltd., 181, High Holborn, London, W.C.1.

These firms issue particularly good catalogues of the toys which they make.

The following books or series of books are recommended :

" Verses for Children." *Harry Golding.* Ward, Lock & Co., London.
" The Book of a Thousand Poems." *J. M. MacBain.* Evans Brothers Ltd., London.
The *Beatrix Potter* Series. F. Warne & Co. Ltd., London.
" Tirra Lirra." *Laura Richards.* George Harrap, London.
The Janet and John Books. *Mabel O'Donnell* and *Rona Munro.* James Nisbet & Co., London.
Gay Colour Books. *Alice Williamson.* E. J. Arnold & Son Ltd., Leeds.
Colour Photo Books. E. J. Arnold & Son Ltd., Leeds.
First Stories. *Margaret Barnes.* E. J. Arnold & Son Ltd., Leeds.
The Little Golden Books. *Various Authors.* Simon Schuster, New York.
" Tales to Read." *Mollie Clarke.* A. Wheaton & Co., Exeter.
Little Things Series. A. Wheaton & Co., Exeter.
My First Little Books Series. Evans Brothers Ltd., London.
Thomas the Tank Engine Series. *W. Awdry.* Edmund Ward, Leicester.
The March of Rhyme. Compiled by *Dorothy Green.* E. J. Arnold & Son Ltd., Leeds.
Listen with Mother Series. Juvenile Productions, London.
Blackberry Farm Books. *Jane Pilgrim.* Brockhampton Press Ltd., Leicester.

Nursery School

The question of whether or not to send a child to a nursery school sometimes arises towards the end of the third year. It is very undesirable that he should be placed in a nursery earlier in order to enable the mother to work in industry or elsewhere. The child in his first two years needs his mother, and separation from her for the major part of each day is unsound psychologically and is very apt to lead to insecurity and other behaviour problems.

In the latter part of the third year, however, it becomes increasingly difficult to keep the only child, if he is a very active one, adequately occupied. The question hardly arises if there are siblings with whom he can play. The decision must be an individual matter. It depends largely on his personality, on his maturity, his ability to mix with other children and his readiness to be separated from home. The convenience of the mother, unless (as often happens) there is economic necessity, is a secondary matter ; the essential factor to be considered is whether it will contribute to the child's happiness. It is valuable for him to play with other children. In general, however, I think that it is too early for most children to be separated from home. It is unfortunate that financial reasons compel many mothers to work in industry and so to leave their children in the charge of others.

CHAPTER 31

THE SICK CHILD. THE CHILD IN HOSPITAL

WHEN a child is poorly discipline should be relaxed, and he is allowed much more of his own way than normally. There should be no fear of spoiling him if the illness is only a short one. It is essential, however, that as soon as he is convalescent, normal discipline should be exerted.

Many children learn bad habits during an illness as a result of some indulgence, and the habit proves difficult to break. The mother may sleep in the child's room or the child in the parent's room, or a warm drink is taken to him every time he cries out at night, and instead of reverting to the normal practice immediately after the acute illness (which in most cases is only one or two days) the parent makes the mistake of continuing the indulgence too long.

Food forcing is never justifiable even in an illness. There is no need to persuade a feverish child to eat. He should be given what he wants and no more. There is something to be said for trying to persuade him to drink more fluid, but even that is uncertain. When he is thirsty he will ask for fluid.

The role of suggestion must always be remembered. Parents make the mistake of repeatedly asking a child if he is going to be sick again, or if he still has a pain or headache, with the result that the symptom is suggested. It is far better to make light of his symptom and distract his attention to other things.

When a child who has recently acquired sphincter control becomes ill " accidents " are very apt to occur. The parents should be warned of this and told not to make any fuss about it and not to scold the child.

It is always difficult to keep a poorly child occupied in bed. The book by Cornelia Stratton Parker entitled " Your Child can be Happy in Bed " (New York, Thomas Crowell) gives useful ideas in this respect. She suggests that periods of illness should be anticipated, books and suitable toys, along with such materials as Christmas calendars, sea shells, and pictures to colour or cut out, should be kept in a box, to be used only when the child is ill.

I have no doubt that many children are kept in bed far too long. Except in the cases of rheumatic fever and infective hepatitis there are very few medical conditions indeed which necessitate a child staying in bed after his temperature has become normal.

The Child in Hospital

Children are sent into hospital very lightly, with little thought of possible psychological trauma. It is just when a child is ill, however, that he most needs his mother to comfort him and give him love and security. At this very time he is separated from his mother for the first time in his life.

As Newman [310] wrote " Admission to a hospital means separation from his parents, his home and all with which he is familiar, to meet a new environment at a time when he is handicapped by illness, confused and anxious." He may interpret his separation as a punishment or desertion, especially if his mother has been foolish enough to threaten to leave him if he does not obey, or if he " is not a good boy." Some mothers even threaten to take their child to hospital if they do not obey.

If he is an infant he is likely to be placed in a cubicle because of the risk of cross-infection. He is visited very occasionally by someone in a white coat and mask, someone he has never seen before. No one picks him up, however much he cries. He is left crying longer than he has ever been left before. He is thought to be " spoilt." No one realizes that this is a normal reaction for a child of his age who has the firm attachment to his mother which he ought to have.

Meals come round at fixed intervals to which he is not accustomed, and he cries from hunger long before these times. They contain items of diet which he has never tasted before, or which he does not like. No one knows anything about his likes or dislikes. His favourite cup and dish are missing. He wants a drink. His mother would know perfectly well, but the nurse does not realize that this is the reason for his fussing.

He has no toys, or perhaps a single teddy, but it is not his favourite one. He is given no chance of practising his newly-learned skills. His personality and individuality are not recognized. He is just left to cry.

A doctor comes in at intervals, and he is held down by a nurse while needles are pushed unexpectedly into his back, neck or thigh, causing great pain. This happens at intervals throughout the day. He is carried away to another room, and there a dark thing is held over his nose and mouth. There is a nasty smell in it and it hurts his nose and throat. He screams in terror, but is held down firmly by two nurses until he goes to sleep.

Bakwin [26] described how infants in hospital may fail to gain weight on a correct diet and in the absence of any infection. This has been ascribed to loss of extra fluid in exhaled air, with a rise in basal metabolic rate, causing weight loss,[81] but probably other factors are involved. Most pædiatricians are fully conversant with such failure to gain weight. The children tend to become listless and apathetic, to sleep less than at home, to eat less well and to have more frequent stools. In another paper [27] Bakwin showed that such infants may have persistent low-grade fever for months, the temperature settling promptly to normal when they return home.

Older children settle down very well in hospital, and many of them thoroughly enjoy themselves. The problem lies with the younger child, who cannot understand why he has been left in hospital, because he is too young for adequate explanation to be given to him. In a study of the effect of admission to hospital at Sheffield [213] we found that only 32 per cent. of the children aged 1–4 were apparently unaffected during the day by the separation, as compared with 59 per cent. of those aged 5–6, and 72 per cent. of those aged 7–14. Only 14 per cent. of those aged 1–4 did not cry when their visitors left them, as compared with 29 per cent. of those aged 5–6, and 62 per cent. of those aged 7–14.

Levy [252] and others have written about the psychological trauma of operations, particularly tonsillectomy. He described children who as a result of such operations in the first 3 years had developed night terrors, negativism, dependency reactions, causing the child to cling to the mother, and various fears—fears of the dark and of strange men. He thought that they were due chiefly to the removal from the mother just at the time when the child most needed her and to painful experiences, such as that of an anæsthetic.

There are other ways in which a period in hospital disturbs a child. It upsets his whole rhythm and he is liable to develop sleep and sphincter disturbances on his return home. Langford [244a] wrote that illness may lead to a "regression to an immature level of social and emotional adaptation. Some react with persistent dependency reactions, rebellion or chronic invalid reactions." Common problems include enuresis, reduced talkativeness, fears of the dark, fears of strange people, and negativism. Wallgren [436] described how a mother said: "I delivered a sprightly child to the hospital and received in return a statue."

Parental attitudes in the convalescent stage are of great importance. A child who has been seriously ill is apt to suffer from parental over-protection when he returns home. The parents should be made aware, by means of a simple discussion on his discharge, of the significance of the behaviour problems, so that they can meet them with extra love and attention, without, however, over-indulgence.

Much can be done to prevent these psychological disturbances.[6, 82] Every effort should be made to avoid admitting a child under 3 years to hospital, for it is just in this period that he most needs his mother. If admission is necessary and it is thought that separation from the mother will be difficult for the child (or that the mother will herself worry unduly), then every effort should be made to admit the mother with the child, so that she can stay with him night and day, helping to look after him, feeding and bathing him. This can be of great psychological help to both mother and child. The child is helped by the mother's constant reassuring presence, and the mother is helped by the feeling that she has contributed to her child's recovery. Unfortunately there are very few hospitals in the country where this is possible. There are facilities for this in both the Babies' Hospital at Newcastle and the Children's Hospital at Sheffield. The difficulty is that the mother may not be able to come in to hospital on account of other children. One must strike a balance between the psychological trauma to the sick child, and that to the other children in the family.

If there are no facilities for the admission of the mother, then frequent visiting is certainly possible. It may be arranged that the mother should stay with him the whole day in the acute stage of his illness and help to look after him. In my opinion the advantages of frequent visiting far outweigh the disadvantages. There is no satisfactory evidence that visiting leads to a greater risk of infection. When visiting was introduced at the Sheffield Children's Hospital there was no increase in the incidence of cross-infection. Many have said that visiting causes troublesome psychological disturbance in the child. I feel that this criticism is largely wishful thinking on the part of those who oppose visiting because of the inconvenience and disturbance of ward routine which it is thought to cause.

In our study at Sheffield, it was certainly clear that many children were disturbed after the departure of their parents. I am sure, however, that it is far better for a child to see his parents every day, even though he is upset when they leave, than to be allowed to become more and more certain that they have deserted him just when he wanted them most. In any case, it is surely the right of parents to see their children when they are ill.

In some hospitals [202] so-called unrestricted visiting has been successfully introduced, whereby parents can visit at any time of the day convenient to them. At others visiting is allowed in the early evening, so that parents can help with the suppers, read to the child, and tuck him up for the night.

When a child is admitted, the admission procedure is important. The mother should be allowed to go up to the ward with him, see him bathed and sit with him for a time when he has got into bed in the ward.

When a child is old enough to understand (e.g. at 3 years of age), his mother should give him an idea of the experiences which he will meet in hospital. He is told about caps and gowns. He is told that he may be put into a cot instead of a bed, to which he is accustomed.

There should always be a balance between the desire to prevent cross-infection and to minimize psychological trauma to the child. It is undesirable for children other than babies to be in cubicles unless it is absolutely necessary because of an infectious disease. With proper precautions nurses should be encouraged to pick up small children who are crying for love and security. The danger of infection from toys must be remembered, but when a little common sense is used they can be given to the child in hospital. Every children's department should have an occupational therapist with assistants, who help to keep children occupied. It is the doctor's responsibility to see that toys suitable for different ages are provided (p. 326).

Adequate premedication should always be given before an anæsthetic, so that the child never experiences the unpleasantness of an anæsthetic mask over the face. If atropine or other injection has to be given, it should be given, if possible, when the child is asleep or under the anæsthetic. When mechanical procedures are necessary the child who is old enough should be told what they involve. It is always wrong to lie to a child, telling him that a needle will not hurt him. After an operation he can be handed to his mother to hold him or to be near him. He should never be allowed to see other children suffering painful procedures. Rectal temperatures should be avoided. Much can be done to reduce his stay in hospital to a minimum.

It is a mistake to suppose that all young children are upset by admission to hospital. They are not. It is very difficult to show just how frequent such disturbances are. In general those children who have been wisely managed at home, and given all the love and security which they need, are much less likely to be disturbed than those who have already suffered some degree of emotional deprivation at home.

Apart from the child's home management, his age, personality and intelligence (and therefore his ability to understand) are relevant factors in determining the amount, if any, of psychological trauma which will result from admission to hospital.

Prolonged Stay in Hospital

There has been a considerable amount of work on the effect of prolonged institutional care in the first 3 years on the subsequent character of the child.[78, 159, 251, 262] In an excellent monograph on the subject, summarizing the world's literature, Bowlby[55] stated that, although many of the papers lack thoroughness, scientific reliability and precision, there is striking unanimity in the various follow-up and retrospective studies by people of many nations. There is a practically unanimous conclusion that prolonged deprivation of maternal care leads to grave physical, intellectual and social retardation, and that some children are damaged for life. He described the abnormal quietness, listlessness and unresponsiveness in infants who have been in institutions for some months. They fail to try to establish contact with strangers. There is a notable regression in toilet training, eating and play behaviour. In other cases the child is easy to manage in the institution ; he is abnormally obedient and well mannered, with a cheerful indiscriminating friendliness. On his return home he is babyish, anxious and difficult to control. Various workers have described the later psychological traits in these children. They show a characteristic inability to give or receive affection, aggressiveness, bad temper, negativeness, selfishness, finger sucking and speech defects. They are liable to develop anti-social behaviour, with a failure to regard the rights of others. There is difficulty in concentrating, difficulty in abstract thought, poor reasoning, cruelty and destructiveness. It was notable that these character traits only developed if the children were in institutions for the first 2 or 3 years of their life ; the traits did not develop in children placed there after that age.

Bowlby's monograph is an effective reply to the review by Orlansky,[322] who concluded that there was no reliable scientific evidence that environment in infancy had a permanent effect on the child's character.

There is interesting experimental work on emotional deprivation in animals. It is said [259] that goslings allowed to hatch in the absence of a goose will follow the experimenter as long as he gives a passable imitation of goose behaviour, and after a few days they are very attached to him, and refuse to become attached to a goose. Lambs removed from a flock and brought up on a bottle take no notice of sheep and refuse to be led by them. Puppies and guinea-pigs behave abnormally if taken from their mother and then returned.

After reading Bowlby's monograph one cannot help feeling that there are very many infants and children who suffer minor degrees of emotional deprivation. The fear of spoiling children is a major factor in causing this, and lack of real love and affection for the child is another. There are too many mothers who are willing to leave their children for prolonged periods almost every day in the first 3 years while they do other things. One wonders what effect such emotional deprivation will have on their future character.

REFERENCES

The more important references are indicated in bold type.

1. Abramson, M. (1947). *Gen. Pract. Clin.*, **4**, 318.
2. Abt., I. A., Adler, H. M., Bartelme, P. (1929). *J.A.M.A.*, **93**, 1351.
3. Acheson, R. M., Jefferson, E. (1954). *Arch. Dis. Childh.*, **29**, 196.
4. Ackerman, N. W., Chidester, L. (1936). *Arch. Pediat.*, **53**, 711.
5. Aisenson, M. R. (1950). *Pediatrics*, **6**, 223.
6. Albany Research Project (1952). " Reducing Emotional Trauma in Hospitalized Children."

6a. Aldrich, C. A. (1928). *Am. J. Dis. Child.*, **35**, 36.

7. Aldrich, C. A., Aldrich, M. M. (1938). " Babies are Human Beings." New York. Macmillan.
8. Aldrich, C. A., Sung, C., Knop, C. (1945a). *J. Pediat.*, **26**, 313.
9. Aldrich, C. A., Sung, C., Knop, C. (1945b). *J. Pediat.*, **27**, 89, 428.
10. Aldrich, C. A., Norval, M. A., Knop, C., Venegas, F. (1946). *J. Pediat.*, **28**, 665.
11. Aldrich, C. A., Hewitt, E. S. (1947). *J.A.M.A.*, **135**, 340.
12. Aldrich, C. A. (1948). *J. Pediat.*, **32**, 109.
13. Alm, I. (1953). *Acta pæd. Uppsala*, **42**, Suppl. 94.
14. American Academy of Pediatrics (1954). " Hospital Care of Newborn Infants." Illinois.
15. American Academy of Pediatrics (1955). " Report of Committee in the Control of Infectious Disease."
16. American Public Health Assn. (1950). " The Control of Communicable Disease in Man." 7th Edn. New York.
17. American Public Health Association (1947). *Am. J. Pub. Health*, **37**, 13.
18. Anderson, A. B., Wickes, I. G. (1954). *Brit. med. J.*, *ii*, 722.
19. Anderson, T. (1955). *Brit. med. J.*, *ii*, 485.
20. Apgar, V., Girdant, B. R., McIntosh, R., Taylor, H. C. (1955). *Pediatrics*, **15**, 653.
21. Apley, J., Laurance, B., Macmath, I. F. (1954). *Lancet*, *ii*, 1048.
22. **Arlitt, A. H.** (1946). " Psychology of Infancy and Early Childhood." New York. McGraw Hill Book Co.
23. Army, Navy, Air Force Motion Sickness Team (1956). *J.A.M.A.*, **160**, 755.
25. Bakwin, H. (1926). *Am. J. Dis. Child.*, **31**, 102.
26. Bakwin, H. (1942). *Ibid.*, **63**, 30.
27. Bakwin, H. (1944). *Ibid.*, **67**, 176.
28. Bakwin, H. (1948a). *J. Pediat.*, **32**, 99.
29. Bakwin, H (1948b) *Ibid.*, **33**, 788.
30. Bakwin, H. (1949a). *Ibid.*, **35**, 786.
31. Bakwin, H. (1949b). *Ibid.*, **35**, 390.
32. **Bakwin, H.** (1949c). *Ibid.*, **35**, 512.
33. Bakwin, H. (1949d). *Ibid.*, **34**, 249.
35. Bakwin, H. (1950). *J. Pediat.*, **36**, 385.
36. Bakwin, H. (1950). *Ibid.*, **37**, 271.
37. **Bakwin, H., Bakwin, R. M.** (1940). *Ibid.*, **16**, 89, 220, 357.
38. Bakwin, H., Bakwin, R. M. (1948). *Ibid.*, **32**, 749.
39. **Bakwin, H., Bakwin, R. M.** (1951). *Ibid.*, **39**, 623.
40. Barats, M. E. (1948). *Akush Ginek*, **5**, 52.
41. Barlow, F. (1951). " Mental Prodigies." London. Hutchinson.

41a. **Bayley, N.** (1933). *Genet. Psychol. Monogr.*, **14**, 1.

42. **Beebe, H. H.** (1951). *The Nervous Child*, **9**, 8.
43. **Benjamin, E.** (1942). *Am. J. Dis. Child.*, **63**, 1019.

43a. Bergman, P. (1946). *The Nervous Child*, **5**, 37.
44. Bille, B. S. V. (1955). *Acta pæd. Uppsala*, **44**, 185.
45. Billig, A. L. (1954). *Genet. Psychol. Monogr.*, **24**, 125.
46. Birch, L. B. (1955). *Brit. J. educ. Psychol.*, **25**, 123.
47. Bisdom, C. J. W. (1936). *Maandschr. Kindergeneesk.*, **6**, 332.
48. Blatz, W. E. (1928). *Genet. Psychol. Monogr.*, **4**, 89.
49. Blatz, W. E. (1933), in Murchison, C. "A Handbook of Child Psychology." Worcester. Clark University Press.
50. Blegen, S. D. (1953). *Acta. pæd. Uppsala.*, **42**, Suppl. 88.
51. Bogert, F. van der, Moravec, C. L. (1937). *J. Pediat.*, **10**, 466.
52. Boissard, J. M., Eton, B. (1956). *Brit. med. J.*, *ii*, 574.
53. Bonar, B. E. (1936). *Am. J. Dis. Child.*, **51**, 255.
53a. Bostock, J., Shackleton, M. G. (1951). *Med. J. Aust.*, **2**, 110.
54. Bound, J. P. (1956). *Brit. med. J.*, *i*, 782.
55. **Bowlby, J.** (1951). "Maternal Care and Mental Health," *Bull. World Health Org.*, **3**, 355.
56. Bowley, A. (1949). *Proc. R. Soc. Med.*, **42**, 905.
56a Boyd, J. D. (1934). *J. Pediat.*, **4**, 263.
57. Boyd, J. D. (1941). *Ibid.*, **18**, 289.
58. Bradley, C. (1950). *J. Pediat.*, **5**, 24.
59. Bragman, L. L., quoted by Kanner (227).
60. **Brennemann, J.** (1932). *J. Pediat.*, **1**, 145.
61. **Brennemann, J.** (1948a). "Practice of Pediatrics," Vol. 1, Ch. 25, p. 18. Hagerstown. W. F. Prior & Co.
62. **Brennemann, J.** (1948b). *Ibid.*, Vol. 1, Ch. 25, p. 1.
63. **Bridge, E. M., Livingston, S., Tietze, C.** (1943). *J. Pediat.*, **23**, 539.
64. Bridges, E. L. (1951). "Uttermost Part of the Earth." London. Hodder and Stoughton.
65. British Dental Assn. (1954). "Proposals for Safeguarding and Improving the Dental Health of Children."
66. *Brit. med. J.* (1948), *ii*, 768.
67. *Brit. med. J.* (1952), *ii*, 766. (Leading Article.)
68. Browne, D. (1950). *Brit. med. J.*, *i*, 181.
69. Browne, D. (1952). *Brit. med. J.*, *ii*, 1144.
70. Bruce, J. W. (1936). *J. Pediat.*, **8**, 651.
71. **Bruch, H.** (1939a). *Am. J. Dis. Child.*, **58**, 457.
72. **Bruch, H.** (1939b). *Ibid.*, **58**, 1001.
73. **Bruch, H.** (1940a). *Ibid.*, **59**, 739.
74. **Bruch, H.** (1940b). *Ibid.*, **60**, 1082.
75. **Bühler, C.** (1930). "The First Year of Life." New York. John Day Co.
76. **Bühler, C.** (1935). "From Birth to Maturity." London. Kegan Paul.
77. Burke, J. (1956). *Brit. med. J.*, *i*, 538.
78. Burlingham, D., Freud, A. (1944). "Infants without Families." London. George Allen and Unwin.
79. Butler, A. M., Wolman, I. J. (1954). Q. Rev. *Pediat.*, **9**, 63.
80. Campbell, M. F. (1951). "Clinical Pediatric Urology." Philadelphia. W. B. Saunders.
81. Campbell, K. (1953). *Med. J. Aust.*, *i*, 201.
82. Capes, M. (1955). *Bull. World Hlth. Org.*, **12**, 427.
83. **Cassidy, J. V.** (1948). *Am. J. Ophth.*, **31**, 773.
84. Castle, O. M. (1950). *Lancet*, *i*, 315.
85. Cathie, I. A. B. (1947). *Ibid.*, *ii*, 442.
86. Cattell, P. (1947). "The Measurement of Intelligence of Infants and Young Children." New York. The Psychological Corporation.
87. Cautley, E. (1905). *Brit. med. J.*, *ii*, 555.
87a. Chant, N., Blatz, W. E. (1928). *Genet. Psychol. Monogr.*, **4**, 13.
88. Chapman, H. (1955). *Lancet*, *i*, 871.
89. Childers, A. T., Hamil, B. M. (1932). *Am. J. Orthopsychiat.*, **2**, 134.
90. Christ, M. A. (1954). *Gynæcologia*, Basel, 37, 32.

91. Clements, F. W. (1955). "The Teeth and Food." Royal Australian Coll. Physicians.
92. Clemetson, C. A. B. (1956). *J. Obst. and Gynæc. Brit. Emp.*, **63**, 1, 9, 15.
93. Clifford, S. H. (1954). *J. Pediat.*, **44**, 1.
94. Colebrook, L., Colebrook, V. (1949). *Lancet, ii*, 181.
95. Colebrook, L. (1956). *Brit. med. J., i*, 1379.
96. Colebrook, L. (1956). *Ibid., ii*, 711.
97. Collins-Williams, C. (1951). *Can. med. Ass. J.*, **65**, 531.
98. Conrad, C. (1943). *J. Pediat.*, **23**, 473.
98a. Conn, J. H., Kanner, L. (1940). *J. Pediat.*, **16**, 337.
99. Croft, P. G. (1951). *J. Ment. Sc.*, **97**, 584.
100. Crump, E. P., Robinson, J. M. (1952). *J. Pediat.*, **40**, 777.
101. Cullumbine, H. (1953). *Lancet, i*, 1193.
102. Danforth, C. H. (1927). *J. Hered.*, **18**, 153.
103. Davidson, W. D. (1953). *J. Pediat.*, **43**, 74.
104. Davies, D. L. (1950). *Brit. med. J., ii*, 869.
105. Debré, R., Mozziconacci, P., Masse, N. P., Lerique-Koechlin, A. (1948). *Sem. Hôp. Paris*, **24**, 1477.
106. Dennis, W. (1941). *Genet. Psychol. Monogr.*, **23**, 143.
107. Despert, J. L. (1946). *The Nervous Child*, **5**, 8.
108. Despert, J. L. (1949). *Ibid.*, **8**, 8.
109. Deutsch, H. (1947). "The Psychology of Women," Vol. 2. London. Research Books Ltd.
110. Dietrich, H. F. (1950). *J.A.M.A.*, **144**, 1175.
111. Dietrich, H. F. (1951). *The Crippled Child*, February.
112. Dix, M. R., Hallpike, C. S. (1947). *Brit. med. J., ii*, 719.
113. Dix, M. R., Hallpike, C. S. (1952). *Ibid., i*, 235.
114. Dodek, S. M., Friedman, J. M., Soyster, P. A., Marcellus, H. L. (1954). *J.A.M.A.*, **154**, 309.
115. Donnally, H. H. (1930). *J. Immunol.*, **19**, 15.
116. Douglas, J. W. B. (1950). *J. Obst. and Gynæc. Brit. Emp.*, **57**, 335.
117. Douglas, J. W. B., Mogford, C. (1953). *Arch. Dis. Childhood*, **28**, 436.
118. Doxiadis, S. A., Goldfinch, M. K., Cole, N. (1952). *Lancet, ii*, 1242.
119. Durdumas, G. (1938). *Kinderärztl. Prax.*, **9**, 243.
120. Eisenson, J. (1956) in "Psychology of Exceptional Children and Youth," by Cruickshank, W. M. London. Staples Press.
121. Elliott, R. A. (1955). *M. Bull. Min Hlth.*, **14**, 72.
122. English, O. S., Pearson, G. H. (1937). "Common Neuroses of Children and Adults." New York. Norton.
123. Escalona, S. K. (1947). "Transactions of the First Conference on Problems of Early Infancy." Josiah Macy Foundation.
124. Fabian, A. A., Bender, L. (1947). *Am. J. Orthopsychiat.*, **17**, 68.
125. Fairbank, R. E. (1933). *Ment. Hyg.*, **17**, 177.
126. Farquhar, H. G. (1956). *Brit. med. J., i*, 1082.
127. Fehily, L. (1944). *Brit. med. J., ii*, 590.
128. Feldman, G. V., Forrester, R. M. (1955). *Brit. med. J., ii*, 722.
128a. Fields, H. Rose, E. K. (1948). *Am. J. Med. Sc.*, **215**, 710.
129. Finch, E., Lorber, J. (1954). *J. Obst. and Gynæc. Brit. Emp.*, **61**, 833.
130. Forssell, P. (1938). *Acta. Pœdiat. Suppl.*, 1, **23**, 1.
131. Foss, G. L., Short, D. (1951). *J. Obst. and Gynæc. Brit. Emp.*, **58**, 35.
132. Frank, L. K. (1945). *Psychosomatic Med.*, **7**, 169.
133. Freeden, R. C. (1948). *Pediatrics*, **2**, 544.
134. Friedman, A. P., Von Storch, T. J. C. (1951). *J.A.M.A.*, **145**, 1325.
135. Freud, A. (1946). *The Psychoanalytic Study of the Child*, **2**, 119.
136. Freud, P. (1947). *J. Pediat.*, **31**, 131.
137. Freud, S. (1938). "Three Contributions to the Theory of Sex." Translated by A. A. Brill. New York. The Modern Library.
138. Furfey, P. H., Muehlenbein, J. (1932). *J. Genet. Psychol.*, **40**, 219.
139. Furuhjelm, U. (1954). *Etudes Neonatal.*, **3**, 93.

140. **Gairdner, D.** (1949). *Brit. med. J.*, *ii*, 1433.
141. GESELL, A. (1929), in " Foundations of Experimental Psychology," by Murchison, C. Worcester. Clark University Press. Quoted by Bakwin, H., and Bakwin, R. M. (1940).
142. GESELL, A. (1929). " Infancy and Human Growth." New York. Macmillan.
143. **Gesell, A., Amatruda, C. S., Castner, B. M., Thompson, H.** (1930). " Biographies of Child Development." London. Hamish Hamilton.
144. **Gesell, A., Ilg, F. L.** (1937). " Feeding Behaviour of Infants." Philadelphia. J. B. Lippincott Co.
145. GESELL, A., THOMPSON, H. (1938). " The Psychology of Early Growth." New York. Macmillan.
146. **Gesell, A., Halverson, H. M., Thompson, H., Ilg, F. L., Castner, B. M., Ames, L. B., Amatruda, C. S.** (1940). " The First Five Years of Life." London. Harper and Bros.
147. **Gesell, A., Ilg, F. L.** (1943). " Infant and Child in the Culture of Today." New York. Harper and Bros.
148. GESELL, A. (1944). *J. Pediat.*, **24**, 585.
149. **Gesell, A., Amatruda, C. S.** (1947). " Developmental Diagnosis." New York. Paul Hoeber.
150. GESELL, A. (1948). " Studies in Child Development." New York. Harper and Bros.
151. GIANELLI, A., *Minerva pediat.*, **3**, 591.
152. GLASER, E. M., HERVEY, G. R. (1951). *Lancet*, *ii*, 749.
153. GLASER, J. (1953). *J. Pediat.*, **42**, 734.
154. GLASER, J. (1954). *Am. J. Dis. Child.*, **88**, 92.
155. GLOVER, E., in Middlemore, M. P. (1941), " The Nursing Couple." London. Hamish Hamilton.
156. GOFFE, A. P., PARFITT, E. M. (1955). *Lancet*, *i*, 1172.
157. GOFFE, A. P., PARFITT, E. M. (1955). *Ibid.*, *ii*, 45.
158. GOLDBLOOM, R. B., GOLDBLOOM, A. (1953). *J. Pediat.*, **43**, 631.
159. GOLDFARB, W. (1943). *Am. J. Orthopsychiat.*, **13**, 2.
160. GORDON, B. L. (1945). " The Romance of Medicine." Philadelphia. F. A. Davis Co.
161. GORDON, H. H., LEVINE, S. Z., MCNAMARA, H. (1947). *Am. J. Dis. Child.*, **73**, 442.
162. GORDON, I. (1951). *Lancet*, *i*, 1203.
163. GORE, A. T., PALMER, W. T. (1949). *Ibid.*, *i*, 385.
164. GRABER, T. M. (1952). *Pediatrics*, **9**, 709.
164a. GREEN, J. B. M., PENFOLD, J. B. (1947). *Ibid.*, *ii*, 89.
165. GREEN, M., RICHMOND, J. B. (1954). " Pediatric Diagnosis." Philadelphia. Saunders.
166. GREENACRE, P. (1944). *Am. J. Orthopsychiat.*, **14**, 204.
167. GRIFFITHS, R. (1954). " The Abilities of Babies." London. Univ. of London Press.
168. GROOM, D., JENKINS, M. (1955). *J.A.M.A.*, **159**, 639.
169. GROSS, R. E., JEWETT, T. C. (1956). *J.A.M.A.*, **160**, 634.
170. GRULEE, C. G., CALDWELL, F. C. (1915). *Am. J. Dis. Child.*, **9**, 374.
171. GRULEE, C. G., SANFORD, H. N., HERRON, P. H. (1934). *J.A.M.A.*, **103**, 735.
172. **Gunther, M.** (1945). *Lancet*, *ii*, 590.
173. GUNTHER, M. (1953). *Univ. Coll. Hosp. Mag.*, London, **38**, 82.
174. GUNTHER, M. (1955). *Lancet*, *i*, 575.
175. GUNTHER, M. (1956). *Ibid.*, *i*, 175.
176. **Guthrie, L.** (1908). *Brit. med. J.*, *ii*, 468.
177. GYORGY, P. (1953). *Pediatrics*, **11**, 98.
177a. HALLOWELL, D. K. (1932). *J. Genet. Psychol.*, **40**, 406.
178. HALLOWELL, D. K. (1941). *J. Genet. Psychol.*, **58**, 265.
179. HALLIDAY, J. L. (1946). *Lancet*, *ii*, 185.
180. HAMMOND, J., MARSHALL, F. H. A. (1925). " Reproduction in the Rabbit." Edinburgh. Oliver and Boyd.
181. HANSEN, J. D. L., SMITH, C. A. (1953). *Pediatrics*, **12**, 99.
182. HARDCASTLE, D. N. (1935). *J. Mental Sc.*, **81**, 317.

183. Hartley, J. B., Burnett, C. W. F. (1944). *Brit. J. Radiol.*, **17**, 33.
184. Haworth, J. C., McCredie, D. (1956). *Arch. Dis. Childhood*, **31**, 189.
185. Haworth, J. C. (1956). *Brit. med. J.*, *ii*, 1286.
185a. Heinemeyer, H. (1941). *Frankfurt. Z. Path.*, **55**, 240.
186. Helmholz, H. F. (1954), in " Modern Problems in Pediatrics," by Hottinger, A., Hauser, F. Vol. 1. Basle. Karger.
186a. Herlitz, G. (1953). *Acta pæd. Uppsala*, **42**, 506.
187. Hess, J. (1940). *J. Pediat.*, **16**, 123.
188. Hess, J. H., Lundeen, E. C. (1941). " The Premature Infant." Philadelphia. Lippincott.
189. Hesseltine, H. C., Bustamente, J., Navori, C. A. (1955). *Am. J. Obst. and Gynec.*, **69**, 686.
190. Higgins, J. M. (1942). *Penn. med. J.*, **45**, 455.
191. Hill, J. (1937). *Psychoanalytic Quarterly*, **11**, 356.
192. Hill, G. (1952). *Am. J. Obst. and Syph.*, **59**, 807.
193. Hill-Young, E. (1944). *Am. J. Dis. Child.*, **68**, 250.
194. Hinman, A., Dickey, L. B. (1956). *Am. J. Dis. Child.*, **91**, 23.
195. Hoefer, C., Hardy, M. C. (1929). *J.A.M.A.*, **92**, 615.
196. **Hollingworth, L. S.** (1929). " Gifted Children." New York. Macmillan.
197. Holt, J. F., Latourette, H. B., Watson, E. H. (1954). *J.A.M.A.*, **154**, 390.
198. Holzel, A. (1953). *Arch. Dis. Childhood*, **28**, 413.
199. Howard, P. J., Bauer, A. R. (1949). *Am. J. Dis. Child.*, **77**, 592.
200. Hughes, R., Todd, R. M. (1953). *Arch. Dis. Childhood*, **28**, 198.
201. Hytten, F. E. (1954). *Brit. med. J.*, *i*, 249.
202. Ievers, M., Campbell, K., Blanch, M. (1955). *Lancet*, *ii*, 971.
203. Ilg, F. L., Ames, L. B. (1955). " Child Behaviour." London. Hamish Hamilton.
204. Illingworth, R. S., Harvey, C. C., Gin, Shan-Yah (1949). *Lancet*, *ii*, 598.
205. Illingworth, R. S. (1950). *Brit. med. J.*, *i*, 96.
206. Illingworth, R. S., Harvey, C. C., Jowett, G. H. (1950). *Arch. Dis. Childhood*, **25**, 380.
207. Illingworth, R. S., Stone, D. (1952). *Lancet*, *i*, 683.
208. Illingworth, R. S., Barlow, J. (1954). *Arch. Dis. Childhood*, **29**, 422.
209. Illingworth, R. S., Kilpatrick, B. (1953). *Lancet*, *ii*, 1175.
210. Illingworth, R. S. (1953). *Practitioner*, **171**, 533.
211. Illingworth, R. S. (1954). *Arch. Dis. Childhood.*, **29**, 165.
212. Illingworth, R. S. (1955). *Acta pæd. Uppsala*, **44**, 203.
213. Illingworth, R. S., Holt, K. (1955). *Lancet*, *ii*, 1257.
214. Illingworth, R. S. (1955). *Brit. med. J.*, *i*, 75.
215. Ingram, M. D., Hamilton, N. M. (1950). *Radiology*, **55**, 503.
216. Irwin, O. C. (1932). *J. Comp. Psychol.*, **14**, 415.
217. Jeans, P. C. (1950). *J.A.M.A.*, **142**, 806.
218. Jelliffe, D. B. (1956). *Courrier du Centre de l'Enfance*, **6**, 191.
219. Joensen, H. D. (1954). *Ann. Soc. Scient. Faeroensis Torshavn.*
220. Johansson and Hansson (1940), quoted by Douglas (116).
221. **Johnson, W.** (1942). *J. Speech Disorders*, **7**, 251.
221a. Johnstone, D. E., Basila, N., Glaser, J. (1955). *J. Pediat.*, **46**, 160.
222. Jorup, S. (1952). *Acta. pæd. Uppsala*, **41**, Suppl. 85.
223. *J.A.M.A.* (1956), **160**, 1472. (Leading Article.)
224. Kagan, B. M., Mirman, B., Calvin, J., Lundeen, E. (1949). *J. Pediat.*, **34**, 574.
225. Kaliski, S. (1941). *Texas State J. Med.*, **37**, 288.
226. **Kanner, L.** (1938). *J. Pediat.*, **13**, 422.
227. **Kanner, L.** (1948). " Child Psychiatry." Springfield. Charles Thomas.
228. Karlin, I. W., Kennedy, L. (1936). *Am. J. Dis. Child.*, **51**, 1138.
229. Keith, H. M. (1955). *Ped. Clin. N. Am.*, May, 595.
230. Kendall, N., Woloshin, H. (1952). *J. Pediat.*, **41**, 125.
231. Kendig, E. L., Guerry, D. (1948). *Arch. Ophth.*, **39**, 193.
232. Kendig, E. L., Guerry, D. (1950). *J. Pediat.*, **36**, 212.
232a. Kennedy, G. C. (1951). *Lancet*, *i*, 1160.
233. Kennedy, D. A. (1953). *Lancet*, *ii*, 734.

234. King, H. L., Bourgeois, G. A. (1947). *Bull. U.S. Army med. Dept.*, **7**, 147.
235. King, Truby M. (1941). "Mothercraft." London. Simpkin Marshall.
236. Kirman, B. (1953). *J. ment. Sci.*, **99**, 416, 531.
237. Klein, M. (1937). "The Psychoanalysis of Children." Translated by A. Strachey. Hogarth Press.
237a. Knott, F. A., Blaikley, J. B. (1944). *J. Obst. and Gynæc. Brit. Emp.*, **51**, 386.
238. Kon, S. K., Mawson, E. H. (1950). "Human Milk." Medical Research Council Special Report, No. 269.
239. Kritzer, M. D. (1952). *Med. Clin. N. Am.*, **36**, 1151.
240. Krost, G. N., Epstein, I. M. (1931). *J. Pediat.*, **10**, 221.
241. Krugman, S., Ward, R. (1951). *J.A.M.A.*, **145**, 775.
242. Krupp, G. R., Friedman, A. P. (1953). *Am. J. Dis. Child.*, **85**, 146.
243. Kugelmass, I. N., Berggren, R. E., Cummings, M. (1933). *Am. J. Dis. Child.*. **46**, 280.
244. *Lancet* (1955), *i*, 1009. (Leading Article.)
244a. Langford, W. S. (1948). *J. Pediat.*, **33**, 242.
245. Lawson, L. J. (1956). *J. Pediat.*, **48**, 477.
246. Lelong, M., Alison, F., Vinceneux, J. (1949). Lait, **29**, 237.
247. Levine, M. I., Bell, A. I. (1950). *J. Pediat.*, **37**, 750.
248. Levy, D. M. (1928). *Am. J. Psychiat.*, **84**, 881.
249. Levy, D. M. (1934). *Am. J. Orthopsychiat.*, **4**, 203.
250. Levy, D. M. (1935). *Psychoanalytic Quarterly*, **4**, 612.
251. Levy, D. M. (1937). *Am. J. Psychiat.*, **94**, 643.
252. **Levy, D. M.** (1945). *Am. J. Dis. Child.*, **69**, 7.
253. Lewis, S. J. (1930). *J. Am. Dent. A.*, **17**, 1060.
254. Lewis, S. J. (1931). *Ibid.*, **18**, 1766.
255. Liddiard, M. (1948). "The Mothercraft Manual." London. Churchill.
256. Linfert, H. E., Hierholzer, H.M., quoted by Goodenough, F. L., in Murchison, C. (1933), "A Handbook of Child Psychology." London. Oxford University Press.
257. Livingston, S. (1954). "Convulsive Disorders in Children." Springfield. Thomas.
258. Looney, J. M., Edsall, G., Ipsen, J., Chasen, W. H. (1956). *New England J. Med.*, **254**, 6.
259. Lorenz (1954), quoted by *Lancet*, *i*, 37. (Leading Article.)
260. Low, N. L., Gibbs, F. A., Gibbs, L. E. (1955). *Pediatrics*, **15**, 595.
261. Lowe, C. R., Gibson, J. R. (1953). *Brit. J. Prev. Soc. Med.*, **7**, 78.
262. Lowrey, L. G. (1940). *Am. J. Orthopsychiat.*, **10**, 576.
263. Luck, J. W., Maddux, R. (1955). *Gen. Practit.*, **12**, 87.
264. Lyon, R. A., Rauh, L. W., Stirling, J. W. (1940). *J. Pediat.*, **16**, 310.
265. Macnamara, J. (1947). *M. J. Australia*, **2**, 720.
266. Macnamara, J. (1948). *Ibid.*, **2**, 592.
267. Macy, I. G., Hunscher, H. A., Donelson, E., Nims, B. (1930). *Am. J. Dis. Child.*, **39**, 1186.
268. Malone, A. J., Massler, M., quoted by Valentine, C. W. (1956). "The Normal Child." London. Penguin Books.
269. Markey, O. B. (1950). *Q. J. Child Behaviour*, **2**, 237.
270. Massler, M. (1950). *M. Clin. North America*, January, p. 13.
271. Massler, M., Malone, A. J. (1950). *J. Pediat.*, **36**, 523.
272. **Massler, M., Savara, B. S.** (1950). *J. Pediat.*, **36**, 349.
273. Massler, M., Wood, A. (1917). *J. Dent. Child.*, **16**, 1.
274. Mayer, J. (1954). 11th M. & R. Pediatric Research Conference.
275. Mazzini, G., quoted by Kanner, L. (227).
276. McCarthy, D., Douglas, J. W. B., Mogford, C. (1952). *Brit. med. J.*, **2**, 755.
277. McGee, W. A. (1950). *South Med. J., Bham. Ala.*, **43**, 335.
278. McKeown, B. J. (1953). *B. J. Prev. and Social Med.*, **7**, 78.
279. McLane, M. (1933), quoted by Clouston, E. C. T., *Brit. med. J.*, *i*, 200.
280. McCoy, G. E. (1950). *J. Indiana State Med. Ass.*, **43**, 1095.
281. Mead, M. (1933), in Murchison, C., "A Handbook of Child Psychology." Worcester. Clark University Press.
282. Mead, M. (1935). "Sex and Temperament." London. Routledge and Kegan Paul.

283. MEAD, M. (1949). "Male and Female." London. Gollancz.
284. Medical Research Council Report (1950). *Lancet, ii*, 732.
285. **Medical Research Council Memo. No. 11** (1951). "The Control of Cross-infection in Hospitals." London. H.M. Stationery Office.
286. Medical Research Council Investigation (1951). *Brit. med. J., i*, 1463.
287. Medical Research Council Investigation (1951). *Brit. med. J., i*, 1463.
288. Medical Research Council and Ind. Hlth. Research Board Report (1946) No. 89.
289. Medical Research Council (1956). "The Hazards to Man of Nuclear and Allied Radiations." London. H. M. Stationery Office.
290. Medical Research Council (1955). Spec. Rep. No. 288.
291. MELIN, K. (1953). *J. Pediat*, **43**, 672 (and Editorial, 746).
292. MEYER, H. F. (1952). "Infant Feeding.' Springfield. Thomas.
293. **Middlemore, M. P.** (1941). "The Nursing Couple." London. Hamish Hamilton.
294. MIGUEL MILLAN, A., SAN MARTIN, S. (1950). *Rev. chil. Pediat.*, **21**, 209.
295. MILLER, C. A., LENNOX, M. A. (1948). *J. Pediat.*, **33**, 753.
295a. MILLER, H., WEETCH, R. S. (1955), *Lancet, ii*, 1013.
296. MILLER, H. G., STANTON, J. B. (1954). *Quart. J. Med.*, **23**, 1.
297. MILLER, R. L., SNYDER, D. C. (1953). *Am. J. Obst. and Gynec.*, **65**, 1.
298. Ministry of Education and of Health. Memorandum on the closure of schools and exclusion from school on account of Infectious Illness (1956). London. H.M. Stationery Office.
299. MOGGI, D. (1940). *Riv. Clin. pediat.*, **38**, 549.
300. MOLONEY, J. C. (1945). *Psychiatry*, **8**, 391.
301. MOLOSHOK, R. E., MOSELEY, J. E. (1956). *Pediatrics*, **17**, 327.
302. MORRISON, S. D. (1952). "Human Milk." Commonwealth Agric. Bureau. Farnham Royal.
303. MOSSBERG, H. O. (1948). *Acta Pædiat.*, **35**, Suppl. 2.
304. MURRAY, A. B. (1956). *Brit. med. J., i*, 1530.
305. NAISH, F. C. (1948). "Breast Feeding." London. Oxford University Press.
305a. NEALE, A. V., PIERCE, M., BRAID, F., CASSIE, E. (1943). *Am. J. Dis. Child.*, **65**, **147**.
306. NEILON, P. (1948). *J. Genet. Psychol.*, **73**, 175.
307. NELIGAN, G. A., STRANG, L. B. (1952). *Lancet, ii*, 1005.
307a. NELSON, V. L., RICHARDS, T. W. (1938). *J. Genet. Psychol.*, **52**, 303.
308. NELSON, W. E. (1954). "Pediatrics." Philadelphia. Saunders.
309. **Newburgh, L. H.** (1942). *Arch. Int. Med.*, **70**, 1033.
310. NEWMAN, J. (1956). "Psychology of Exceptional Children and Youth." Cruikshank, W. M. London. Staples Press.
311. NEWTON, M., NEWTON, N. R. (1948). *J. Pediat.*, **33**, 698.
312. NEWTON, M., NEWTON, N. R. (1951). *Am. J. Obst. and Gynec.*, **61**, 664.
313. NEWTON, N. R. (1951). *J. Pediat.*, **38**, 28.
314. NEWTON, N. (1952). *J. Pediat.*, **41**, 411.
315. New York State Sanitary Code (1948) quoted in *Pediatrics*, **2**, 116.
316. NORTON, E. W. D., COGAN, D. G. (1954). *A.M.A. Arch. Ophth.*, **52**, 442.
317. NORVAL, M. (1951). *Hum. Biol.*, **23**, 273.
318. OGDEN, K. M., MACKEITH, R. (1955). *J. Pediat.*, **46**, 210.
319. OLDFIELD, M. C. (1955). *Lancet, i*, 528.
320. OLSEN, A. (1940). *Acta. obstet. gynec. scand.*, **20**, 313.
321. OLSEN, A. (1941). *Ugeskr. Læg.*, **103**, 897.
322. **Orlansky, H.** (1949). *Psychol. Bull.*, **46**, 1.
323. ORTON, S. T. (1939). *J. Pediat.*, **15**, 453.
324. OSNATO, M. (1920). "Aphasia and Associated Speech Problems." New York. Paul Hoeber.
325. PARISH, H. J. (1955). *Brit. med. J., ii*, 631.
326. PARMELEE, A. H. (1936). *J. Pediat.*, **8**, 646.
327. PARMELEE, A. H. (1952). "Management of the Newborn." Chicago. Year Book Publishers Inc.
328. PATERSON, A. S. (1953). *Practitioner*, **170**, 677.
329. PEARCE, R. (1953). *Arch. Dis. Childhood*, **28**, 247.
330. PEARSON, G. H. J. (1931). *Am. J. Orthopsychiat.*, **1**, 284.

331. PENNINGTON, A. W. (1953). *New England J. Med.*, **248**, 959.
332. PETERSEN, W. E. (1955). *Q. Rev. Pediat.*, **10**, 90.
333. PETERSON, C. H., SPANO, F. L. (1941). *Character and Personality*, **10**, 62.
334. PHAER, quoted by Still (403).
335. PIERCE, P. P. (1948). *Am. J. Dis. Child.*, **75**, 190.
336. PLANTENGA, P., FILIPPO, J. (1916). *Z. Kinderheilk.*, **14**, 166.
337. PLATT, B. S., GIN, S. Y. (1938). *Arch. Dis. Childhood*, **13**, 343.
338. PRATT, A. G., READ, W. T. (1955). *J. Pediat.*, **46**, 539.
339. PRESS, E. (1947). *J.A.M.A.*, **135**, 824.
340. PRICE, E. E. (1949). *M. J. Australia*, **2**, 589.
341. *Q. Rev. Pediat.* (1949), **4**, 295.
341a. RAND, W., SWEENEY, M. E., VINCENT, L. (1930). "Growth and Development of the Young Child." Philadelphia. W. B. Saunders.
342. RANK, quoted by Ruja, H. (1948). *J. Genet. Psychol.*, **73**, 53.
343. RAPPAPORT, E. M. (1946). *Ann. Int. Med.*, **25**, 1.
344. RASMUSSEN, V., quoted by Arlitt (1946).
345. REINHOLD, J. D. L. (1948). *Brit. med. J.*, *i*, 981.
346. RENDLE-SHORT, J. (1956). *Lancet*, *ii*, 1189.
347. RICHARDS, M. R., SAMUELS, M. H., MERRITT, K. K., LANGMANN, A. G. (1955). *Pediatrics*, **15**, 169.
348. RICHARDSON, F. H. (1925). *J.A.M.A.*, **85**, 668.
349. RICHARDSON, F. H. (1950). *Ibid.*, **142**, 863.
350. RICHARDSON, K. C. (1950). *Brit. med. J.*, *ii*, 350.
351. RICHMOND, J. B., GROSSMAN, H. J., LUSTMAN, S. L. (1953). *Pediatrics*, **11**, 635.
352. RICHTER, C. P. (1942). *J. Pediat.*, **20**, 230.
353. ROBERTS, K. E., SCHOELLKOPF, J. A. (1951). *Am. J. Dis. Child.*, **82**, 121 *et seq.*
354. ROBERTSON, J. (1952). (Film) "A Two-Year-Old goes to Hospital." London. Tavistock Clinic.
355. **Robinson, M.** (1951). *Lancet*, *i*, 788.
356. ROBINSON, P., HIRSCH, W. (1952). *Courrier du Centre de l'enfance*, **2**, 318.
357. RODDA, F. C., STOESSER, A. V. (1938). *Wisconsin med. J.*, **37**, 547.
358. ROGERSON, B. C. F., ROGERSON, C. H. (1939). *J. Ment. Sc.*, **85**, 1163.
359. ROSAMOND, E. (1921). *Southern med. J.*, **14**, 768.
360. ROSS, C. A. C., DAWES, E. A. (1954). *Lancet*, *i*, 994.
361. ROSS, Pediatric Research Conf., 1956 (17th).
362. ROURKE, A. J. J. (1947). *Hospitals*, **21**, May, No. 5.
363. ROWNTREE, G. (1950). *J. Hyg.*, **48**, 323.
364. **Rubenstein, A. D., Foley, G. E.** (1947). *New England J. Med.*, **236**, 87.
365. RYLE, J. A. (1942). *Brit. med. J.*, **2**, 745.
366. **Sabin, A. B.** (1951). *J. Pediat.*, **39**, 519.
367. SANFORD, H. N. (1937). *Ibid.*, **11**, 68.
368. SANFORD, H. N. (1939). *J.A.M.A.*, **113**, 470.
369. SCHORER, E. H., LAFFOON, F. L. (1935). *J. Pediat.*, **7**, 613.
370. SCORER, C. G. (1956). *Arch. Dis. Childhood*, **31**, 198.
371. **Sedgwick, J. P.** (1917). *J.A.M.A.*, **69**, 417.
372. SEDGWICK, J. P., FLEISCHNER, E. C. (1921). *Am. J. Pub. Health*, **11**, 153.
373. SEDGWICK, J. P. (1921). *Am. J. Dis. Child.*, **21**, 455.
374. SELBER, E. J. (1955). M. D. Thesis Univ. of Cape Town.
375. SEWELL, W. H., MURSEN, P. H. (1952). *Child Development*, **23**, 185.
376. SHANNON, W. B. (1921). *Am. J. Dis. Child.*, **22**, 223.
376a. SHANNON, W. B. (1921). *Arch. Pediat.*, **38**, 756.
377. SHARPEY-SCHAFER, E. P., HOWARD, P., LEATHART, G. L., DORNHURST, A. C. (1951). *Brit. med. J.*, *ii*, 382.
378. SHERRY, S. N., KRAMER, I. (1955). *J. Pediat.*, **46**, 158.
379. **Shirley, H. F.** (1948). "Psychiatry for the Pediatrician." New York. The Commonwealth Fund.
380. **Shirley, M. M.** (1931). "The First Two Years of Life." Minneapolis. University of Minnesota Press.
381. SILLMAN, J. H. (1951). *J. Pediat.*, **39**, 424.

382. SIMON, A. J., BASS, L. G. (1956). *Am. J. Orthopsychiat.*, **26**, 340.
383. SIMPSON, E. (1953). *Med. Officer*, **89**, 133.
384. SIMPSON, S. L. (1952). *Brit. med. J.*, *i*, 725.
385. SIMPSON, S. L. (1955). *J.A.M.A.*, **158**, 423.
386. SKODAK, M. (1938). *Child Development*, **9**, 303.
387. **Smith, C.** (1951). " Physiology of the Newborn." Springfield. Charles Thomas.
388. **Smith, C. H.** (1937). *J. Pediat.*, **10**, 719.
389. SMITH, L. H. (1935). *Am. J. Dis. Child.*, **49**, 1177.
390. SMITH, R. E. (1947). *Lancet*, *ii*, 1.
391. SMITH, R. E. (1952). *Brit. med. J.*, *ii*, 34.
392. SPENCE, J. C. (1938). *Brit. med. J.*, *ii*, 729.
393. SPENCE, J., WALTON, W. S., MILLER, F. J. W., COURT, S. D. M. (1954). " A Thousand Families in Newcastle-on-Tyne." London. Oxford Univ. Press.
394. SPERLING, M. (1949). *The Nervous Child*, **8**, 28.
395. SPITZ, R. A. (1951). *Psychoanal. Study Child.*, **6**, 255.
396. **Spock, B.** (1946). " Baby and Child Care." New York. Pocket Books Inc.
397. **Spock, B.** (1948). *J.A.M.A.*, **136**, 811.
398. **Spock, B.** (1949). *Pediatrics*, **4**, 89.
399. SPOCK, B. (1950). *M. Clin. North America*, July, 1079.
400. STEINER, M. M. (1950). *Ibid.*, **34**, 223.
401. STEVENSON, S. S. (1947). *J. Pediat.*, **31**, 616.
402. STEVENSON, S. S. (1949). *J. Am. Dietet. A.*, **25**, 752.
403. STILL, G. H. (1931). " The History of Pædiatrics." London. Milford.
404. STILL, G. F. (1930). *Practitioner*, **125**, 49.
405. STOTT, D. H. (1950). " Delinquency and Human Nature." Dunfermline. Carnegie United Kingdom Trust.
406. **Stuart, H. C., Meredith, H. V.** (1946). *Am. J. Pub. Health*, **36**, 1365.
407. STUART, H. (1955). *Q. Rev. Pediat.*, **10**, 131.
408. SYMES, E. (1933). *Am. J. Orthopsychiat.*, **3**, 409.
409. TALBOT, F. (1931). *Am. J. Dis. Child.*, **42**, 965.
410. TALBOT, F. (1948), in Brennemann's " Practice of Pediatrics," Vol. 1, Ch. 5, p. 3. Hagerstown. W. F. Prior Co.
411. TANNER, J. M. (1953). " Prospects in Psychiatric Research." Oxford. Blackwell Scientific Publications.
412. TERMAN, L. M. (1926). " Genetic Studies of Genius." London. George Harrap.
413. TERMAN, L. M., ODEN, M. H. (1947). " The Gifted Child Grows Up." Stanford. Stanford University Press.
414. THELANDER, H. E., FITZHUGH, M. L. (1942). *J. Pediat.*, **21**, 306.
415. **Tilney, F., Casamajor, L.** (1924). *Arch. Neurol. and Psychiat.*, **12**, 1.
416. TRAINHAM, G., PILAFIAN, G. J., KRAFT, R. M. (1945). *J. Pediat.*, **27**, 97.
417. TURNER, C. E. H. (1947). *J. Mental Sc.*, **93**, 522.
418. TURNER, T. B., STAFFORD, E. S., GOLDMAN, L. (1954). *Johns Hopk. Hosp. Bull.*, **94**, 204.
419. TYSON, R. M. (1927). *Am. J. Dis. Child.*, **34**, 979.
420. UNGAR, R. (1949). *Kinderärztl Praxis*, **17**, 285.
421. VAHLQUIST, B. (1949). *Acta Pædiat. Suppl.*, **77**, 56.
422. VAHLQUIST, B., HACKZELL, G. (1949). *Acta Pædiat.*, **38**, 622.
423. VALENTINE, C. W. (1946). " The Psychology of Early Childhood." London. Methuen.
424. VAN NOORDEN, C. (1909). *Med. Klin.*, **5**, 1.
425. VAN RIPER, H. E. (1956). 8th International Congress of Pædiatrics. 127.
426. VAN THAL, J. H. (1955). *Lancet*, *i*, 871.
427. **Vining, C. W.** (1950). *Univ. Leeds med. Mag.*, **20**, 1.
428. VINING, C. W. (1952). *Lancet*, *ii*, 99.
429. VON REUSS, A. (1921). " The Diseases of the Newborn." London. John Bale, Sons, and Danielsson.
430. VON SYDOW (1952). *Acta pæd. Uppsala*, **41**, 449.
431. VULLIAMY, D., MACKEITH, R. (1954). *Practitioner*, **173**, 271.
432. WALKER, A. R. P., ARVIDSSON, U. B., DRAPER, W. L. (1952). *Lancet*, *i*, 317.

433. Wallace, L. R. (1948). *J. Agric. Sc.*, **38**, 93.
434. **Waller, H.** (1946). *Arch. Dis. Childhood*, **21**, 1.
435. Waller, H. (1950). *Lancet*, *i*, 53.
435a. Wallgren, A. (1945). *Acta pæd. Uppsala*, **32**, 778.
436. Wallgren, A. (1955). *J. Pediat.* **46**, 458.
437. Wallis, H. R. E. (1956). "Masked Epilepsy." London. Livingstone.
438. Walser, H. C. (1945). *Psychosomatic Med.*, **7**, 174.
439. Wanning, P. (1948). *J. Pediat.*, **32**, 107.
440. Watson, J. B. (1925). "Behaviourism." London. Kegan Paul.
441. Watson, J. B., Morgan, J. J. B. (1917). *Amer. J. Psychol.*, **28**, 163.
442. Wechsler, D. (1931). *Psychoanal. Rev.*, **18**, 201.
443. Wegman, M. E. (1948). *Pediatrics*, **2**, 110.
444. Weinfeld, G. F., Floore, F. B. (1930). *Am. J. Dis. Child.*, **40**, 1208.
445. Weinfeld, G. F. (1950). *M. Clin. North America*, January, p. 33.
446. Weiss, P. (1939). "The Principles of Development." New York. Henry Holt.
447. Wessel, M. A., Cobb, J. C., Jackson, E. B., Harris, G. S., Detwiler, A. C. (1954). *Pediatrics*, **14**, 421.
448. Westrop, C. K., Barber, C. R. (1956). *J. Neurol. Psychiat.*, **19**, 52.
449. Wetzel, N. C. (1946). *J. Pediat.*, **29**, 439.
450. Wetzel, N. C. (1948), in Litchfield and Dembo's "Pediatric Progress." Philadelphia. F. A. Davis.
451. "Whiddon," D. (1953). *Lancet*, *ii*, 337.
452. White, P. J. (1929). *Am. J. Dis. Child.*, **38**, 935.
453. Wickes, I. G. (1952). *Brit. med. J.*, *ii*, 1178.
454. Wickes, I. G. (1952). *Arch. Dis. Childhood*, **27**, 449.
455. Wickes, I. G. (1953). *J. Pediat.*, **43**, 74.
456. Wickes, I. G. (1953). *Arch. Dis. Childhood*, **28**, 151, 232, 332, 416, 495.
457. Wieschhoff, H. A. (1940). *Bull. Hist. Med.*, **8**, 1403.
458. Wilkins, L. (1954). 11th M. & R. Pediatric Research Conference.
459. Williams, R. H., Kay, G. H., Jandorf, B. J. (1944). *J. clin. Invest.*, **23**, 613.
460. Wilson, J. G. (1951). *Arch. Dis. Childhood*, **26**, 452.
461. Wilson, J. L., Dickinson, D. G. (1955). *J.A.M.A.*, **158**, 261.
462. Woods, G. E. (1953). *Arch. Dis. Childhood*, **28**, 450.
463. Wright, H. P. (1934). "Essentials of Infant Feeding and Pædiatric Practice." London. Oxford Medical Publications.
463a. Wright, J. (1947). *Lancet*, *ii*, 121.
463b. Wright, J. (1951). *Brit. med. J.*, *ii*, 138.
464. **Young, P. T.** (1941). *Psychol. Bull.*, **38**, 129.
465. Zausmer, D. M. (1954). *Arch. Dis. Childhood*, **29**, 537.
466. Zeiss, F. R. (1955). *Ped. Clin. N. Am.*, Nov., 957.
467. Ziman, E. (1950). "Jealousy in Children." London. Gollancz.
468. Zlocisti, quoted by Von Reuss (1921).

ADDITIONAL READING RECOMMENDED

Feeding Problems

British Medical Bulletin (1947), **5,** 120–220. (Symposium on Lactation.)
Evans, P., Mackeith, R. (1954). " Infant Feeding and Feeding Difficulties." London. Churchill.

Physical Problems

Physical Development

WATSON, E. H., LOWREY, G. H. (1954). " Growth and Development of Children." Chicago. The Year Book Publishers Inc.

Tongue Tie

McENERY, E. T., GAINES, F. P. (1941). *J. Pediat.*, **18,** 252.

Prevention of Infection

ABRAMSON, H. (1944). *J. Pediat.*, **24,** 684. (The Value of Masks.)
" Control of Communicable Diseases in Man " (1950). New York. American Public Health Association.
CONYBEARE, E. T. (1948). *Monthly Bull. Min. Health,* **7,** 72. (Incidence of Post-vaccinial Encephalopathy.)
ROSENSTERN, I. (1948). *Am. J. Dis. Child.*, **75,** 193. (Physical Arrangements in the Nursery to prevent Infection.)
WEYMULLER, C. A., BECK, A. C., ITTNER, E. J. (1947). *J.A.M.A.*, **133,** 78. (Prevention of Infection in Newborn Babies.)

Developmental Problems

General Development

BARKER, R. G., KOUNIN, J. S., WRIGHT, H. F. (1943). " Child Behaviour and Development." New York. McGraw Hill Book Co.
DARWIN, C. (1877). *Mind,* **2,** 285. (Accurate Observation of a Child's Development.)
DEWEY, E. (1935). " Behaviour Development in Infants." New York. Columbia University Press.
GESELL, A. (1945) " The Embryology of Behaviour." New York. Harper.
McGRAW, M. B. (1943). " The Neuromuscular Maturation of the Human Infant." New York. Columbia University Press.

Measurement of Intelligence

STUTSMAN, R. (1948). " Mental Measurement of Preschool Children." World Book Co.
TERMAN, L. M., MERRILL, M. A. (1946). " Measuring Intelligence." London. Harrap.

Speech

DESPERT, J. L., KOPP, H., KRUGMAN, S. (1946). *Am. J. Orthopsychiat.*, **16,** 110–127. (Symposium on Stuttering.)
STINCHFIELD, S. M., YOUNG, E. H. (1938). " Children with Delayed or Defective Speech." London. Oxford University Press.
WEISS, D. A. (1951). *The Nervous Child,* **9,** 21. (Symposium on Speech Problems.)

Behaviour Problems

BAUER, W. W. (1947). "Stop Annoying your Children." New York. Bobbs Merrill Co.

BRENNEMANN, J. (1930). *Am. J. Dis. Child.*, **40**, 1. (Eating Problems.)

BRENNEMANN, J. (1931). *Am. J. Dis. Child.*, **42**, 376. (The Menace of Psychiatry.)

CAMERON, H. C. (1946). "The Nervous Child." London. Oxford Medical Publications.

HEMMING, J., BALLS, J. (1949). "The Child is Right." London. Longmans Green & Co.

JOSEPH, H., ZERN, G. (1954). "The Emotional Problems of Children." New York. Crown Publications.

KANNER, L. (1939). *J. Pediat.*, **15**, 583. (Infant Sexuality.)

KANNER, L. (1941). "In Defence of Mothers." New York. Dodd Mead & Co.

LAWTON, G. (1938). *Child Development*, **9**, 151. (Fears.)

MURCHISON, C. (1933). "A Handbook of Child Psychology." Worcester. Clark University Press.

NIXON, N. K. (1934). *J. Pediat.*, **4**, 295. (Obesity.)

RICH, G. J., SELLING, L. S. (1936). *The Nervous Child*, **5**, 222, 226. (Punishment.)

RIDENOUR, N., JOHNSON, I. (1949). "Some Special Problems of Children." Philadelphia. National Mental Health Foundation Inc.

SHIRLEY, H. F. (1954). "The Child, His Parents and the Physician." Springfield. Thomas.

INDEX

The principal references are printed in heavy type.

PRINTED IN GREAT BRITAIN BY THE WHITEFRIARS PRESS LTD.
LONDON AND TONBRIDGE